1986
YEAR BOOK OF
CARDIOLOGY®

The Year Book Series

Anesthesia: Drs. Miller, Kirby, Ostheimer, Saidman, and Stoelting

Cancer: Drs. Hickey, Clark, and Cumley

Cardiology: Drs. Harvey, Kirkendall, Laks, Resnekov, Rosenthal, and Sonnenblick

Critical Care Medicine: Drs. Rogers, Allo, Dean, Gioia, McPherson, Michael, Miller, and Traystman

Dentistry: Drs. Cohen, Hendler, Johnson, Jordan, Moyers, Robinson, and Silverman

Dermatology: Drs. Sober and Fitzpatrick

Diagnostic Radiology: Drs. Bragg, Keats, Kieffer, Kirkpatrick, Koehler, Miller, and Sorenson

Digestive Diseases: Drs. Greenberger and Moody

Drug Therapy: Drs. Hollister and Lasagna

Emergency Medicine: Dr. Wagner

Endocrinology: Drs. Schwartz and Ryan

Family Practice: Dr. Rakel

Hand Surgery: Drs. Dobyns and Chase

Hematology: Drs. Spivak, Bell, Ness, Quesenberry, and Wiernik

Infectious Diseases: Drs. Wolff, Gorbach, Keusch, Klempner, and Snydman

Medicine: Drs. Rogers, Des Prez, Cline, Braunwald, Greenberger, Wilson, Epstein, and Malawista

Neurology and Neurosurgery: Drs. DeJong, Currier, and Crowell

Nuclear Medicine: Drs. Hoffer, Gore, Gottschalk, Sostman, and Zaret

Obstetrics and Gynecology: Drs. Pitkin and Zlatnik

Ophthalmology: Drs. Ernest and Deutsch

Orthopedics: Dr. Coventry

Otolaryngology–Head and Neck Surgery: Drs. Paparella and Bailey

Pathology and Clinical Pathology: Dr. Brinkhous

Pediatrics: Drs. Oski and Stockman

Plastic and Reconstructive Surgery: Drs. McCoy, Brauer, Haynes, Hoehn, Miller, and Whitaker

Podiatric Medicine and Surgery: Dr. Jay

Psychiatry and Applied Mental Health: Drs. Freedman, Lourie, Meltzer, Nemiah, Talbott, and Weiner

Pulmonary Disease: Drs. Green, Ball, Menkes, Michael, Peters, Terry, Tockman, and Wise

Rehabilitation: Drs. Kaplan and Szumski

Sports Medicine: Drs. Krakauer, Shephard, and Torg, Col. Anderson, and Mr. George

Surgery: Drs. Schwartz, Jonasson, Peacock, Shires, Spencer, and Thompson

Urology: Drs. Gillenwater and Howards

Vascular Surgery: Drs. Bergan and Yao

Editors

W. Proctor Harvey, M.D.
Professor of Medicine, Georgetown University School of Medicine; Division of Cardiology, Georgetown University Hospital

Walter M. Kirkendall, M.D.
Professor of Internal Medicine and Director of the Hypertension Section, University of Texas Medical School at Houston

Hillel Laks, M.D.
Professor and Chief, Cardiothoracic Surgery, Department of Surgery, UCLA Center for the Health Sciences

Leon Resnekov, M.D., F.R.C.P.
Frederick H. Rawson Professor of Medicine, Section of Cardiology, University of Chicago

Amnon Rosenthal, M.D.
Professor of Pediatrics and Communicable Diseases, The University of Michigan Medical School; and Director of Pediatric Cardiology, C. S. Mott Children's Hospital, Ann Arbor

Edmund H. Sonnenblick, M.D.
Olson Professor of Medicine; Chief, Division of Cardiology; and Director, Cardiovascular Center, Department of Medicine, Albert Einstein College of Medicine

1986

The Year Book of CARDIOLOGY®

Editors

W. Proctor Harvey, M.D.
Walter M. Kirkendall, M.D.
Hillel Laks, M.D.
Leon Resnekov, M.D. F.R.C.P.
Amnon Rosenthal, M.D.
Edmund H. Sonnenblick, M.D.

Year Book Medical Publishers, Inc.
Chicago • London

The editor for this book was Marcia Bottoms and the production manager was H. E. Nielsen. The Editor-in-Chief for the Year Book series is Nancy Gorham.

Table of Contents

The material covered in this volume represents literature reviewed through November 1985.

Journals Represented

Acta Medica Scandinavica
American Heart Journal
American Journal of Cardiology
American Journal of Epidemiology
American Journal of Medicine
American Journal of Obstetrics and Gynecology
American Journal of Physiology
American Journal of Public Health
Annals of Neurology
Annals of Surgery
Annals of Thoracic Surgery
Archives of Disease in Childhood
Archives of Internal Medicine
Arthritis and Rheumatism
British Heart Journal
British Medical Journal
Chest
Circulation
Circulation Research
Clinical Endocrinology
Clinical Science
Deutsche Medizinische Wochenschrift
European Journal of Respiratory Diseases
Fortschritte auf dem Gebiete der Rontgenstrahlen und der Nuklear Medizin,
    Erganzungsband
Hypertension
International Journal of Cardiology
Indian Heart Journal
Journal of the American College of Cardiology
Journal of the American Geriatrics Society
Journal of the American Medical Association
Journal of the Applied Physiology; Respiratory, Environmental
    and Exercise Physiology
Journal of Cardiac Rehabilitation
Journal of Cardiovascular Surgery
Journal of Clinical Endocrinology & Metabolism
Journal of Clinical Investigation
Journal of Clinical Pathology
Journal of Hypertension
Journal of Neurology, Neurosurgery and Psychiatry
Journal of Pediatrics
Journal of Physiology
Journal of Thoracic and Cardiovascular Surgery
Journal of Vascular Surgery
Lancet
Mayo Clinic Proceedings
Nature
Nephron
New England Journal of Medicine
New Zealand Medical Journal
Pediatrics

Pfluger's Archiv: European Journal of Physiology
Quarterly Journal of Medicine
Science
Seminars in Perinatology
South African Medical Journal
Stroke
Surgery
Texas Heart Institute Journal
Transplantation
Wiener Klinische Wochenschrift
World Journal of Surgery

Publisher's Preface

Publication of the 1986 YEAR BOOK OF CARDIOLOGY marks the end of an outstanding era of YEAR BOOK editorship by W. Proctor Harvey, M.D., Walter M. Kirkendall, M.D., Edmund H. Sonnenblick, M.D., and Leon Resnekov, M.D., F.R.C.P. During Dr. Harvey's 26 years of editorship, Dr. Kirkendall's 15 years, Dr. Sonnenblick's 13 years, and Dr. Resnekov's 2 years, the volume's readers have been treated to perceptive commentary of the highest caliber. While the editorship by Hillel Laks, M.D., and Amnon Rosenthal, M.D., has spanned only 1 year, their literature selections and editorial commentary have matched the standards set for past YEAR BOOKS. We extend our deepest appreciation for the service provided by all of the editors and for their support and enthusiasm for the YEAR BOOK.

In the preface to the inaugural YEAR BOOK edition published in 1961, Dr. Harvey and his colleagues wrote, "Perhaps this volume can stand as evidence of another step inserted in the step staircase of scientific advancement." On publication of the 1986 edition, we applaud Dr. Harvey, his colleagues through the years, and the current Editors for the many steps they have inserted on that staircase. We have been enriched by the opportunity to work with such outstanding individuals. All will be missed by the staff of Year Book Medical Publishers, Inc.

Succeeding this distinguished group beginning with the 1987 edition will be Robert C. Schlant, M.D., Director of the Division of Cardiology at the Emory University School of Medicine, who will serve as Editor-in-Chief for a team of associate editors, all of whom will cover the field of cardiology as comprehensively and authoritatively as their predecessors have. While we welcome Dr. Schlant and his associate editors, we wish to extend our sincere thanks and appreciation to Drs. Harvey, Kirkendall, Sonnenblick, Resnekov, Laks, and Rosenthal for their years of excellent service.

1 Normal and Altered Cardiovascular Function

Heart Failure

Tachycardia Induced Myocardial Dysfunction: A Reversible Phenomenon?
Christopher J. McLaran, Bernard J. Gersh, Declan D. Sugrue, Stephen C. Hammill, James B. Seward, and David R. Holmes, Jr. (Mayo Clinic and Found.)

Br. Heart J. 53:323–327, March 1985   1–1

Four patients were encountered with chronic or frequent episodes of supraventricular tachycardia that resulted in severely impaired left ventricular (LV) function. Electrophysiologic studies showed reentrant supraventricular tachycardia using an accessory atrioventricular connection. Serial studies of LV function by echocardiography before and after control of the tachycardia showed varying degrees of reversibility of ventricular dysfunction. Three patients ultimately were well clinically, and the fourth was improving when last evaluated. Endomyocardial biopsy specimens in two cases showed only nonspecific histologic changes, including interstitial fibrosis and edema and focal degenerative change.

Reversible impairment of myocardial cellular function appeared to be related to supraventricular tachycardia in these patients. A mild increase in diastolic dimension can persist despite normal cardiac function at rest and during exercise. Two of the four patients were young infants; the immature left ventricle may be especially vulnerable to the demands of rapid tachycardia. Chronic or frequent episodes of supraventricular tachycardia can adversely affect LV function to a significant degree, and chronic ventricular dysfunction is a possibility. Prompt treatment is required in the presence of tachyarrhythmia and systemic desaturation of arterial oxygen. Further study is needed to identify the mechanisms of tachycardia-induced LV dysfunction.

▶ In dogs under experimental conditions, rapid tachycardia can result in persistent reductions in ventricular function that are associated with a decrease in total myocardial energy stores (Coleman, H. N., et al.: *Am. Heart J.* 81:790–798, 1971). That LV failure can be produced by persistent tachycardia is supported by the present study and the articles it refers to. It is also possible that the tachycardia that occurs when heart failure is present for other reasons may further amplify the process, and control of such tachycardia may be one of the beneficial effects that β blockers have had in the treatment of congestive cardiomyopathy. Administering drugs that can lower the heart rate without producing further ventricular depression may be useful in testing whether tachycardia is contributing to the problem per se. At present, it is reasonable to conclude that control of the heart rate is a useful additional measure in the treatment of heart failure and may primarily benefit the failing myocardium as well.—Edmund H. Sonnenblick, M.D.

Plasma Atrial Natriuretic Peptide in Cardiac Disease and During Infusion in Healthy Volunteers

Ilkka Tikkanen, Frej Fyhrquist, Kaj Metsärinne, and Raoul Leidenius (Helsinki Univ. Central Hosp.)
Lancet 2:66–69, July 13, 1985   1–2

Mammalian atria contain peptides with potent diuretic, natriuretic, and vasorelaxing actions that may have a role in the regulation of sodium and volume homeostasis and possibly in the development of heart failure and hypertension. Synthetic human α-atrial natriuretic peptide (α-ANP) causes natriuresis and diuresis, but it is not clear whether ANP is released into the circulation during volume expansion in man.

Three healthy men received an infusion of synthetic human α-ANP in physiologic saline solution after an overnight fast. The level of plasma immunoreactive ANP was measured in 17 patients with congestive heart failure, 9 controls, and 8 healthy persons. The sensitivity of the radioimmunoassay was less than 10 pg/ml with 95% confidence limits.

Healthy persons had undetectable or very low levels of ANP; levels up to 330 pg/ml were present during infusion of ANP. After infusion, levels

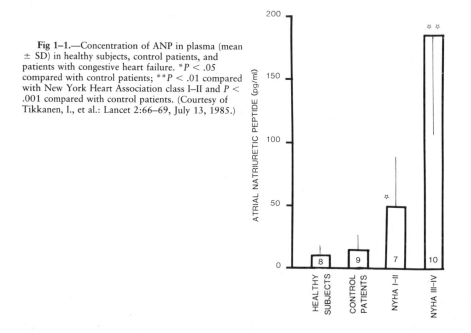

Fig 1–1.—Concentration of ANP in plasma (mean ± SD) in healthy subjects, control patients, and patients with congestive heart failure. *P < .05 compared with control patients; **P < .01 compared with New York Heart Association class I–II and P < .001 compared with control patients. (Courtesy of Tikkanen, I., et al.: Lancet 2:66–69, July 13, 1985.)

returned to normal in 15 minutes. A brisk natriuresis and diuresis were observed. Urine osmolality tended to decrease. With ANP infusion, plasma renin activity decreased insignificantly; the plasma aldosterone level and antidiuretic hormone activity were unchanged, as was potassium excretion. Patients with severe congestive heart failure had elevated levels of ANP (Fig 1–1). Controls had levels similar to those in healthy persons. Elevated levels were found in two patients with paroxysmal supraventricular tachycardia.

It appears that ANP is a circulating hormone in human beings, at least in the presence of severe congestive heart failure and supraventricular tachycardia. Future studies of ANP infusion in human beings may confirm the decrease in production of aldosterone that is observed in animal studies.

▶ Atrial natriuretic peptide has important actions to enhance sodium excretion, produce peripheral vasodilation, and inhibit the renin-angiotensin system that leads to a decrease in plasma aldosterone activity. These salutory effects would be helpful in the treatment of hypertension and in the definition of the receptors involved in this activity that form the basis for the development of new antihypertensive medications. In addition, the role of ANP in problems such as heart failure requires further exploration.—Edmund H. Sonnenblick, M.D.

Myocardial Perfusion in Compensated and Failing Hypertrophied Left Ventricle

Debora G. Parrish, W. Steves Ring, and Robert J. Bache (Univ. of Minnesota)
Am. J. Physiol. 249:H534–H539, September 1985   1–3

It has been proposed that, as myocardial hypertrophy progresses, coronary vasodilator reserve may be exhausted, leading to myocardial hypoperfusion and cardiac decompensation. Most previous studies have concerned compensated left ventricular (LV) hypertrophy; however, if the perfusion abnormality is progressive, abnormal flow should be found most readily when overt cardiac failure develops. Left ventricular hypertrophy was produced in dogs by banding the ascending aorta at age 6–7 weeks or in adulthood. Sixteen dogs with compensated hypertrophy and four with cardiac failure, manifested by LV dilatation and end-diastolic pressures of more than 18 mm Hg, were available for study. Blood flow was estimated by the labeled microsphere technique.

Dogs with compensated hypertrophy and those in failure had similar degrees of LV hypertrophy and similar LV systolic pressures. The mean LV blood flow per minute was 0.89 ml/gm in control dogs, 1.34 ml in those with compensated hypertrophy, and 1.86 ml in dogs with failure. The LV wall thickness-to-cavity diameter ratio was 0.63 in dogs with compensated hypertrophy and 0.4 in those with failure.

Significantly higher resting LV blood flow was observed in dogs with LV hypertrophy and failure than in those with compensated hypertrophy in this study. Increased cavity diameter in failure presumably results in increased systolic wall stress that increases myocardial oxygen needs. The need for increased blood flow at rest in dogs with failure would reduce the capacity for further coronary vasodilation during periods of stress. Right ventricular hypertrophy probably results from the mechanical stimulus of the increased LV filling pressure transmitted back through the lungs to cause elevated right ventricular systolic pressure.

▶ Whether coronary blood flow limitation leads to further failure in the presence of severe hypertrophy has yet to be established, even though the maximum blood flow that can be obtained under these circumstances is relatively reduced.—Edmund H. Sonnenblick, M.D.

Endogenous Catecholamine Levels in Chronic Heart Failure: Relation to the Severity of Hemodynamic Abnormalities
Christian E. Viquerat, Paul Daly, Karl Swedberg, Cathy Evers, Deirdre Curran, William W. Parmley, and Kanu Chatterjee (Univ. of California at San Francisco)
Am. J. Med. 78:455–460, March 1985   1–4

Increased levels of circulating catecholamines which are not infrequent in patients in heart failure, have been ascribed to a reflex increase in systemic sympathetic activity in response to depressed left ventricular function. Levels of endogenous catecholamines and their correlation with the severity of hemodynamic impairment were determined in a series of 63 patients with clinical chronic congestive heart failure. Twenty-six patients without clinical heart failure also were studied. The group with heart failure included 9 in New York Heart Association class II, 9 in class III, and 45 in class IV. Ischemic heart disease was the cause of heart failure in 35 patients, and dilated primary congestive cardiomyopathy in 25. The mean age of patients with and without clinical heart failure was 61 years.

Arterial levels of norepinephrine and dopamine were significantly higher in the patients with heart failure than in the control group, but levels of epinephrine were normal in both groups. Levels of plasma norepinephrine did not correlate with any hemodynamic markers of heart failure. Weak, probably clinically insignificant, correlations were found between levels of epinephrine and dopamine and various hemodynamic parameters.

Levels of plasma norepinephrine and dopamine often are elevated in patients with congestive heart failure, probably reflecting heightened adrenergic activity, but levels of catecholamines did not correlate with hemodynamic abnormalities in the present series. Patients with high levels of catecholamines may benefit more from measures that reduce release of norepinephrine, e.g., inhibition of angiotensin II activity.

▶ The present study shows that, although circulating norepinephrine levels may be elevated in congestive heart failure, these levels do not correlate with the hemodynamic abnormality reflecting the severity of the heart failure.—Edmund H. Sonnenblick, M.D.

The Relationship Between Intracellular Calcium and Contraction in Calcium-Overloaded Ferret Papillary Muscles

D. G. Allen, D. A. Eisner, J. S. Pirolo, and G. L. Smith (Univ. College, London)
J. Physiol. 364:169–182, July 1985   1–5

An increased concentration of extracellular calcium ion ($[Ca^{++}]_o$) can reduce tension that has developed in cardiac muscle, particularly when the tissue is already calcium loaded by inhibition of the sodium-potassium pump. The mechanism of the decline in tension in calcium overload is uncertain. The photoprotein aequorin was used to measure myoplasmic concentrations of calcium ($[Ca^{++}]_i$) in calcium-overloaded conditions in papillary muscles of ferrets. The concentrations of $[Ca^{++}]_i$ and tension were measured during stimulated contractions and also during the spontaneous oscillations that occurred in diastole.

Small increases in the concentration of $[Ca^{++}]_o$ led to the expected increase in both systolic light signal and developed tension, but a high concentration of $[Ca^{++}]_o$ led to a fall in developed tension. The decrease in tension occurred at a lower concentration of $[Ca^{++}]_o$ if strophanthidin was present. Oscillations in diastolic light were always present under conditions of calcium overload and were accompanied by small aftercontractions. The variance in amplitude of the systolic light signal during calcium overload was greater than could be explained by the random arrival of photons. The findings could not be ascribed to a simple change in calcium sensitivity.

If the sarcoplasmic reticulum spontaneously releases its calcium content, as shown by a diastolic $[Ca^{++}]_i$ oscillation, the stimulated systolic calcium signal that occurs within the next second is smaller, possibly because the sarcoplasmic reticulum requires longer to reload with calcium. Overall developed tension will be reduced, because cells with a small release of calcium act as a compliance in series with cells that have a large release

▶ This study shows that an increase in extracellular calcium induces an increase in the intracellular levels of calcium availability and resultant contraction. Moreover, when very high levels of calcium are present, the calcium release within cells remains the same and tension may decline as a function of this so-called calcium overload. These elegant methods reveal important relationships between intracellular calcium release and resultant contraction, which is a general principle in activation of the heart muscle. Moreover, calcium overloads may lead to a secondary release of calcium after the initial contraction (aftercontractions), which may be related to arrhythmogenesis.—Edmund H. Sonnenblick, M.D.

The Effects of Ryanodine on Calcium-Overloaded Sheep Cardiac Purkinje Fibers

M. Valdeolmillos and D. A. Eisner (Univ. College, London)
Circ. Res. 56:452–456, March 1985   1–6

The slow decline in twitch tension after prolonged inhibition of the sodium-potassium pump, which is accompanied by an increase in tonic tension and aftercontraction, has been described as "calcium overload," but the mechanism is uncertain. Assessment was made of the effects of the plant alkaloid ryanodine on sheep cardiac Purkinje fibers. Ryanodine interferes with excitation-contraction coupling and depresses contraction in various cardiac preparations. It also inhibits calcium release from the sarcoplasmic reticulum.

Application of strophanthidin to achieve calcium overload was followed by twitch from a depolarizing pulse, and tonic components of tension and repolarization produced an aftercontraction. A corresponding increase in emission of aequorin light was observed, which reflected an increased concentration of intracellular calcium. Ryanodine administration led to a transient increase in twitch tension and then a reduction in twitch to very low levels. The aftercontraction and aequorin light signal decreased monotonically after application of ryanodine.

These findings can be explained if ryanodine decreases the diastolic release of calcium. The transient positive inotropic effect of ryanodine is consistent with the hypothesis that the fall of force in calcium overload results from diastolic oscillations of calcium. It remains possible that part of the fall in force of calcium overload is caused by intracellular acidification.

Systemic and Regional Hemodynamic Effects of Captopril and Milrinone Administered Alone and Concomitantly in Patients With Heart Failure

Thierry H. LeJemtel, Carol S. Maskin, Donna Mancini, Lawrence Sinoway, Harry Feld, and Brian Chadwick (Albert Einstein College of Medicine, Bronx)
Circulation 72:364–369, August 1985   1–7

Certain patients with advanced heart failure fail to respond to captopril or experience serious side effects from it. The effect of milrinone, a selective phosphodiesterase inhibitor having both positive inotropic and vasodilatory properties, was compared with that of captopril in 16 men and 2 women (mean age, 60 years) with severe chronic congestive heart failure. Ten patients had ischemic heart disease and eight had cardiomyopathy of unknown origin. All patients had been in New York Heart Association functional class III or IV for at least 3 months, and all had a resting left ventricular ejection fraction of less than 20%. Patients received 7.5 mg of milrinone and 12.5 mg of captopril orally, or a bolus of 25 µg/kg or 50 µg/kg of milrinone intravenously.

Orally administered milrinone produced more improvement in cardiac performance than did captopril. Systemic arterial pressure was reduced more by captopril. The peak effect of captopril on cardiac index was less than that of milrinone. Resting femoral oxygen content was increased only by milrinone. Intravenously administered milrinone, added at the peak captopril effect, further augmented the stroke volume index and tended to reduce pulmonary capillary wedge pressure even more. In addition, the femoral venous oxygen content was increased.

Captopril and milrinone have synergistic effects on cardiac performance and complementary effects on the peripheral circulation in patients with advanced chronic heart failure. The increased cardiac output resulting from milrinone treatment may be shunted to vascular beds (e.g., skeletal muscle) where conductance can be improved.

▶ This study illustrates that all peripheral vasodilators do not produce the same alterations in peripheral blood flow. For example, captopril leads to renal vasodilatation but does not alter the flow to skeletal muscles acutely. On the other hand, milrinone, which is a phosphodiesterase inhibitor and thus an inotropic vasodilator, causes an increase in skeletal muscle blood flow that is superimposed on the increase in renal blood flow that occurs with the administration of captopril, an angiotensin-converting enzyme inhibitor. Given these concepts, the addition of drugs that affect the peripheral beds differently may have salutory effects that are additive when used concomitantly.—Edmund H. Sonnenblick, M.D.

Physiologic Assessment of the Inotropic, Vasodilator, and Afterload Reducing Effects of Milrinone in Subjects Without Cardiac Disease
Kenneth M. Borow, Patricia C. Come, Alexander Neumann, Donald S. Baim, Eugene Braunwald, and William Grossman (Brigham and Women's Hosp., Beth Israel Hosp., and Harvard Univ., Boston, and Univ. of Chicago)
Am. J. Cardiol. 55:1204–1209, April 15, 1985   1–8

Milrinone increases left ventricular (LV) shortening while augmenting cardiac output and reducing systemic vascular resistance. It is not known whether these changes result from vasodilation alone or from a combination of vasodilatory and positive inotropic effects. Load-independent end-systolic indices of the LV contractile state were used to evaluate contractility at baseline and during infusion of milrinone in 11 normotensive males aged 18–31 years who had no history of cardiopulmonary disease and no echocardiographic evidence of abnormality in LV regional wall motion. Two-dimensional targeted M-mode studies were done after premedication with atropine. The results of phonocardiographic studies, ECGs, carotid pulse tracings, and blood pressure readings also were recorded. Methoxamine was given by infusion for afterload augmentation of the left ventricle. The loading dose of milrinone per kg was 30 μg, 45 μg, or 60 μg, followed by an infusion of 0.66 μg/kg/minute or 0.99 μg/kg/minute for 15 minutes before methoxamine challenge was repeated.

The heart rate remained stable. Aortic diastolic and mean pressures declined, as did LV preload and LV end-systolic dimension. The percent of LV fractional shortening increased significantly. Total systemic resistance decreased by 10%, and LV end-systolic wall stress decreased by 32%. End-systolic indices of LV contractile state changed to indicate a positive inotropic effect, with no associated change in ventricular shape. All indices of contractility indicated a greater inotropic effect at higher plasma concentrations of milrinone.

Milrinone exerts a dose-related positive inotropic effect that is distinct from its vasodilatory and afterload-reducing actions in normal human beings. Further studies are needed to define the effects of the drug in patients with depressed cardiac output.

▶ This study clearly demonstrates that the effects of milrinone produce augmentation of myocardial contractility with enhanced ventricular performance while causing peripheral vasodilatation that further increases cardiac output. The net effect of these two actions is to enhance cardiac output while reducing peripheral resistance. These methods have been beautifully demonstrated in the normal ventricle. However, when there is substantial ventricular dilatation and decreases in wall motion, such measurements may be harder to make, and differentiation between peripheral and central effects may be more difficult under such circumstances using noninvasive techniques. Nevertheless, the present study shows how noninvasive techniques can be used to demonstrate the heart's mechanical activity and the relative influence of preload, afterload, and contractility.—Edmund H. Sonnenblick, M.D.

Effects of Enalapril, A New Angiotensin-Converting Enzyme Inhibitor, in a Controlled Trial in Heart Failure

Joseph A. Franciosa, Mary M. Wilen, and Randy A. Jordan (VA Med. Ctr., Little Rock, and Univ. of Arkansas)
J. Am. Coll. Cardiol. 5:101–107, January 1985   1–9

Enalapril, an orally active angiotensin-converting enzyme inhibitor that is more potent and longer acting than captopril is, lowers blood pressure in hypertensive patients and improves hemodynamics in patients in heart failure. The results of long-term enalapril therapy were compared with those of a placebo in a double-blind, randomized trial in 17 patients with chronic left ventricular (LV) failure that had been present for at least 3 months despite digitalis-diuretic therapy. All patients were in New York Heart Association functional classes II–IV and had a recent LV ejection fraction of less than 41%. The initial dose of enalapril, 5 mg twice daily, was increased as indicated clinically. The nine enalapril-treated patients and the eight who received placebo were clinically comparable.

Exercise capacity increased significantly during enalapril therapy, as did maximal oxygen consumption and duration of exercise. The LV ejection fraction did not change significantly in either group during the study. Yale scale scores declined significantly only in the enalapril group. No major clinical events or side effects occurred in either group.

Enalapril produces sustained vasodilation and significantly improves symptoms in patients with chronic LV failure. Exercise capacity is significantly increased. Major side effects did not occur in the present series.

Treatment with enalapril may prove superior to captopril therapy in this setting, especially in patients who experience side effects when taking captopril.

▶ The efficacy of enalapril appears similar to that of captopril, but its duration of action is considerably longer.—Edmund H. Sonnenblick, M.D.

Effects of a New Cardiotonic Agent, MDL-17,043, on Myocardial Contractility and Left Ventricular Performance in Congestive Heart Failure

Janet Strain, Richard Grose, Carol S. Maskin, and Thierry H. LeJemtel (Albert Einstein College of Medicine)
Am. Heart J. 110:91–96, July 1985   1–10

A newly synthesized imidazole derivative, MDL-17,043, has a potent positive inotropic effect and also direct vasodilatory activity in dogs. Its inotropic effect is additive to that of digitalis glycosides, and treatment with this drug improved left ventricular (LV) performance in patients in congestive heart failure. After intravenous injection, the effects of MDL-17,043 on myocardial contractility were examined in seven patients with severe congestive heart failure; all were in New York Heart Association functional classes III and IV. The mean level of digoxin at the time of study was 1.2 ng/ml. Four patients had ischemic heart disease, two had alcoholic cardiomyopathy, and one had hypertensive heart disease. The drug was given in an intravenous bolus of 0.25 mg/kg, followed by boluses of 0.5 mg/kg at 15-minute intervals to achieve the maximum increase in cardiac output.

The rate of rise in LV pressure increased almost immediately after injection of MDL-17,043. The mean cardiac index increased from 1.87 L/minute/sq m to 2.04 L/minute/sq m, whereas the mean pulmonary capillary wedge pressure fell from 23.7 mm Hg to 18.7 mm Hg. The mean aortic pressure did not change significantly. The peak rise in cardiac index coincided with the maximum fall in mean pulmonary capillary wedge and mean aortic pressures (Fig 1–2). The decline in mean right atrial pressure was not significant. The rate of rise in LV pressure was near baseline at peak cardiac performance.

Intravenous injections of MDL-17,043 improve myocardial contractility and LV performance in patients with severe congestive heart failure. The improved LV performance probably results from both the positive inotropic and direct vasodilatory effects of the agent. Improved blood flow to the renal vasculature at rest and to muscles during exercise contributes to the successful treatment of chronic congestive heart failure.

▶ This agent might be viewed as an inotropic vasodilator and has major effects to inhibit specific type III phosphodiesterase activity, thus augmenting intracellular cyclic adenosine monophosphate (*J. Cardiovasc. Pharmacol.* 4:509, 1982). Such effects are similar to those of other agents such as amrinone (*Am.*

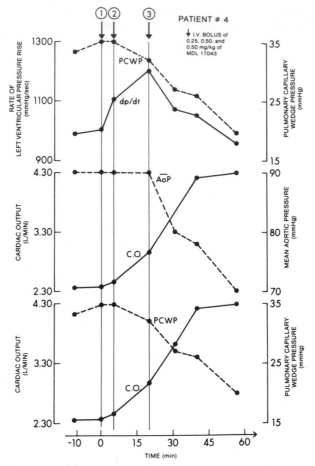

Fig 1–2.—Time course of changes in rate of increase in LV pressure, pulmonary capillary wedge pressure (PCWP), cardiac output (C.O.), and mean aortic pressure (AōP) after three successive intravenous boluses of MDL-17,043. (Courtesy of Strain, J., et al.: Am. Heart J. 110:91–96, July 1985.)

J. Cardiol. 45:123, 1980) and milrinone (*Circulation* 67:1065, 1983). It is of interest that the initial increase in the differential LV pressure (dP/dt) produced by the inotropic action of the agent may be offset by a decrease in the filling pressure, so that the dP/dt may appear unchanged because of the balance of an increase in contractility and a decrease in LV filling pressure.—Edmund H. Sonnenblick, M.D.

Relative Attenuation of Sympathetic Drive During Exercise in Patients With Congestive Heart Failure
Gary S. Francis, Steven R. Goldsmith, Susan Ziesche, Hisayoshi Nakajima, and Jay N. Cohn (Univ. of Minnesota and VA Med. Ctr., Minneapolis)
J. Am. Coll. Cardiol. 5:832–839, April 1985   1–11

Patients in chronic congestive heart failure have altered sympathetic responsiveness to certain types of stress. An augmented response to exercise despite a reduced heart rate-blood pressure response suggests a lack of myocardial responsiveness to stimulation by catecholamines. Cardiovascular responses to exercise were assessed as a function of both absolute work intensity, measured as total body oxygen uptake, and relative work intensity in 31 men aged 32–71 years with chronic, stable, New York Heart Association clinical classes II–III heart failure.

Eighteen patients had idiopathic or alcoholic cardiomyopathy and 13 had coronary artery disease. No patient had sustained an infarct in the preceding 4 months. The average left ventricular ejection fraction, as determined by radionuclide ventriculography at rest before exercise, was 24%. Ten healthy males aged 15–54 years also were examined. Exercise studies were done by using a bicycle ergometer at a starting workload of 25 W for patients with heart failure and 50 W for normal persons. The load was increased to the symptomatic maximum.

Patients in heart failure had significantly greater heart rate responses to exercise for any given comparable oxygen consumption, but they had a smaller incremental increase in heart rate than found in controls. Responses of blood pressure to exercise were reduced in the patient group on comparison at equivalent exercise levels. The maximum achievable heart rate and systolic blood pressure responses were blunted as the severity of heart failure increased, but peak plasma levels of norepinephrine did not distinguish between mild and severe heart failure.

The mechanism of the attenuated sympathetic response to exercise in patients in heart failure is uncertain, but it resembles that seen after orthostasis and infusion of nitroprusside. The attenuated response probably reflects the severity of congestive failure to some extent. It may contribute to intolerance of exercise in patients with heart failure.

▶ Attenuation of the heart rate and blood pressure responses in heart failure in relation to the severity of failure has been well demonstrated. To what extent depletion of myocardial catecholamines in heart failure, despite remaining β receptors within the myocardial cells per se, contributes to this difference is unknown. The interrelationship between peripheral catecholamine levels and cardiac responses is also complex. Normally, catecholamines mediate their effect in the heart through primarily local release from cardiac nerves, producing a high transient concentration of catecholamines in the cleft between cardiac nerves and the myocardial cell. In heart failure, the catecholamines are largely depleted from the myocardium, leaving the heart effectively denervated. Thus, circulating catecholamines from peripheral vascular stores can return to the myocardium, but are not absorbed by the nerves there; rather, the catecholamines are left free to act on the myocardium. This produces "down-regulation," in which the β_1 receptors in the myocardium are effectively reduced. Keeping all of these considerations in mind, it is not surprising that the interrelationship between peripheral catecholamines and cardiac responses is complex. Nevertheless, this may be an important consideration relative to the course of heart failure and its treatment.—Edmund H. Sonnenblick, M.D.

Ventricular Arrhythmias in Severe Heart Failure: Incidence, Significance, and Effectiveness of Antiarrhythmic Therapy

C. Simon Chakko and Mihai Gheorghiade (VA Med. Ctr. and Univ. of Virginia, Salem)
Am. Heart J. 109:497–504, March 1985   1–12

Antiarrhythmic therapy has been suggested for patients in severe heart failure who have asymptomatic nonsustained ventricular tachycardia. A trial of antiarrhythmic therapy based on the presence of a low left ventricular ejection fraction (LVEF) alone may be indicated, rather than reliance on results of 24-hour ambulatory ECGs. Monitoring was carried out in 43 patients receiving maximum medical treatment for severe chronic heart failure in whom premature ventricular beats were detected on 12-lead ECG. Twenty-eight patients had ischemic and 15 had idiopathic dilated cardiomyopathy. Twenty-three of the 43 patients received long-term antiarrhythmic therapy, 20 with procainamide and 3 with quinidine. Treatment decisions were made by the primary care physicians.

Baseline ECG studies showed sinus rhythm in 37 patients, atrial fibrillation with a controlled ventricular response in 5, and atrial tachycardia with block in 1. Twenty-two patients had ventricular tachycardia. Ten sudden deaths occurred during an average follow-up period of 16 months. Six other patients died of intractable congestive heart failure. Total mortality and sudden death were comparable in the treated and untreated groups, even when data on those with complex premature ventricular beats were analyzed separately. Sudden death was relatively frequent in patients whose LVEF was 20% or less (Fig 1–3). Among patients who had nonsustained ventricular tachycardia, those who died suddenly had more marked left ventricular dysfunction than occurred in those who survived.

Asymptomatic complex ventricular arrhythmias are frequent in patients with severe heart failure caused by dilated cardiomyopathy. Mortality is high and many sudden, unexpected deaths occur, especially in patients with nonsustained ventricular tachycardia and a low LVEF. Conventional antiarrhythmic therapy does not seem to prevent sudden death in this population.

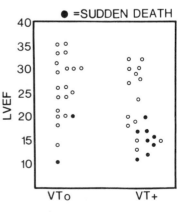

Fig 1–3.—Relationship among absent ventricular tachycardia (VT0) and present ventricular tachycardia (VT +), percent of left ventricular ejection fraction (LVEF), and sudden death. (Courtesy of Chakko, C.S., and Gheorghiade, M.: Am. Heart J. 109:497–504, March 1985.)

▶ The approach to arrhythmias in severe heart failure remains controversial. Nevertheless, it is apparent that routine antiarrhythmic therapy does not seem to alter the incidence of sudden death. Whether further subgroups who are at risk relative to arrhythmias in the presence of heart failure can be identified and treated appropriately requires further exploration. At the present time, the best treatment of ventricular arrhythmias in heart failure appears to be treatment of the heart failure per se.—Edmund H. Sonnenblick, M.D.

Postoperative Regression of Left Ventricular Dimensions in Aortic Insufficiency: A Long-Term Echocardiographic Study
Paolo Fioretti, Jos Roelandt, Mariagrazia Sclavo, Stefano Domenicucci, Max Haalebos, Egbert Bos, and Paul G. Hugenholtz (Erasmus Univ. and Academic Hosp. Dijkzigt, Rotterdam, and Interuniversity Cardiology Inst., Utrecht)
J. Am. Coll. Cardiol. 5:856–861, April 1985   1–13

Left ventricular (LV) dysfunction appears not to preclude a favorable clinical course in most patients who have valve replacement for chronic aortic insufficiency, but persistent LV enlargement in the first months after operation may indicate irreversible dysfunction. Changes in LV dimension were assessed up to 3 years after operation in 42 consecutive patients whose median age was 45 years; all underwent uncomplicated valve replacement for symptomatic aortic insufficiency between 1973 and 1981. The peak transvalvular gradient was less than 20 mm Hg. The most frequent known causes of insufficiency were rheumatic disease and endocarditis. A Björk-Shiley tilting disk prosthesis was used in 30 patients and a Hancock xenograft bioprosthesis was used in 8.

Twenty-four of the 37 patients who were evaluated 3 years after operation had a normal LV end-diastolic diameter and cross-sectional area; 13 had persistent LV enlargement. The median clinical follow-up period was 5 years. The functional status of all patients was improved after valve replacement. One patient died of progressive heart failure 2 years after valve replacement. On average, end-diastolic diameter decreased by 22% and cross-sectional area decreased by 16% within a year after operation. Persistent LV enlargement was not predicted by age, functional class, or duration of symptoms before surgery. End-diastolic diameter was the most predictive parameter. The combination of an end-diastolic diameter of at least 75 mm and an end-systolic diameter of at least 50 mm had a negative predictive value of 92%, but a 50% false positive rate.

Patients with symptomatic aortic insufficiency without other disease have a favorable long-term prognosis after uncomplicated valve replacement. The LV dimensions may regress after the first postoperative year and are normal in most patients 3 years after operation. Early operation is not necessary in patients with initial echocardiographic signs of LV dysfunction if appropriate symptoms are not present.

▶ The present article argues against early valve replacement in asymptomatic or mildly symptomatic patients with early signs of left ventricular dysfunction in the presence of aortic insufficiency. Although improvement in surgical techniques and perioperative myocardial protection has reduced the surgical risk, the subsequent morbidity related to an implanted prosthetic valve remains a long-term problem. The excellent long-term outcome with a return to normal LV size in most patients with aortic insufficiency suggests that patients with early LV dysfunction need not be operated on if the operation is not indicated by symptoms. In general, a very large end-diastolic diameter preoperatively is probably associated with persistence of LV enlargement postoperatively, although this is not always the case. Moreover, persistence of moderate LV enlargement after surgery does not indicate a poor clinical prognosis: reduction of LV size may continue even beyond the first postoperative year.—Edmund H. Sonnenblick, M.D.

Effects of Intravenous Infusion of Esmolol and Propranolol on Biventricular Performance at Rest and During Exercise as Assessed by Quantitative Radionuclide Angiography
Abdulmassih S. Iskandrian, A-Hamid Hakki, Atul Laddu, James Steck, Roy Saunders, Sally Kane-Marsch, and Joel Morganroth (Hahnemann Univ.)
Am. J. Cardiol. 55:1287–1292, May 1, 1985   1–14

Esmolol is a β-blocker found in animal studies to have both cardiac selectivity and a short duration of action. The drug also suppressed sinus tachyarrhythmias and slowed the ventricular rate in patients with supraventricular tachycardias. The effects of infusion of esmolol and intravenous injections of propranolol on cardiovascular performance at rest and during upright bicycle exercise were examined in 12 men and 3 women with stable angina. The mean age was 54 years. Four patients had significant coronary artery disease and four had evidence of past myocardial infarction.

A double-blind, crossover design was used. Biventricular function was evaluated by radionuclide ventriculography. Esmolol was given in a loading dose of 500 μg/kg/minute for 2 minutes, followed by 200 μg/kg/minute. Propranolol was given in four doses of 1 mg each.

No significant adverse reactions developed. Significant differences in hemodynamic variables occurred with the two drugs, both at rest and during exercise. There were no significant differences between average esmolol and average propranolol measurements at rest and during exercise except for systolic blood pressure during exercise, which was lower during infusion of esmolol. Blood levels of esmolol declined markedly within 30 minutes after infusion.

The effects of esmolol on biventricular function are similar to those of propranolol. Its major advantage is the short duration of action, which permits management of adverse effects by terminating the infusion. Esmolol may be useful in patients with AMI and unstable angina, as well as in the postoperative period. The safety of the drug should be confirmed in patients with poor left ventricular function. The required 1:10 dilution for infusion may limit use of the drug in patients whose fluid intake is restricted.

▶ Esmolol is a cardioselective β blocker that has a very short duration of activity; thus, it may be used in circumstances in which β blockade would be useful, but safety would dictate the presence of a very short-acting agent.—Edmund H. Sonnenblick, M.D.

Catecholamines and Adrenergic Receptors

Mechanisms of Supersensitivity to Sympathomimetic Amines in the Chronically Denervated Heart of the Conscious Dog

Dorothy E. Vatner, Michel Lavallee, Jun Amano, Auris Finizola, Charles J. Homcy, and Stephen F. Vatner (Harvard Univ., Massachusetts Gen. Hosp., and Brigham and Women's Hosp., Boston, and New England Primate Res. Ctr., Southboro, Mass.)
Circ. Res. 57:55–64, July 1985   1–15

Knowledge of the mechanisms of denervation supersensitivity is important in relation to clinical cardiac transplantation. Further, transmural myocardial infarction interrupts the sympathetic nerves and leads to local cardiac denervation. Cardiac responses to catecholamines were compared in chronically instrumented, conscious, intact dogs and dogs subjected to total surgical cardiac denervation by an intrapericardial approach. Sympathomimetic amine responses were also studied after ganglionic blockade with hexamethonium and atropine in conscious dogs. β-Adrenergic receptor-binding saturation was studied with ^{3}H-dihydroalprenolol (DHA) and the muscarinic, cholinergic receptor with ^{3}H-quinuclidinyl benzilate (QNB).

Norepinephrine increased the differential left ventricular pressure (dP/dt) more in dogs with cardiac denervation than in intact dogs, but responses to isoproterenol were similar unless opposing reflex effects were blocked, when treatment with isoproterenol and prenalterol led to 40% to 50% greater increases in dP/dt and heart rate in denervated dogs. The density of β-adrenergic receptors was increased in denervated left ventricles, and enhanced isoproterenol-mediated adenylate cyclase activity was found. Muscarinic cholinergic receptor density was decreased in denervated ventricles.

Chronic cardiac denervation in the dog leads to up-regulation of the β-adrenergic receptor and down-regulation of the muscarinic receptor. The chief mechanism of denervation supersensitivity to norepinephrine appears to involve a lack of norepinephrine reuptake. Up-regulation of the β-adrenergic receptor is responsible for only a fraction of the supersensitivity response to norepinephrine. Concomitant parasympathetic denervation results in down-regulation of the muscarinic receptor.

Mechanisms of β-Adrenergic Receptor Regulation in Cultured Chick Heart Cells: Role of Cytoskeleton Function and Protein Synthesis

James D. Marsh, Daniel Lachance, and Donghee Kim (Brigham and Women's Hosp. and Harvard Univ., Boston)
Circ. Res. 57:171–181, July 1985   1–16

The mechanism by which cardiac β-adrenergic receptors are regulated probably is important in the pathophysiology of states including congestive heart failure and acute myocardial ischemia, in which local catecholamine concentrations are altered. The effects of cytoskeletal disrupting agents and inhibition of protein synthesis on receptor properties and contractile responses to isoproterenol were examined in cultured ventricular cells from the embryonic chick heart. Monolayer cultures of beating ventricular cells were used. Contractility was monitored directly by an optical apparatus with magnification and a television camera.

Exposure of intact cells to 1 μM of isoproterenol for 30 minutes led to loss of the high-affinity state of the receptor in cell membranes, with no loss of receptors. The contractile response to isoproterenol fell to 41% of baseline, and it recovered to 78% 1 hour after agonist removal. The high-affinity receptor state recovered at the same time. These effects were markedly reduced by preincubation with cytochalasin B. A colchicine-sensitive loss of receptors from intact cells was observed after prolonged exposure. Recovery of receptor number was blocked by cycloheximide.

Rapid desensitization and resensitization of the β-receptor-mediated contractile response of chick embryo ventricular cells are associated with changes in high-affinity agonist binding and appear to be modulated by microfilaments. Receptor down-regulation depends on functional microtubules, and recovery of receptors after agonist removal requires protein synthesis. Other hormones and neurotransmitters (e.g., acetylcholine, thyroid hormone, and cortisol) probably modulate the β-receptor as well.

▶ "Down-regulation" of β receptors in cardiac tissue may be an important mechanism by which the sensitivity of this tissue is modulated when catecholamines are released in increased quantity. For example, in heart failure there is depletion of norepinephrine from its stores in cardiac nerves, and the ability of these nerves to sequester circulating catecholamines is markedly reduced or absent. Thus, the β receptors on cardiac tissue are exposed to circulating catecholamines and subject to "down-regulation." The mechanisms by which this down-regulation takes place are physiologic once it has occurred, and the rates at which it either recurs or recovers are of considerable interest. The present study supports the view that down-regulation occurs in two dynamic stages: a rapid initial desensitization, which appears to require microfilament function, followed by a slower process of microtubule-modulated down-regulation with loss of receptors. Recovery of receptors is relatively slow and requires protein synthesis. The physiologic consequences of these alterations in tissue that is effectively denervated (as occurs in heart failure) is as yet unclear. Moreover, in the absence of denervation, the importance of down-regulation also requires further definition.—Edmund H. Sonnenblick, M.D.

Stimulation of Hypertrophy of Cultured Neonatal Rat Heart Cells Through an α₁-Adrenergic Receptor and Induction of Beating Through an α₁- and

β₁-Adrenergic Receptor Interaction: Evidence for Independent Regulation of Growth and Beating

Paul Simpson (Univ. of California at San Francisco)
Circ. Res. 56:884–894, June 1985   1–17

In vitro studies have suggested that catecholamines may be molecular signals that link increased circulatory demand with myocardial hypertrophy. Norepinephrine stimulates hypertrophy of cultured cells of the heart muscle of the neonatal rat through an α_1-adrenergic receptor. The fact that catecholaminergic stimulation of contractility presumably is under β-adrenergic control suggests that the cells may have dual pathways regulating growth and contractility through α-receptors and β-adrenergic receptors, respectively. The effects of adrenergic agents on beating and hypertrophy of myocytes were examined in serum-free cultures of heart cells obtained from day-old rats.

Norepinephrine and epinephrine were equally potent stimulants of hypertrophy, assessed radioisotopically, and chronotropic activity. Cell protein and area were increased by up to twofold, and the proportion of beating cells increased from 5% or less to 95%. Maximal response occurred within 24–48 hours after exposure. Studies with various agonists and antagonists indicated that hypertrophy was mediated through an α_1-adrenergic receptor, but induction of beating required activation of both α_1-receptor and β_1-receptors. α-Stimulation alone produced hypertrophied cells with minimal beating. With the use of cycloheximide to inhibit protein synthesis, α stimulation plus β stimulation produced maximum beating without hypertrophy.

Growth and beating of cardiac cells can be regulated independently via separate cellular pathways in a neonatal rat model. Excessive hypertrophy, as in hypertrophic cardiomyopathy, may reflect excessive α-mediated growth, whereas inadequate growth can produce a lack of adequate hypertrophy in valvular heart disease or congestive cardiomyopathy.

▶ While catecholamines may stimulate hypertrophy through stimulation of α_1 receptors, this may not be the only mechanism by which hypertrophy may be induced and facilitated. For example, in the presence of α blockade, cardiac growth still occurs and hypertrophy in response to loading has not been shown to require catecholamines. Whether mechanical and hormonal effects are additive or facilitative requires further analysis.—Edmund H. Sonnenblick, M.D.

Direct Analysis of β-Adrenergic Receptor Subtypes on Intact Adult Ventricular Myocytes of the Rat

Iain L. O. Buxton and Laurence L. Brunton (Univ. of California at San Diego)
Circ. Res. 56:126–132, January 1985   1–18

There is evidence for the coexistence of β_1 receptors and β_2 receptors for catecholamines in the mammalian myocardium. Radioligand binding and cell purification techniques were used to measure the distribution of β-receptor subtypes on purified cardiomyocytes from the ventricle of adult rats and also on the nonmyocyte elements of the ventricle to determine whether β_1 receptors and β_2 receptors coexist on the myocytes. In these studies the subtype nonselective β-adrenergic antagonist ^{125}I-iodocyano-pindolol, the β_1-subtype-selective antagonists betaxolol and practolol, and the β_2-selective antagonist zinterol were used.

Iodine-125-iodocyanopindolol bound to 2×10^5 receptors per purified adult rat cardiomyocyte, with a dissociation constant of 70 pM. Betaxolol, practolol, and zinterol competed for ^{125}I-iodocyanopindolol-binding sites on intact myocytes in a monophasic manner, with respective dissociation constants of 46, 845, and 923 nM. Binding of ^{125}I-iodocyanopindolol to membranes prepared from nonmyocyte elements of the ventricle occurred with a dissociation constant of 43 pM and a capacity of 88 fmole/mg of membrane protein.

These findings indicate that purified adult rat ventricular myocytes possess only β_1 receptors and that the β_2 receptors present in the rat ventricle are located on nonmyocyte cells. It would seem that the metabolic and contractile responses of rat ventricular muscle to β-agonists result exclusively from occupation of β_1 receptors.

Positive Inotropic Effect of Acetylcholine in Canine Cardiac Purkinje Fibers
Robert F. Gilmour, Jr., and Douglas P. Zipes (Indiana Univ. and VA Med. Ctr., Indianapolis)
Am. J. Physiol. 249:H735–H740, October 1985 1–19

Acetylcholine increases developed tension in canine cardiac Purkinje fibers. It seemed possible that it increases tension directly, and is also capable of antagonizing the positive inotropic effects of isoproterenol. Action potentials and developed tension were recorded from canine Purkinje fibers in vitro using microelectrodes and a force transducer. The fibers were exposed to acetylcholine in concentrations ranging from 10^{-9} to 10^{-4} M, with and without pretreatment with atropine, hexamethonium, propranolol, phentolamine, and a combination of propranolol and phentolamine. Fibers exposed to verapamil or isoproterenol were superfused with acetylcholine.

Acetylcholine produced a dose-dependent increase in tension that was blocked by atropine administration; however, it was not blocked by propranolol, phentolamine, hexamethonium, or verapamil. Acetylcholine at 10^{-5} M increased the action potential duration at 50% of repolarization, but did not alter the resting membrane potential or action potential amplitude. Isoproterenol at 10^{-7} M increased developed tension and shortened the action potential duration. Superfusion with acetylcholine countered both effects of isoproterenol. An increased extracellular Ca^{--} increased tension and shortened the action potential duration; addition of acetylcholine increased tension further and prolonged the action potential duration. High levels of acetylcholine restored excitability to K-depolarized fibers, but lower concentrations suppressed slow responses induced by isoproterenol.

The effects of acetylcholine on canine cardiac Purkinje fibers are mediated by muscarinic receptors and are independent of catecholamine release. It is unclear whether the effect of acetylcholine on action potential duration results from a change in calcium or potassium conductance.

▶ It is of interest that acetylcholine increases developed tension in canine cardiac Purkinje fibers. It is well known that acetylcholine leads to a substantial decrease in tension in atrial tissue and has only minimal effects on ventricular tissue aside from its secondary effects to increase catecholamines, which may augment contractility slightly. The significance of the ability of an acetylcholine to antagonize the positive inotropic effects of β-adrenergic agonists requires further study.—Edmund H. Sonnenblick, M.D.

Phorbol Ester- and Diacylglycerol-Mediated Desensitization of Cardiac β-Adrenergic Receptors
Constantinos J. Limas and Catherine Limas (Univ. of Minnesota)
Circ. Res. 57:443–449, September 1985   1–20

Phorbol esters modify hormone-receptor interactions, presumably through binding to specific receptors that may be identical to the Ca^{--}/ phospholipid-dependent protein kinase C. They substitute for unsaturated diacylglycerols, the endogenous activators of protein kinase C, in lowering Ca^{++} requirements for enzymatic activity. Protein kinase C, which is present in myocardium, influences Ca^{++} transport by the cardiac sarcoplasmic reticulum and sarcolemma through phosphorylation of phospholamban. The effects of phorbol esters and a synthetic diacylglycerol, 1-oleyl-2-acetyl diglycerol (OADG), on cardiac myocytes obtained from adult rats were investigated.

Incubation of dissociated cardiac myocytes with biologically active phorbol esters led to a time-dependent and concentration-dependent loss of β-adrenergic receptors, as identified with the hydrophilic ligand ^{3}H-CGP-12177. Both maximum β receptor numbers and their affinity were reduced. Desensitization of β receptors also occurred with OADG, which activates protein kinase C. Both phorbol dibutyrate and OADG were additive to isoproterenol. Their effects were countered by colchicine, suggesting microtubular dependence. The loss of membrane-bound β-receptors on preincubation with phorobol dibutyrate or OADG was accompanied by an increase in β receptors associated with a cytosol-derived vesicular fraction that is devoid of plasma membrane markers, indicating a process of internalization.

Activation of protein kinase C by diacylglycerols that are derived from receptor-linked phosphoinositide hydrolysis may be one mechanism of cardiac β-receptor desensitization. There is early evidence that phorbol ester binding is altered in the course of cardiac hypertrophy. The functional effects of β-receptor desensitization mediated via protein kinase C probably are different from those mediated via β agonists.

▶ "Down-regulation" has been demonstrated in the presence of chronic heart failure when catecholamine stores within the myocardium are lost and serum levels of circulating catecholamines are elevated. How this is mediated has yet to be defined. The present study shows that there may be multiple mechanisms for down-regulation of β receptors under such circumstances.—Edmund H. Sonnenblick, M.D.

The Mechanism by Which Adenosine and Cholinergic Agents Reduce Contractility in Rat Myocardium: Correlation With Cyclic Adenosine Monophosphate and Receptor Densities
Joel Linden, Cathy E. Hollen, and Amrat Patel (Oklahoma Med. Res. Found., Oklahoma City)
Circ. Res. 56:728–735, May 1985   1–21

The cardiac muscle response to cholinergic muscarinic agents closely resembles the response to adenosine. Adenosine deaminase was used to deaminate endogenous adenosine in the isolated rat left atrium, and the contractile effects of the adenosine analogue l-N^6-(R-phenyl-isopropyl)-adenosine (PIA) were examined. Radioligand binding assays were done with ^{125}I-aminobenzyladenosine, ^{125}I-pindolol, and ^{3}H-quinuclidinyl benzilate.

The analogue PIA decreased both the basal and the isoproterenol-stimulated contractile state of the isolated rat left atrium, with closely similar ED_{50} levels. It decreased the cyclic adenosine monophosphate (cAMP) content of atria and inhibited isoproterenol-stimulated adenylate cyclase activity in membranes from atria and ventricles, although less than methacholine did. The effects of PIA and methacholine were greatly attenuated in the presence of both isoproterenol and the phosphodiesterase inhibitor Ro7-2956. The densities of adenosine, muscarinic, and β-adrenergic receptors in rat atrial membranes were 30 fmole/mg, 551 fmole/mg, and 24 fmole/mg of protein, respectively.

The direct and antiadrenergic contractile effects of PIA and methacholine appear to result primarily from their effects on cAMP metabolism. The greater effectiveness of methacholine as a negative inotropic agent and an inhibitor of adenylate cyclase in atria may be related to the relative densities of muscarinic and adenosine receptors. The likelihood of an interaction between agonist-occupied receptors and inhibitory guanine nucleotide-binding proteins is enhanced as the receptor density increases.

Lateral Border Zone: Quantitation of Lateral Extension of Subendocardial Infarction in the Dog

Robert Forman, Sangho Cho, Stephen M. Factor, and Edward S. Kirk (Albert Einstein College of Medicine)

J. Am. Coll. Cardiol. 5:1125–1131, May 1985 1–22

There is a border zone at the epicardial aspect of a subendocardial infarct, but the existence of a lateral border zone is uncertain. Subendocardial infarcts were produced in 12 dogs by 40-minute occlusion of the left anterior descending coronary artery distal to the first large diagonal branch. Extension of the infarct was induced a week later by permanently occluding the same vessel. Regional myocardial blood flow was estimated by the labeled microsphere method, and the vascular boundaries between normally perfused and ischemic regions were defined by perfusion with variously colored Microfil solutions. The extent of transmural and lateral extension was documented by point counting histologic specimens.

Temporary occlusion produced a mean transmural infarct of 30% and later permanent occlusion produced a mean transmural extension of 29% in a mean risk region of 39 gm. Mean measured lateral extension of the infarct in eight evaluable animals was 1.7% of the cross-sectional area of the risk region as determined planimetrically. Analysis of a model of the risk region indicated a mean lateral extension that amounted to 3.5% of the region at risk.

These findings suggest that a border zone exists at the lateral margin of a subendocardial infarct. A significant mass of myocardium cannot be salvaged at this site. Significant lateral extension would not be expected, because collateral blood flow is distributed via epicardial collateral vessels rather than by intramyocardial vascular connections from the normal myocardium to the region at risk.

▶ This study supports the view that the area at risk in AMI is determined by anatomy and that lateral extension of infarction does not contribute greatly to the extent of infarction; however, rather than transmural extension, lateral extension remains the most important consideration in the enlargement of a given area of infarction.—Edmund H. Sonnenblick, M.D.

Vagal Chemoreflex Coronary Vasodilation Evoked by Stimulating Pulmonary C-Fibers in Dogs

J. P. Clozel, A. M. Roberts, J. I. E. Hoffman, H. M. Coleridge, and J. C. G. Coleridge (Univ. of California at San Francisco)
Circ. Res. 57:450–460, September 1985 1–23

A parasympathetic vasodilator nerve supply exists in the coronary vascular bed. It is engaged reflexly when the carotid body chemoreceptors are stimulated, or when carotid baroreceptors or afferent vagal nerve endings in the heart are stimulated. An attempt was made to determine whether the canine cholinergic coronary vasodilator pathway is activated by stimulating chemosensitive vagal nerve endings in the lung. The circumflex coronary artery was perfused at constant pressure, and pulmonary C fibers were stimulated by injecting capsaicin into the right atrium. The heart rate was kept constant in some studies. Coronary flow distribution was examined using radioactive microspheres.

Stimulation of pulmonary C fibers with capsaicin decreased arterial blood pressure and heart rate and increased circumflex blood flow by up to 109%. Circumflex blood flow increased comparably when the heart rate was kept constant by pacing. Coronary vasodilation could not be ascribed to the reflex reduction in arterial blood pressure. Injection of capsaicin into the left atrium did not increase circumflex blood flow. Reflex coronary vasodilation was abolished by cooling the cervical vagi to 0 C, cutting the pulmonary vagal branches, and giving atropine. Reflex vasodilation occurred despite low coronary perfusion pressure. The endocardial:epicardial flow ratio declined as perfusion pressure was reduced, but it was not altered by stimulation of the pulmonary C fibers at any perfusion pressure.

Stimulation of pulmonary C fibers leads to reflex cholinergic vasodilation in all layers of the canine myocardium. Autoregulatory vasodilation is the basic means of maintaining coronary blood flow in the face of decreased perfusion pressure, but neurally induced vasodilation can provide additional protection to the myocardium.

▶ Pulmonary C fibers are known to be stimulated in a variety of pathophysiologic conditions, including embolization, inflammation, congestion, and edema of the lung, as well as inhalation of irritant gases (Coleridge, J. C. G., and Coleridge, H. M.: *Rev. Physiol. Biochem. Pharmacol.* 99:1–110, 1984). The role that these chemoreflexes play in providing additional coronary blood flow under pathologic conditions in man has yet to be determined.—Edmund H. Sonnenblick, M.D.

Signal-Averaged Electrocardiographic Late Potentials in Patients With Ventricular Fibrillation or Ventricular Tachycardia: Correlation With Clinical Arrhythmia and Electrophysiologic Study
Roger A. Freedman, Anne M. Gillis, Andre Keren, Vivian Soderholm-Difatte, and Jay W. Mason (Stanford Univ.)
Am J. Cardiol. 55:1350–1353, May 1, 1985   1–24

Low-amplitude, high-frequency potentials at the end of the QRS complex are sometimes detected during sinus rhythm in patients with ventricular tachycardia by signal-averaged ECG. The findings of signal-averaged ECG were compared in 27 patients with spontaneous, sustained ventricular tachycardia and 24 with spontaneous ventricular fibrillation. Nineteen normal persons were also studied. Sustained arrhythmias lasted for at least 15 seconds. Patients with myocardial infarction in the preceding week and those with bundle-branch block were excluded. Forty-six patients underwent electrophysiologic study while not taking antiarrhythmia drugs other than digitalis and β blockers.

The mean amplitude in the terminal 40 msec of the QRS complex (V40) was lower in patients with ventricular tachycardia than in those with ventricular fibrillation or normal individuals. Half of the patients with tachycardia had a V40 of 25 μV or less. The lowest values were in patients with reproducibly inducible sustained ventricular tachycardia or fibrillation. This was correctly predicted by a V40 of 25 μV or less in 88% of instances. The relationship was evident in each patient group considered separately. Past myocardial infarction was not a significant determinant of V40, nor was V40 related to ejection fraction or New York Heart Association functional class.

Different electrophysiologic mechanisms may underlie ventricular tachycardia and ventricular fibrillation. Correlation of inducibility of arrhythmia with low late-potential amplitude suggests that the presence or degree of slowed conduction may predispose to arrhythmia inducibility. Signal-averaged ECG may have a role in the management of patients with ventricular tachycardia or fibrillation.

▶ Signal-averaged ECG measurement of late potentials following the QRS complex provides another method to use in attempts to define the etiology of ventricular fibrillation and ventricular tachycardia under various circumstances. The mechanisms by which these high-frequency, low-level potentials are created requires further physiologic definition, and their role in the initiation of various arrhythmias requires more investigation. The usefulness of such measurements in the management of patients remains to be determined.—Edmund H. Sonnenblick, M.D.

The Impact of Aging on Adrenergic Receptor Function: Clinical and Biochemical Aspects
James A. Heinsimer and Robert J. Lefkowitz (Duke Univ.)
J. Am. Geriatrics Soc. 33:184–188, March 1985   1–25

The physiologic changes that accompany advancing age presumably reflect changes in biochemical adaptive mechanisms. The decreased resting and exercise cardiac output that is observed despite an increase in left ventricular mass has been ascribed in part to impaired adrenergic nervous system function. Decreased sympathetic reserve has been proposed. Inotropic responses to catecholamines are reduced in aging animals. Tolerance ("desensitization") to increasing basal catecholamine concentrations may be responsible, or adrenergic denervation supersensitivity may be reduced with aging. Studies of changes in receptor density with aging have given conflicting results. Most data indicate that lymphocyte from elderly human beings have decreased isoproterenol responsiveness in terms of cyclic adenosine monophosphate production, but no decrease in receptor density. Certain animal studies confirm these findings.

Cardiovascular responsiveness is reduced with advancing age. Catecholamine-stimulated chronotropic and inotropic responses both decline. β-Adrenergic receptor density appears to be unaltered, although measurements of β-receptor concentration in various animal cells have given ambiguous results. Circulating lymphocytes may not accurately reflect the catecholamine environment to which other tissues are exposed. Age-related changes in adrenergic function may result from changes in the coupling of receptors to the adenylate cyclase system. The clinical implication is that geriatric patients may be at risk of unusual sensitivity to sympathetic agonists and antagonists. Further studies of drug pharmacokinetics and adrenergic drug dose schedules are needed in the geriatric population.

Atherosclerosis and Coronary Heart Disease

Atherosclerosis: Progression, Regression, and Resolution
M. Rene Malinow (Oregon Health Sciences Univ.)
Am. Heart J. 108:1523–1537, December 1984   1–26

Despite clinical impressions that atherosclerosis is a progressive disease, animal studies have shown that atherosclerotic plaques can decrease in size when atherogenic stimuli are removed. Sequential angiographic studies in human beings also suggest that atherosclerotic stenoses may enlarge under certain circumstances. The concept of anatomical progression of atherosclerosis is based mainly on static microscopic studies and autopsy findings.

Withdrawal of dietary cholesterol has been associated with shrinkage of induced atherosclerotic lesions in several animals species, including nonhuman primates. Most anatomical evidence for regression in man is circumstantial. Some studies have indicated that patients with malignant disease have less severe atherosclerosis than others have. Reported rates of regression in human beings vary widely. Up to 20% of patients in serial angiographic studies reportedly have regression of lesions. Intensive treatment to reduce the plasma cholesterol level has led to regression of femoral arterial disease.

Depletion of lipids and a reduction in both cell numbers and extracellular material could account for angiographically observed regression of atherosclerosis in human beings. Other mechanisms could include lysis or retraction of superimposed thrombi incorporation of thrombi into the arterial wall, followed by organization, contraction, or channel formation; release of spasm; arterial ectasia or dilatation; medial thinning with outward bulging of the plaque; and plaque ulceration. Various animal studies have suggested the importance of local mechanisms in regression. The hemodynamic consequences of regression remain to be determined, and studies are needed to learn how to influence the course of regression. Prevention remains the best course until it is learned how atherosclerosis regression can be induced consistently.

▶ This review, together with the results of the study by Arntzenius and others and the Leiden Intervention Trial, supports the view that dietary intervention may not only prevent the progression of coronary artery disease, but may play a role in regression of atheromatous lesions. This concept remains controversial but highly challenging.—Edmund H. Sonnenblick, M.D.

Diet, Lipoproteins, and the Progression of Coronary Atherosclerosis: The Leiden Intervention Trial

Alexander C. Arntzenius, Daan Kromhout, Jacques D. Barth, Johan H. C. Reiber, Albert V. G. Bruschke, Beert Buis, Coen M. van Gent, Noes Kempen-Voogd, Sipke Strikwerda, and Edo A. van der Velde (Leiden Univ., The Netherlands)
N. Engl. J. Med. 312:805–811, March 28, 1985   1–27

The Leiden Intervention Trial is a study of the effect on coronary atherosclerosis of reducing the blood cholesterol level. Lipid levels were reduced by dietary measures alone, unlike in other studies. The patients, 35 men and 4 women (mean age, 49 years), had stable angina at baseline and at least one major coronary artery with 50% obstruction. A vegetarian diet with a polyunsaturated:saturated fatty acid ratio of at least 2 was given. Considerable emphasis was placed on dietary instruction and continuous supervision. The diet contained less than 100 mg of cholesterol daily.

A significant increase in the linoleic acid content of cholesteryl esters occurred, with significant reductions in body weight, serum total cholesterol level, and ratio of total cholesterol to high-density lipoprotein (HDL) cholesterol. Systolic blood pressure decreased significantly. Visual and computer-assisted analysis of angiograms after 2 years showed no lesion growth in 18 of the 39 patients. Significant progression was noted in patients having relatively high total:HDL cholesterol ratios during the trial. Lesion growth tended not to occur in patients with ratios below 6.9 or in those with initially higher ratios that fell significantly during dietary intervention. Progression of coronary disease was not related to blood pressure, smoking status, alcohol intake, weight, or drug treatment.

A low total:HDL cholesterol ratio was associated with relatively less progression of coronary atherosclerosis in this dietary intervention trial. Such intervention may be effective when a high total:HDL cholesterol ratio is present and the fatty acid and cholesterol content of the current diet is high. However, dietary intervention alone may not control coronary atherosclerosis in most heterozygous patients with familial hypercholesterolemia.

▶ The present study attempts to show that the ratio of serum total cholesterol to HDL cholesterol is directly related to the growth of obstructive coronary lesions. Moreover, dietary improvement in this ratio, albeit studied in a relatively small group of patients, appears to slow the progression of the process. These effects were demonstrated with the use of diet alone; if the diet is used with other measures to lower the cholesterol level more substantially, one might obtain even more dramatic results. The hypothesis presented here is challenging and deserves further support so that the implications can be applied to patient care with vigor. Early identification of patients with high cholesterol ratios should be made and their vigorous treatment undertaken, with results of therapy verified. Ultimately, one would hope that treatment of coronary artery disease would be preventive rather than palliative once the damage has occurred.—Edmund H. Sonnenblick, M.D.

Reduction of Plasma Lipids, Lipoproteins, and Apoproteins by Dietary Fish Oils in Patients With Hypertriglyceridemia
Beverley E. Phillipson, Douglas W. Rothrock, William E. Connor, William S. Harris, and D. Roger Illingworth (Oregon Health Sciences Univ.)
N. Engl. J. Med. 312:1210–1216, May 9, 1985   1–28

Dietary fish oils rich in omega-3 fatty acids reduce plasma lipid levels in normolipidemic individuals. The effects of a fish oil diet, a polyunsaturated vegetable oil diet, and a control low-fat, low-cholesterol diet were compared in 20 hypertriglyceridemic patients, 10 with type IIb hyperlipidemia and 10 with type V hyperlipidemia. The initial mean levels of plasma cholesterol and triglyceride were 337 mg/dl and 355 mg/dl, respectively. The eucaloric experimental diets were given for 4-week periods. In patients with type IIb hyperlipidemia, the fish oil and vegetable oil diets provided between 20% and 30% of the total calories as fat and 325 mg of cholesterol daily. In those with type V hyperlipidemia, the two diets contained between 20% and 30% of the total calories as fat and 350 mg of cholesterol daily. The control diet had a ratio of polyunsaturated to saturated fat of 1.4.

The fish oil diet led to a mean reduction of 27% in the plasma cholesterol level and a mean decline of 64% in the triglyceride level in patients with type IIb hyperlipidemia, compared with values derived from the control diet. A marked reduction in the very-low-density lipoprotein level also was noted. The vegetable oil diet had much lesser effects. Patients with type V hyperlipidemia experienced a mean decline of 45% in total cholesterol and a mean reduction of 79% in the triglyceride level associated with the fish oil diet, as well as pronounced lowering of very-low-density lipoprotein and apoprotein E levels. The level of plasma triglycerides rose significantly with the vegetable oil diet in this group.

A fish oil or fish-containing diet may be helpful in the management of hypertriglyceridemia. Further study is needed to determine the minimum amounts necessary to achieve the optimal hypolipidemic effect in hyperlipidemic patients.

Epidemiologic Assessment of the Role of Physical Activity and Fitness in Development of Cardiovascular Disease
W. B. Kannel, P. Wilson, and S. N. Blair (Boston Univ.; NHLBI; and Inst. for Aerobic Research, Dallas)
Am. Heart J. 109:876–885, April 1985   1–29

The level of physical activity is considered by some to be an important cardiovascular risk factor, but epidemiologic studies of this factor are difficult to carry out. There are suggestions for protection against coronary mortality in general, but the role of physical activity in the occurrence of sudden death is less certain. A close relationship was found between cardiovascular morbidity and mortality in the Framingham Study and in various surrogates for physical activity. Most studies indicate a weak or moderate association between the level of activity and the occurrence of cardiovascular disease. Activity rather than fitness has been measured in most studies. Reported associations are less convincing for women than for men. Exercise appears to be most beneficial in increasing the angina threshold and cardiac functional capacity. Many factors confound secondary prevention trials of physical fitness. There is evidence that exertion may precipitate sudden death in persons with heart disease.

There are many reasons to consider an independent causal role for physical inactivity on the rate of occurrence of coronary heart disease, but there are other reasons for skepticism. Epidemiologic evidence generally supports an association between regular exercise and a lower incidence of coronary heart disease. It seems unlikely that exercise programs can have as great an impact on cardiovascular disease as can control of major cardiovascular risk factors. Many clinicians nevertheless prescribe exercise for health reasons.

The overall evidence supports a life-style that emphasizes regular physical activity. Regular exercise helps to control other cardiovascular risk factors, improves the quality of life, and may encourage coronary candidates to take their health more seriously. Modest exercise programs that most persons accept and that do not cause orthopedic problems may suffice. It appears that physical exercise and conditioning are best included in a comprehensive program of multiple risk factor intervention.

▶ This article summarizes the benefits of exercise and a trained state to reduce the incidence of cardiovascular events. The argument is well supported that physical exercise and conditioning are best included as part of a comprehensive program of multiple risk factor intervention (Paffenbarger, R. S., Jr., and Hyde, R. T.: *Prev. Med.* 13:3, 1984). The reader is referred to the primary article for a detailed listing of literature in support of this argument.—Edmund H. Sonnenblick, M.D.

Plaque Fissuring: The Cause of Acute Myocardial Infarction, Sudden Ischaemic Death, and Crescendo Angina
Michael J. Davies and Anthony C. Thomas (St. Mary's Hosp. Med. School, London)
Br. Heart J. 53:363–373, April 1985   1–30

Recent pathologic studies of patients dying of AMI have shown that virtually all coronary thrombi were related to rupture or fissuring of atheromatous plaques. Dissection by blood from the lumen into the plaque can produce a large intraintimal thrombus that is rich in platelets. Thrombus can develop within the lumen over the site of rupture and propagate distally into arterial segments without significant intimal disease. Acute evolving coronary artery lesions in patients who die suddenly of ischemic heart disease also represent atheromatous plaques that are undergoing fissure or rupture. Rupture of the fibrous cap of the plaque with dissection of blood into the intima may be the initial event. The intraluminal thrombus may become totally occlusive or be completely lysed with resealing of the plaque fissure, thus stabilizing a larger plaque.

Patients with established regional infarction are those in whom thrombus has occluded the lumen at least long enough for myocardial necrosis to occur. Those with crescendo angina or those who die suddenly have coronary lesions in the earlier stages of plaque fissuring. Sudden death may sometimes result from a high incidence of platelet emboli in small myocardial vessels. Tearing of the intima, with resultant deposition of thrombus, could invoke local arterial spasm and infarction. It is likely that many patients survive plaque fissuring without experiencing symptoms. Patients with numerous plaques are at higher risk of repeated episodes of plaque fissuring.

Failure to view these events dynamically may make it difficult to understand how atheromatous disease produces acute clinical symptoms. The important process underlying acute infarction and sudden ischemic death is plaque fissuring with related intraintimal thrombosis, which progresses to formation of an intraluminal thrombus.

▶ This study provides a rational basis for explaining the development of unstable obstruction of a coronary artery when this event is superimposed on what had previously been a stable atherosclerotic plaque. Thus, bleeding into the plaque with extravasation into the bloodstream in the presence of thromboplastic material would explain many of the dynamic phenomena that are currently observed and whose control by thrombolytic therapy may provide a new approach to AMI.—Edmund H. Sonnenblick, M.D.

Simultaneous Therapy With Antiplatelet and Anticoagulant Drugs in Symptomatic Cardiovascular Disease
Arnold Miller and Robert S. Lees (New England Deaconess Hosp. and Massachusetts Inst. of Technology, Boston)
Stroke 16:668–675, July–August 1985   1–31

Twenty patients seen between 1970 and 1983 with advanced atherosclerosis received simultaneous aspirin and warfarin therapy. Nineteen had symptomatic atherosclerotic disease, and one had rheumatic heart disease. The 16 male and 4 female patients (mean age, 55 years) were treated for 6 years on the average. Aspirin was given in a dose of 0.6 gm twice daily, and warfarin in the dose necessary to maintain a prothrombin time of 16–20 seconds.

Thirteen patients had CNS symptoms and five had symptoms of peripheral vascular disease. All 20 patients became asymptomatic or were markedly improved clinically during treatment, and only 6 continued to take combined treatment when last seen. Six patients were withdrawn after acute bleeding occurred; two of these had intracranial bleeding and four had gastrointestinal tract hemorrhage. Both sudden deaths that occurred during treatment were consistent with acute myocardial ischemia. Seven patients in all had complications of treatment. One patient required evacuation of an intracranial hematoma. One required emergency operation for graft embolism.

Simultaneous aspirin and anticoagulant therapy may be warranted in patients with advanced atherosclerosis in whom alternative methods are not feasible or have proved ineffective. There is, however, an increased risk of hemorrhage with this treatment, and extreme caution is necessary. Prospective randomized studies are needed to quantify the risk-benefit ratio of this approach.

▶ In transient cerebral ischemia, antiplatelet drugs have been shown to provide symptomatic relief. A benefit has also been demonstrated with the use of combined dipyridamole and aspirin in early postoperative vein graft patency after coronary artery bypass surgery (Chesebro, J. H., et al.: *N. Engl. J. Med.* 307:73–78, 1982). Currently, there is increased enthusiasm for the use of aspirin to prevent recurrent closure of coronary arteries after AMI, especially during periods of unstable angina and intermediate syndromes. The broadened claims for the use of aspirin in specific occlusive syndromes require more specific delineation of those patients who are at risk and the underlying pathophysiology involved; double-blind, carefully controlled studies are needed to demonstrate both benefits and specific utilization. At present, it seems reasonable to conclude that aspirin may have very specific areas for use, but when this drug is combined with anticoagulant therapy (e.g., warfarin), the dangers of bleeding must be strongly considered. —Edmund H. Sonnenblick, M.D.

Prevalence and Significance of Residual Flow to the Infarct Zone During the Acute Phase of Myocardial Infarction

Heiner Blanke, Marc Cohen, Karl R. Karsch, Richard Fagerstrom, and K. Peter Rentrop (Mt. Sinai Hosp., New York, and Univ. of Goettingen, Federal Republic of Germany)

J. Am. Coll. Cardiol. 5:827–831, April 1985   1–32

Residual flow into an infarct zone can be present in an anterograde fashion if the infarct-related coronary vessel is incompletely obstructed, or in a retrograde fashion via intercoronary collateral channels. Residual flow was evaluated by coronary angiography in the acute phase of infarction in 130 patients seen from 1977 through 1980 at the University of Goettingen Hospital. All patients except those in cardiogenic shock received intravenous injections of nitroglycerin and heparin. Twenty-one patients had intra-aortic balloon counterpulsation before coronary angiography.

Incomplete obstruction of the infarct-related vessel was found in 36 patients (group I). Another 56 patients (group II) had complete obstruction with collateral flow to the infarct zone, and 38 others (group III) had complete obstruction of the infarct vessel without residual flow. The interval from onset of angina to infarction was longer in group II than in group III patients. Both group I and group II patients were more likely to be receiving antianginal drugs than those in group III were. The left ventricular ejection fraction in the acute phase was significantly higher in group I patients than in the other groups. The ejection fraction fell significantly during the follow-up period in group III patients. In group II patients the ejection fraction improved only when spontaneous recanalization occurred.

Repeat angiography showed patency of the initially completely obstructed infarct vessel in 7 of 16 group II patients and in 4 of 9 group III patients. In 2 of 12 group I patients the infarct progressed to total occlusion.

The availability of residual coronary flow to infarcting myocardium influences the extent of damage and may also be a factor in the efficacy of interventions that are designed to limit the size of an infarct. Very early thrombolysis is necessary for improvement in patients with an avascular infarct. When there is residual coronary flow, function may improve even with later treatment. Counterpulsation and β-blockade may control ischemia only in patients with residual coronary flow.

▶ This study emphasizes the importance of residual collateral blood flow into an area at risk in determining the subsequent size of the myocardial infarction. The other important factor is the length of time after deprivation of flow. How these two factors interact requires further definition.—Edmund H. Sonnenblick, M.D.

Effects of Reestablishing Blood Flow on Extent of Myocardial Infarction in Conscious Dogs

Robert H. Murdock, Jr., Alan Chu, Marjorie Grubb, and Frederick R. Cobb (Duke Med. Ctr. and Durham VA Med. Ctr.)
Am. J. Physiol. 249:H783–H791, September 1985   1–33

Conflicting data have been reported concerning the effects of longer periods of transient coronary occlusion compared with permanent occlusion on the extent of myocardial infarction in acute surgical preparations. The effects of reestablishing blood flow at 2 hours and at 6 hours were compared with those of permanent proximal circumflex occlusion in chronically instrumented awake dogs. The extent of left ventricular (LV) ischemia was determined by the microsphere method.

The mean degree of histologic infarction after permanent circumflex coronary occlusion was 21% of the LV weight. The mean extent of infarction after 2 hours and 6 hours of occlusion was 19% and 13%, respectively. The values did not differ significantly. Histologic infarction was less extensive when blood flow was reestablished at 2 hours, as determined by data grouped according to epicardial and endocardial layers and ischemic blood flow ranges. Analysis of findings in individual dogs, using total ischemic region blood flow to the epicardial and endocardial layers, indicated that reestablishment of blood flow at 2 hours, but not at 6 hours, was associated with less extensive infarction in most instances, although not in some animals with the most extensive ischemia.

The relative vulnerability of the endocardium to ischemic injury is influenced by factors other than the degree of ischemia itself. Eng et al. found that necrosis begins in the endocardium even when collateral flow is diverted from the ischemic region.

▶ This study supports and extends the concepts of the time dependency of necrosis after AMI (Reimer, K. W., et al.: *Circulation* 56:786–794, 1977), and emphasizes the need to reperfuse the myocardium in less than 4 hours if significant amounts are to be salvaged after acute coronary obstruction. Indeed, most salvage of tissue takes place within 2 hours or less. These findings are of great importance when considering problems of clinical thrombolysis to reperfuse the human heart.—Edmund H. Sonnenblick, M.D.

Interruption of Sympathetic and Vagal-Mediated Afferent Responses by Transmural Myocardial Infarction
Michael J. Barber, Thomas M. Mueller, Becky G. Davies, Robert M. Gill, and Douglas P. Zipes (Indiana Univ. and VA Med. Ctr., Indianapolis)
Circulation 72:623–631, September 1985   1–34

Sympathetic and vagal afferents, which follow an apical-to-basal course in the heart, can be stimulated selectively by epicardial application of bradykinin and nicotine, respectively. Transmural myocardial infarction might interrupt these fibers, leading to regions of afferent denervation apical to the infarct. This possibility was examined in open-chest dogs in which transmural infarcts were created by embolizing a diagonal branch of the left anterior descending coronary artery with vinyl latex solution. Epicardial applications of 5 μg of bradykinin and 50 μg of nicotine were made before and 90 minutes after the production of transmural infarction.

Epicardial bradykinin produced a peak pressor response of 13 mm Hg when applied before infarction, and topically administered nicotine produced a maximum depressor response of 14 mm Hg. Epicardial sites basal to the infarct continued to respond normally to both agents, but sites within the area of infarction and apical to it no longer responded to either one. Responses to bradykinin were eliminated by bilateral stellectomy, whereas those to nicotine were eliminated by transecting the cervical vagi. Epicardial mapping studies showed that sites were not consistently denervated in a homogeneous manner; some sites medial and apical to the infarct continued to respond to bradykinin, but not to nicotine.

Both sympathetic and vagal afferent denervation may occur after transmural myocardial infarction, within and apical to the site of infarction. Areas of denervation could modify reflexes that influence blood pressure, muscle contractility, and heart rate. The production of autonomic imbalance may dispose to the development of arrhythmias.

▶ The production of autonomic imbalance in AMI, resulting from the mechanisms described above, may also contribute to abnormalities of ST segment deviation that are beyond what is occurring from this simple ischemia alone. This imbalance may also contribute importantly to the development of ischemic-related arrhythmias.—Edmund H. Sonnenblick, M.D.

Hypoxia Releases a Vasoconstrictor Substance From the Canine Vascular Endothelium

Gabor M. Rubanyi and Paul M. Vanhoutte (Mayo Clinic and Found.)

J. Physiol. 364:45–56, July 1985   1–35

Anoxia augments contractile responses of isolated canine arteries and veins to vasoconstrictor agents; removal of the endothelium usually attenuates or abolishes this response. It is not clear whether this anoxic effect results from interruption of the production of a vasodilator substance or from generation of a vasoconstrictor mediator from anoxic endothelial cells. An attempt was made to determine whether the endothelium is involved in anoxic facilitation of contractile responses of canine coronary arteries. Left circumflex coronary and femoral arteries and femoral veins were used. Both ring and strip preparations were examined. Strips without endothelium were layered with strips that contained endothelium to identify the release of any vasoactive substance from endothelial cells.

Anoxia augmented contractile responses of prostaglandin F_2 in both ring preparations and preparations layered with endothelium. Hypoxia, with 5% or 10% oxygen, produced contractions in the presence of indomethacin. Removal of endothelium abolished both anoxic facilitation and hypoxic contractions. The response to anoxia was not prevented by inhibitors of cyclo-oxygenase, lipoxygenase, or phospholipase A_2, or by inhibitors of adrenergic, serotonergic, or histaminergic receptors. Inhibitors of endothelium-derived factors (e.g., quinacrine and phenidone) also did not influence anoxic facilitation. Anoxia and hypoxia produced contraction of coronary arteries when vessels without endothelium were layered with femoral arteries and veins with endothelium. Anoxic facilitation occurred in femoral arteries with endothelium, but not in femoral veins.

Hypoxia and anoxia appear to cause release of a diffusible vasoconstrictor substance from endothelial cells. There would seem to be differences in the responsiveness of arterial and venous smooth muscle to the vasoconstrictor mediator or mediators.

► The relationship between these results and vascular spasm remains to be explored, and the nature of the vasoconstrictor substance needs to be defined. Nevertheless, the fact that systemic arteries and veins have endothelial vasoconstrictor substances that may potentiate constrictor activity may be an important factor in maintaining vascular tone.—Edmund H. Sonnenblick, M.D.

Effects of Peptide Leukotrienes on Cardiac Dynamics in Rat, Cat, and Guinea Pig Hearts

David M. Roth, David J. Lefer, Carl E. Hock, and Allan M. Lefer (Thomas Jefferson Univ.)

Am. J. Physiol. 249:H477–H484, September 1985   1–36

Some peptide-containing leukotrienes, including leukotrienes C_4 (LTC_4) and D_4 (LTD_4), are potent coronary artery constrictors. They also have been reported to exert a direct negative inotropic effect on the myocardium, but the mechanism is unclear. The potentially direct inotropic effects of leukotrienes were examined in relation to their constricting activity on the coronary arteries of the adult male cat, male guinea pig, and male Sprague-Dawley rat. Both the isolated perfused Langendorff preparation and the isolated papillary muscle preparation were used.

Neither LTC_4 nor LTD_4 in concentrations of 50 ng/ml had an effect on papillary muscles from any species despite their responsiveness to known negative inotropic agents, e.g., pentobarbital and methanol. Both leukotrienes increased perfusion pressure in coronary arteries and decreased cardiac contractile force in isolated hearts that were perfused at constant flow. These changes were seen in all three species. With constant-pressure perfusion both LTC_4 and LTD_4 decreased coronary artery flow and contractile force. The leukotriene antagonist FPL 55712 blocked both the coronary artery constrictor and cardiodepressant effects of LTC_4 and LTD_4. Pentobarbital reduced cardiac contractile force without inducing coronary vasoconstriction.

The leukotrienes LTC_4 and LTD_4 appear not to have direct negative inotropic activity in cardiac muscle from the cat, guinea pig, or rat, They are, however, potent coronary vasoconstrictors and can secondarily reduce myocardial contractile force in this way. The greater reduction in contractile force at constant flow than at constant-pressure perfusion may reflect alterations in actual oxygen delivery, shunting of flow, or local heterogeneities in regional perfusion.

▶ This study clearly shows that the leukotrienes can produce marked coronary vasoconstriction that can then lead to secondary depression of myocardial contractility. This may contribute to the cardiac depression noted in endotoxic shock.—Edmund H. Sonnenblick, M.D.

Excitation Contraction and Biochemistry of Contractility

The Effects of Shortening on Myoplasmic Calcium Concentration and on the Action Potential in Mammalian Ventricular Muscle

Max J. Lab, David G. Allen, and Clive H. Orchard (Charing Cross and Westminster Med. School, and Univ. College, London)
Circ. Res. 55:825–829, December 1984   1–37

The time course of mechanical activity during contraction of cardiac muscle depends on the mechanical conditions under which it contracts. Relationships between prolongation of the calcium transient and the action potential were examined in isolated preparations of papillary muscle obtained from cats and ferrets by measuring the concentration of free myoplasmic calcium during isometric contractions, lightly loaded contractions, and contractions in which sudden releases at varying velocity were imposed on the muscle. Action potentials were recorded under similar conditions in parallel experiments. The concentration of myoplasmic calcium was measured with calcium-sensitive aequorin.

The effects of isometric and lightly loaded contractions on calcium transient and the action potential are shown in Figure 1–4. The concentration

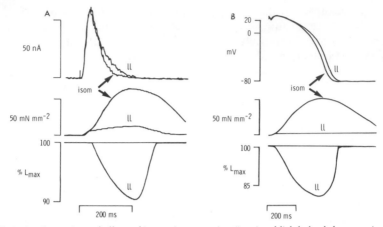

Fig 1–4.—Comparison of effects of isometric contraction *(isom)* and lightly loaded contraction *(11)* on calcium transients *(panel A)* and action potential *(panel B)*. Panel **A** shows superimposed isometric and lightly loaded contractions from aequorin-injected papillary muscle of ferret. Traces show (from top) aequorin light (function of $[Ca^{2+}]_1$), tension, and muscle length. Panel **B** shows action potential measurements from papillary muscle of cat made with "floating" microelectrode. Traces show (from top) membrane potential, tension, and muscle length. (Courtesy of Lab, M.J., et al.: Circ. Res. 55:825–829, December 1984.)

of myoplasmic calcium was increased when shortening occurred, and the membrane potential was more positive than in isometric contractions. Changes in the calcium concentration appeared to precede depolarization. Changes in the calcium transient and those in the action potential under differing mechanical conditions exhibited similar characteristics.

Shortening the cardiac muscle appears to reduce calcium binding to contractile proteins and results in a rise in the concentration of myoplasmic calcium, which activates an inward current that leads to observed alterations in the action potential, possibly through activation of an electrogenic sodium-calcium exchange that is combined with the opening of nonspecific channels carrying sodium and potassium. Under some circumstances, the resulting depolarization can trigger new action potentials, and may be involved in the production of arrhythmias.

▶ This interesting study demonstrates how the course of shortening may alter the affinity of the contractile system for calcium, and how this alteration of affinity may affect the subsequent course of contraction.—Edmund H. Sonnenblick, M.D.

Real-Time Kinetics of Sarcomere Relaxation by Laser Diffraction
Yves Lecarpentier, Jean-Louis Martin, Victor Claes, Jean-Paul Chambaret, Arnold Migus, André Antonetti, and Pierre-Yves Hatt (ENSTA-Ecole Polytechnique, Palaiseau, and Hôpital Léon Bernard, Limeil-Brévannes, France)
Circ. Res. 56:331–339, March 1985   1–38

Sarcomere motion in intact cardiac muscle usually has been examined under isometric conditions in the relaxation phase. The intracellular mechanisms that regulate the slow decline in isometric tension under conditions of low sarcoplasmic concentration of calcium remain uncertain. In the present study the kinetics of the motion of sarcomeres were examined during cardiac relaxation in both isotonic and isometric contractions. A laser diffraction method was used to measure instantaneous shortening of sarcomeres during afterloaded twitches simultaneously with instantaneous shortening and tension of the entire trabecula excised from the right ventricle of ten rats.

The average resting length of sarcomeres at optimal length was 2.2 μm. Maximum average amplitudes of shortening were 0.30 μm and 0.16 μm, respectively, in twitches with preload only and in isometric twitches. The maximum average velocity of relaxation decreased when the isotonic load was increased. Relaxation of sarcomeres appeared to be delayed progressively when the total load was increased from preload only up to isometric load. Rapid and slower phases of relaxation were evident. The former increased and the latter decreased when the total load increased.

Two mechanisms apparently are involved in relaxation of sarcomeres. A relatively rapid initial phase predominates at low load, but a slower phase predominates at high load. It is possible that the affinity of calcium for troponin C is higher at high load or slight amplitude of shortening of sarcomeres than at low load, and vice versa.

▶ These direct measurements of sarcomere dynamics support the view that the affinity of troponin C for calcium is load dependent and, as in the previous study, helps to explain the load dependency of duration of contraction.—Edmund H. Sonnenblick, M.D.

Calcium Exchange in the Resting and Electrically Stimulated Canine Myocardium

Nicholas J. Lodge, Arthur L. Bassett, and Henry Gelband (Univ. of Miami)
Pflugers Arch. 405:37–45, September 1985   1–39

Studies with $^{45}Ca^{++}$ have established that calcium ion exchange in the heart is a complex, multicompartmental system. An attempt was made to resolve intracellular from extracellular $^{45}Ca^{++}$ using thin tissue slices and ice-cold 6.8 mM Ca^{++} in Tyrode's solution with 5 mM ethyleneglycol tetra-acetate added. Left ventricular tissue from adult dogs was used.

Loss of $^{45}Ca^{++}$ from equilibrated tissue into ice-cold wash medium best fitted a model containing at least three compartments. Uptake of $^{45}Ca^{++}$ into and efflux from the most slowly exchanging compartment at 37 C allowed its subdivision into two fractions, a rapidly exchanging one and a slowly exchanging one, with respective half-times of about 1.25 minutes and 50 minutes. The total Ca^{++} content of compartment[3] was enhanced by isoproterenol but was little affected by caffeine. This compartment contains some Ca^{++} of intracellular origin. Action potentials elicited by electric stimulation produced large changes in the Ca^{++} content of compartment 3, up to 170 μmole/kg.

Compartment 3 may have a significant role in the normal cardiac contraction-relaxation cycle. The finding that the rapidly exchanging part of compartment 3 can be preserved by cooling the tissue to 4 C indicates that rapidly exchanging Ca^{++} compartments can be studied in superfused cardiac preparations by this method.

▶ This study further emphasizes the importance of intracellular calcium stores on the mediation of myocardial contractility, and helps to elucidate the interrelations of transmyocardial calcium fluxes with the release of such stores to mediate contractile activity (Fabiato, A.: *Am. J. Physiol.* 245:C1–C14, 1983).—Edmund H. Sonnenblick, M.D.

Aequorin Measurements of Free Calcium in Single Heart Cells
P. H. Cobbold and P. K. Bourne (Univ. of Liverpool)
Nature 312:444–446, Nov. 29, 1984   1–40

Cardiac performance depends on the concentration of free calcium ions in the cytoplasm of myocytes; however, it is difficult to measure the concentration of free calcium concentration that occur in physiologic and pathologic events. The calcium-sensitive photoprotein aequorin was used to study single ventricular myocytes isolated from the rat heart. Signals were detected from resting and contracting cells, and from cells exposed to media with increased concentrations of potassium and lowered concentrations of sodium, as well as to metabolic inhibitors.

Free calcium was stable in metabolically poisoned myocytes. Severe injury to cells occurred before the concentration of free calcium rose to more than $1–3 \times 10^{-7}$M. Blockade of either oxidative phosphorylation or glycolysis alone usually did not affect the free calcium concentration.

This technique should help to elucidate relationships among free calcium metabolic inhibition, altered excitability of heart cells, and injury to structural cells. The present findings indicate that control of free calcium is not critically dependent on an abundant supply of metabolic energy and is more resistant to disturbances than is the maintenance of normal cell structure. Cell damage in this model appears to be a cause, rather than a result, of a rise in the free calcium concentration.

The Effect of pH on Cellular and Membrane Calcium Binding and Contraction of Myocardium: A Possible Role for Sarcolemmal Phospholipid in EC Coupling
G. A. Langer (Univ. of California at Los Angeles)
Circ. Res. 57:374–382, September 1985   1–41

A rapidly exchangeable component of cellular calcium (Ca^{++}) has an important role in controlling force development in cardiac muscle. A large fraction of this Ca^{++} appears to be bound to sites on or within the sarcolemmal membrane. The effects were assessed of altered pH in the range of (5.5–8.5 on Ca^{++} binding to cultured myocardial cells, sarcolemma from these cells, and sarcolemma from canine myocardium.) The effect of pH change on the contraction amplitude of cultured cells also was studied. Membranes of cultured whole cell monolayers were prepared by "gas dissection."

Both calcium binding and contraction responses to pH were well described by a relationship in which calcium binding is primarily dependent on the extent of ionization of sarcolemmal binding sites. Phospholipid extracted from sarcolemmal vesicles accounted for at least 75% of the calcium binding. The extent of ionization of the binding sites was pH dependent. Membranous calcium binding, cellular calcium uptake, and contraction amplitude all increased proportionally as the pH increased. Most of the increase in cellular calcium uptake was rapidly exchangeable and lanthanum-displaceable, indicating sarcolemmal localization. The rest entered a slowly exchangeable pool not directly related to support of contraction.

Calcium bound to sarcolemmal sites appears to have a critical role in regulating myocardial contraction. The sites in question may be amino groups located on a zwitterionic phospholipid. Neutralization of these groups as the pH increases would expose the negatively charged phospholipid acidic groups, which then would be available to bind calcium.

▶ Alterations of pH affect virtually all cellular systems that play a role in excitation contraction coupling in cardiac muscle. This includes the sarcoplasm reticulum, the myofilaments, the cellular calcium exchange in the sarcolemma, transmembrane sodium currents, and the calcium current that is associated with hydrogen-sodium exchange. The present study demonstrates an additional effect. With these considerations in mind, it is clear why acidosis may strongly affect the contractile behavior of heart muscle, and emphasizes a possible direct role for sarcolemmal-bound calcium in myocardial excitation contraction coupling.—Edmund H. Sonnenblick, M.D.

Ryanodine as a Tool to Determine the Contributions of Calcium Entry and Calcium Release to the Calcium Transient and Contraction of Cardiac Purkinje Fibers

Eduardo Marban and W. Gil Wier (Univ. of Maryland at Baltimore and Johns Hopkins Univ.)
Circ. Res. 56:133–138, January 1985   1–42

A rise in the intracellular calcium concentration initiates cardiac muscle, contraction, but the sources of calcium remain unclear, especially in mammalian tissues. An attempt was made to assess the relative roles of the transsarcolemmal entry of calcium and its intracellular release in the contraction of cardiac Purkinje fibers obtained from adult dogs. Intracellular calcium transients, membrane potentials, and contraction were monitored in aequorin-injected fibers that were exposed to selective modifiers of excitation-contraction coupling. The plant alkaloid ryanodine was used to influence the release of calcium from the sarcoplasmic reticulum; calcium entry was modified by the use of the calcium-channel antagonist nitrendipine and the agonist Bay K 8644.

Ryanodine alone reduced both components of the intracellular aequorin luminescence signal. Mean twitch tension was 2% of baseline, whereas the action potential was prolonged. The remaining aequorin signal and twitch were abolished by nitrendipine, which also lowered the action potential plateau. The calcium-channel agonist increased aequorin luminescence and contraction in the presence of ryanodine, but only to a small fraction of baseline levels. Sodium withdrawal in ryanodine-containing, potassium-free solution produced large, slow elevations in calcium and tension. Caffeine increased the intracellular calcium concentration, indicating that calcium stores were not depleted.

The negative inotropic effect of ryanodine can be ascribed to a decrease in release of calcium from internal stores. Calcium entry ordinarily contributes only a small fraction of total activator calcium.

► Activation of mammalian cardiac tissue apparently depends on a small amount of calcium entering the cell via slow channels in the sarcolemma with the release of further amounts of calcium from the sarcoplasm reticulum within the cell (Fabiato, A.: *J. Physiol.* [Lond.] 245:C1–C14, 1983). These specific mechanisms have now been well demonstrated, but the relative importance of the source of calcium, be it across the external membrane or from internal calcium stores, may vary between different types of cardiac tissue and different species. This may have significant implications for the pathophysiology of mechanisms that have a negative inotropic effect on contractility and the development of drugs that augment activation of the failing heart muscle.—Edmund H. Sonnenblick, M.D.

Sodium Pump Inhibition, Enhanced Calcium Influx Via Sodium-Calcium Exchange, and Positive Inotropic Response in Cultured Heart Cells
William H. Barry, Yonathin Hasin, and Thomas W. Smith (Brigham and Women's Hosp. and Harvard Univ., Boston)
Circ. Res. 56:231–241, February 1985   1–43

Altered sodium-calcium (Na-Ca) exchange seems causally related to the positive inotropic effect of digitalis, but it is not clear whether changes in intracellular Ca^{++} result from an enhanced influx of calcium or from a decreased efflux via the Na-Ca exchange system. The relative importance of inhibition of the sodium pump and superficial binding of Ca^{++} also is unknown. The effects of inhibition of the sodium pump on contractile state and Na-Ca exchange were examined in cultures of the primary monolayer of ventricular cells of chick embryos. Inhibition of the pump was produced by exposure to ouabain or dihydroouabain, or by a reduction in extracellular potassium to 1 mM.

All three means of inhibiting the sodium pump induced prominent positive inotropic effects that were accompanied in each case by inhibition of up to 50% of active uptake of potassium and a similar increase in the steady-state content of sodium. The same measures stimulated uptake of ^{45}Ca on exposure to zero extracellular sodium. Reactivation of the sodium pump with 4 mM of extracellular potassium was associated with hyperpolarization of the membrane and slowing the rate of spontaneous beating. The time course of the disappearance of stimulation of the Na-Ca exchange on exposure to zero extracellular sodium was similar to that of loss of the positive inotropic effect. Inotropic concentrations of drug produced a small increase in unidirectional influx of calcium but no discernible change in efflux of calcium under physiologic conditions.

Inhibition of the sodium pump, which results in an increase of intracellular sodium, appears to be chiefly responsible for the positive inotropic effects of digitalis and low extracellular potassium in this model. The increased influx of calcium via Na-Ca exchange may be the chief means by which increased intracellular sodium produces enhanced availability of calcium to myofibrils. An effect on calcium efflux also may be a factor.

A Novel Type of Cardiac Calcium Channel in Ventricular Cells
B. Nilius, P. Hess, J. B. Lansman, and R. W. Tsien [Martin Luther Univ., Halle (Saale), German Democratic Republic, and Yale Univ.]
Nature 316:443–446, August 1985   1–44

A single type of calcium channel has been identified in patch-clamp studies of unitary current, but whole-cell recordings in cardiac cells and unitary recordings in other cells suggest that there is more than one type of channel. A new type of channel was recognized that has several properties distinguishing it from the previously identified calcium channel in cardiac cells. Conductance of the channel in isotonic barium is small and is no greater in barium than in calcium. The channel activates and deactivates at relatively negative potentials, and it remains functional long after patch excision. It is insensitive to dihydropyridines (e.g., nimodipine and the Ca agonist Bay K 8644), and is more resistant than the previously described channel to blockade by external cadmium.

This new calcium channel is termed "T" because of its markedly transient time course, which resembles that of the T-type calcium channel in neurons of the dorsal root ganglion. The previously described type of cardiac calcium channel, which is large in unitary conductance and is long lasting, is referred to as "L." The current of the T channel is much smaller than the current of the L channel, and it decays much more rapidly in ventricular cells. It probably contributes relatively little to calcium influx during the action potential plateau and contraction. Cardiac T-type channels may be most significant in pacemaker depolarization and initiation of the action potential, phenomena that are critically dependent on small inward currents at relatively negative potentials.

▶ The existence of various calcium channels in cardiac muscle may provide a therapeutic opportunity for blockade of activation within various groups of cardiac cells. As yet, this has not been delineated.—Edmund H. Sonnenblick, M.D.

Ultrastructural Morphometric Analysis of Myocardium From Dogs, Rats, Hamsters, Mice, and From Human Hearts
Jutta Schaper, Eckhardt Meiser, and Gerhard Stämmler (Bad Nauheim, Federal Republic of Germany)
Circ. Res. 56:377–391, March 1985   1–45

The quantitative distribution of various cellular organelles in myocytes can be used in calculating the biochemical composition of myocytes when quantitative biochemical data are available. Volume densities of mitochondria, myofibrils, and unspecified cytoplasm were measured by ultrastructural morphometry in samples of myocardium obtained from dogs, rats, hamsters, and mice, and in biopsy specimens from human hearts.

Human myocardium consisted of 23% mitochondria, 62% myofibrils, and 15% unspecified cytoplasm. Volume densities of mitochondria were 22% in dogs, 28% in rats and hamsters, and 32% in mice. Myofibrillar volume density was highest in dogs (63%), followed by rats and hamsters (57%), and mice (49%). Analysis of canine myocardium showed an identical quantitative composition of tissues from the left ventricular free wall and the papillary muscles. There also were no differences between subepicardium, subendocardium, and midmyocardium. Volume densities were identical in longitudinal and transverse sections. Fixation with glutaraldehyde by perfusion and immersion yielded identical results. Volume densities did not differ in samples from the left ventricular free wall of rats, hamsters, and mice.

These findings indicate that each mammalian species has a characteristic quantitative myocardial composition. An increase in mitochondrial volume correlates with an increase in heart rate and consumption of oxygen in smaller animals. These quantitative data seem to be the morphological correlates of differing functional cardiac capacity in various species.

▶ The quantitative morphological analysis of the heart in various pathologic states is an important consideration that will warrant further study. The question of whether specific components of the heart, and indeed the myocardial cells themselves, may be reduced quantitatively under certain pathologic states remains a clear possibility.—Edmund H. Sonnenblick, M.D.

Fiber Types and Myosin Types in Human Atrial and Ventricular Myocardium: An Anatomical Description
Patrice Bouvagnet, Jocelyne Leger, Françoise Pons, Claude Dechesne, and Jean J. Leger (Biological Inst., Montpellier, France)
Circ. Res. 55:794–804, December 1984   1–46

Cardiac myosins exhibit molecular heterogeneity in the ventricles andatria of some mammals. Molecular variants of myosin heavy chains have a role in controlling myocardial function under both normal and pathologic conditions. Hybridomas were prepared from mice immunized with myosin obtained from the enlarged left ventricle of a patient with obstructive cardiomyopathy. The specificity of 15 monoclonal antibodies to myosin heavy chains was evaluated through the reactivity of muscle extracts and of chymotryptic myosin fragments of varying size with the antibodies. The immune replicate technique was used.

Certain monoclonal antibodies cross-reacted only with ventricular V_3-type myosin from hypothyroid rats; other antibodies cross-reacted with ventricular V_1-type myosins from normal young rats as well. Some of the antimyosin antibodies demonstrated immunologic heterogeneity in fibers from human atrial and ventricular muscle when the indirect immunofluorescence technique was used. Fiber heterogeneity also was observed by adenosine triphosphatase (ATPase) staining of the same tissues. Small zones of myosin variation were scattered within large areas of myocardium in which the cellular distribution of myosin was constant.

At least three distinct types of myosin may exist in the human ventricle, including a V_1-type myosin that presumably corresponds to rare fibers with alkaline-stable ATPase activity and two other V_3-type myosins that correspond to immunologically different fibers, each of which has alkaline-labile ATPase activity. The physiologic significance of regional variations in the distribution of the various molecular forms of myosin remains uncertain.

▶ Myosin appears to exist in the human heart as in other mammalian hearts in a V_3(slow) and V_1(fast) isoenzyme with the V_2 isoenzyme being a dimer between these two extremes. The present study shows that these fast and slow myosins are located in a heterogeneous pattern in both the atrium and ventricle. Moreover, any given cell would appear to have a fast or a slow type of myosin. The interaction between two adjacent cells that contain myosins of different speeds of contractile activity of the overall tissue is not at all clear. Indeed, the implications of these variable isoenzymes for ventricular function remain to be worked out, although it is clear that in conditions such as hypothyroidism and hyperthyroidism, the speed of contraction correlates with the presence of the dominant type of isoenzyme. Moreover, in hypertrophy, the V_3 form appears to predominate. Current data would indicate that in adult man, the V_3 is the dominant isoenzyme with very little V_1 persisting.—Edmund H. Sonnenblick, M.D.

Effect of Swimming Training on Cardiac Function and Myosin ATPase Activity in SHR
Ram V. Sharma, Robert J. Tomanek, and Ramesh C. Bhalla (Univ. of Iowa)
J. Appl. Physiol. 59:758–765, September 1985   1–47

It is not clear whether biochemical changes lead to functional alterations in the spontaneously hypertensive rat (SHR), but animals with severe cardiac hypertrophy reportedly have lower myocardial myofibrillar adenosine triphosphatase (ATPase) activity. An attempt was made to learn whether contractile protein ATPase activity and cardiac function in the male SHR are altered by strenuous training started during the prehypertensive stage. Both male SHR and Wistar-Kyoto normotensive rats (WKY) were subjected to swimming training 6 days a week, starting at age 4 weeks. The total duration of exercise was 190 hours. Myofibrillary ATPase activity was assayed at free Ca^{++} concentrations ranging from 10^{-7} to $10^{-5}M$. Actin-activated myosin ATPase activity of purified myosin was determined at various concentrations of actin purified from rabbit skeletal muscle.

Contractile protein ATPase activity was comparable in trained and untrained WKY and SHR under all conditions. A single myosin band corresponding to the V_1 isoenzyme was found, with no differences in relation to training. Both cardiac index and stroke index responses to intravenous volume overloading were increased in trained rats of both species, compared with untrained animals.

Moderate left ventricular (LV) hypertrophy in either exercise-trained rats or SHR is not associated with altered ATPase activity or an altered distribution of myosin isoenzymes. The findings are comparable to those obtained in treadmill-trained rats. Cardiac adaptations to training could result from alterations in plasma membrane Ca^{++} permeability. The SHR has LV mass and cardiac output responses to training similar to those of normotensive WKY.

▶ Physical training may have effects on the excitation contraction coupling system (Tibbits, G. F., et al.: *Am. J. Physiol.* 240:H472–H480, 1981), and these effects may be summated with the effects that occur with severe hypertrophy to reduce actin-activated myosin ATPase.—Edmund H. Sonnenblick, M.D.

Heterogeneity of Myosin Isozyme Content of Rabbit Heart
R. Z. Litten, B. J. Martin, R. H. Buchthal, R. Nagai, R. B. Low, and N. R. Alpert (Univ. of Vermont)
Circ. Res. 57:406–414, September 1985   1–48

Changes in the proportions of the various myosin isozymes with advancing age have created problems in designing experiments. The relative content of the V_1 and V_3 isozymes of myosin was measured in different regions of the rabbit ventricle as a function of age; also, individual variability was examined. A cardiac biopsy method was developed whereby the composition of myosin isozymes could be followed over time in the same animal.

The V_1 isozyme predominated over the V_3 isozyme in hearts of rabbits aged 2 weeks, but V_1 was a minor component in animals aged 10 weeks. There was, however, considerable variability in the relative isozyme content of whole ventricular tissue among different animals of the same age. Less variability was present in littermates and when cardiac biopsy specimens were used to measure changes in isozymes in the same animal over time. Small but significant differences in percent of the V_1 isozyme were found in different regions of a given heart. The proportion was highest in right ventricular papillary muscle, followed by the right ventricular free wall and left ventricle. The percent of V_1 correlated with that of myofibrillar myosin calcium-stimulated adenosine triphosphatase (ATPase) in both the right and left ventricles in normal and developing hearts. The regression slope of calcium-stimulated ATPase vs. the percent of V_1 was steeper in the left than in the right ventricle.

The content of myosin isozymes in cardiac tissues of the rabbit is dependent on age and on cardiac region. Serial biopsies and the use of littermates may help to control for interanimal variability in content. It remains to be determined why the linear relationship between myofibrillar myosin calcium-stimulated ATPase and percent of V_1 isozyme differs in the right and left ventricles.

► Isoenzyme composition can be affected by numerous factors including insulin, diet, and sex hormones. It is also greatly affected by pressure overloads. The role of these isoenzymatic changes in normal and abnormal physiology is as yet unclear.—Edmund H. Sonnenblick, M.D.

Effects of Thyroid Hormone on Calcium Handling in Cultured Chick Ventricular Cells
Donghee Kim and Thomas W. Smith (Brigham and Women's Hosp. and Harvard Univ., Boston)
J. Physiol. 364:131–149, July 1985   1–49

Hyperthyroidism increases the rate of tension development, peak developed tension, and rate of diastolic depolarization in mammalian heart muscle. There is some evidence that thyroid hormone may alter Ca^{++} flux across the sarcolemmal membrane and Ca^{++} movements within the cells, contributing to altered contractility. The direct effects of thyroid hormone on Ca^{++} movements and parameters of contraction were examined in spontaneously beating cultured chick embryo ventricular cells. Monolayers of cells were exposed to triiodothyronine (T_3) at a concentration of 10^{-8}M. Calcium ion kinetics were studied using $^{45}Ca^{++}$.

Cell contraction occurred more rapidly in the presence of T_3 at extracellular Ca^{++} levels of 0.6 mM and 1.2 mM, but not at higher Ca^{++} concentrations. The rapid phase of Ca^{++} uptake was affected by T_3; the increment in total Ca^{++} content was ascribed to the rapidly exchangeable Ca^{++} pool. Verapamil partly inhibited the T_3-increase in the rapidly exchangeable Ca^{++} pool. The rate of calcium ion efflux was greater in the presence of T_3. Caffeine in the efflux medium increased Ca^{++} efflux more in cells grown in the presence of T_3. The cellular content of sarcoplasmic reticulum Ca^{++}-ATPase was increased more than twofold in cells grown in the presence of T_3.

The T_3-induced increase in contractility of cultured cardiac cells probably results, at least in part, from an increase in the rapidly exchangeable

Ca^{++} content thought to reside in the sarcoplasmic reticulum. The results are consistent with the view that increased Ca^{++} influx occurs via both slow Ca^{++} channels and $Na^{+}-Ca^{++}$ exchange, whereas increased Ca^{++} efflux occurs chiefly via sarcolemmal Ca^{++}-ATPase.

▶ Thyroid hormone appears to have multiple effects on cardiac muscle, including an increase in calcium-activated myosin ATPase activity with a shift from the slower V_3 to the more rapid V_1 isoenzyme. (*Prog. Cardiovasc. Dis.* 25:435–464, 1983; *Circ. Res.* 48:498–501, 1981.) This leads to increased turnover at the contractile sites per se. The present study shows that these augmented rates of mechanical interaction of myofilaments are further enhanced by increased activity of the calcium-activating system. These two systems working in parallel would serve to increase the speed of activation as well as the speed of contraction. Moreover, loss of thyroid hormone would produce the converse effects.—Edmund H. Sonnenblick, M.D.

The Economy of Isometric Force Development, Myosin Isoenzyme Pattern, and Myofibrillar ATPase Activity in Normal and Hypothyroid Rat Myocardium
Ch. Holubarsch, R. P. Goulette, R. Z. Litten, B. J. Martin, L. A. Mulieri, and N. R. Alpert (Univ. of Tubingen, Federal Republic of Germany, and Univ. of Vermont, Burlington)
Circ. Res. 56:78–86, January 1985   1–50

It has been proposed that the intrinsic enzymatic properties of actomyosin regulate the velocity of cardiac muscle shortening. An attempt was made to link biophysical and biochemical parameters in hypothyroid rats that were given propylthiouracil. Initial heat, total activity-related heat, and resting heat rate were measured in preparations of left ventricular (LV) papillary muscle obtained from treated and control animals. Isometric contraction was 12 beats per minute at 21 C. Planar thermopiles of vacuum-deposited bismuth and antimony were used.

Time to peak tension increased in the propylthiouracil preparations, and peak twitch tension and maximum differential LV pressure decreased. Initial heat was significantly reduced in propylthiouracil preparations. When the papillary muscles were tetanized, the slope of the linear function of total activity-related heat vs. tension-time integral was reduced by 43% in propylthiouracil preparations. The predominant myosin isoenzyme was V_3 in the propylthiouracil preparations and V_1 in controls. The activity of myofibrillar actomyosin calcium-magnesium-stimulated adenosine triphosphatase (ATPase) was significantly reduced in propylthiouracil preparations as was the activity of myofibrillar myosin calcium-stimulated ATPase.

Improved economy in maintaining isometric tension was apparent in propylthiouracil preparations in this study. The myothermal data reflect slowed cross-bridge cycling in hypothyroid myocardium, which is not necessarily detrimental in view of the increased economy of force generation that results. The fast normal rat heart apparently sacrifices economy of tension development for ability to eject blood at high velocity. In the slow hypothyroid rat heart, the oxygen demand for force development is low and can be met at a slower heart rate and velocity of shortening.

▶ The slowed mechanical speed of contraction and lowered ATPase activity of the myofibrils are manifestations of slowing of the cross-bridge cycling rate, as has been claimed previously. Moreover, as shown in the previous paper, slowing at the myofilament level of contractile proteins is paralleled by a slowing of calcium availability in the excitation contraction coupling system, and these two phenomena are at least additive. In and of themselves, these two basic changes in the biochemistry of contraction help to explain the slowing of the heart in hypothyroidism and the marked speeding of contraction that is observed in the presence of hyperthyroidism.—Edmund H. Sonnenblick, M.D.

2 Heart Disease in Infants and Children

Congenital and Acquired Heart Disease

Spontaneous Closure of Isolated Secundum Atrial Septal Defects in Infants: An Echocardiographic Study

Renzo P. Ghisla, David W. Hannon, Richard A. Meyer, and Samuel Kaplan (Children's Hosp. Med. Ctr., Cincinnati)
Am. Heart J. 109:1327–1333, June 1985   2–1

The incidence and timing of spontaneous closure of isolated secundum atrial septal defects are not known. To determine these, as well as the role of echocardiography in predicting spontaneous closure of secundum defects, 29 consecutive infants under 12 months of age with clinical evidence of significant left-to-right shunting through isolated secundum atrial septal defects were evaluated by M-mode and two-dimensional echocardiography. All had right ventricular hypertrophy as determined by ECG. Right ventricular and left atrial dimensions were obtained, and right ventricular, right atrial, and left atrial areas were measured in all children.

Between 15 and 30 months of age, 4 children had evidence of spontaneous closure of the defect by normalization of clinical, ECG, and chest x-ray findings and documented by two-dimensional and M-mode echocardiography. Seven children underwent surgical closure of the defect between 12 and 28 months of age. Those who underwent spontaneous closure did not differ from those without spontaneous closure in right ventricular or right atrial areas, or in right ventricular dimension, at the time that the atrial defect was diagnosed. However, right ventricular and right atrial areas and dimensions became normal on sequential studies in all 4 children after spontaneous closure. Left atrial areas were normal in all 4 whose defects closed spontaneously, but were large in all but 3 who did not experience spontaneous closure. The mean diameter of the defect was similar in all children. An atrial septal flap was found in all children whose defect closed spontaneously, but in only 4 of 16 whose defect did not undergo spontaneous closure.

The 14% incidence of spontaneous closure observed in this study may underestimate the true incidence, because 7 children had surgical closure prior to age 30 months, the oldest age at which spontaneous closure was documented. Surgical closure should not be performed before age 30 months unless medical management fails to control symptoms. Sequential two-dimensional echocardiography may detect those infants likely to undergo spontaneous closure, including those who are symptomatic and who may be considered for early surgery. The presence of an atrial septal tissue flap may relate to the mechanism of spontaneous closure. Other previously proposed mechanisms of spontaneous closure include septal aneurysm formation, differential growth of the secundum septum, and formation of a thrombotic or fibrous plug.

▶ The study provides a reaffirmation of current practice for elective surgical closure of atrial septal defect secundum some time between 3 and 6 years of age. Clinical evaluation and noninvasive studies are sensitive, and specific means for the diagnosis and follow-up of these patients and cardiac catheterization can usually be avoided. However, it must be remembered that infants presenting with the clinical findings of a large left-to-right shunt at the atrial level frequently have associated underlying cardiac abnormalities (especially left ventricular disease) that result in earlier and larger left-to-right shunt through an atrial defect. There may be associated cardiomyopathy, left ventricular outflow obstruction, anomalous origin of the coronary artery, or patent ductus arteriosus. Whereas cardiac catheterization is not required in the asymptomatic child with an apparent isolated atrial septal defect secundum, the procedure is advisable in the infant with intractable failure or evidence of pulmonary artery hypertension.—Amnon Rosenthal, M.D.

Hemodynamic Effects of Dynamic Exercise in Children and Adolescents With Moderate-to-Small Ventricular Septal Defects
Carel Bendien, Klaas K. Bossina, Arie E. Buurma, Alie M. Gerding, Jaap R. G. Kuipers, Martin L. J. Landsman, Gerrit A. Mook, and Willem G. Zijlstra (Univ. of Groningen, Groningen, The Netherlands)
Circulation 70:929–934, December 1984   2–2

Children with small ventricular septal defects have a nearly normal life expectancy and often are not operated on when they are asymptomatic, but the hemodynamic effects of exercise in this setting are uncertain. To assess the effects of maximal exercise during cardiac catheterization, 20 boys and 15 girls with moderate to small septal defects and a left-to-right shunt not exceeding 50% were studied. All had normal pulmonary artery pressures. Films showed that 12 patients had slight cardiomegaly, and 9 had signs of pulmonary engorgement. Patients were exercised at 25%, 50%, or 60% of their maximum workloads.

The hemodynamic sequelae of exercise were qualitatively comparable at different work loads but were more marked at a higher percentage of maximal work load. Pulmonary vascular resistance did not change on exercise, but systemic vascular resistance declined. Both pulmonary and systolic blood flows increased, with no change in the left-to-right shunt fraction. The shunt volume per beat decreased during exercise. The level of pulmonary arterial oxygen saturation decreased and the level of arterial lactic acid increased significantly with exercise. The level of arterial oxygen saturation was unchanged.

Dynamic exercise has favorable hemodynamic effects in patients with small to moderate ventricular septal defects. The normal rise in systemic blood flow occurs without a corresponding rise in left-to-right shunt flow.

Children and adolescents with such defects should not be restricted in their activities. Running and free cycling probably have hemodynamic sequelae that are similar to those seen on controlled cycle exercise in the present study. Shunt flow may, however, increase on static exercise, since the increase in pressure difference between the left and right ventricles may be substantially greater.

▶ The authors have demonstrated that in children with a small membranous ventricular septal defect (Qp/Qs less than 1.5) and normal pulmonary artery pressure, the left-to-right shunt does not change with dynamic exercise. This hemodynamic observation supports the long-standing clinical practice of permitting children with a small ventricular septal defect to participate fully in all physical activities. One such young man was recently a star on the University of Michigan football team.—Amnon Rosenthal, M.D.

Acute Hemodynamic Effects of Increasing Hemoglobin Concentration in Children With a Right to Left Ventricular Shunt and Relative Anemia
Robert H. Beekman and Dwight T. Tuuri (Wright State Univ. and Children's Med. Ctr., Dayton, Ohio)
J. Am. Coll. Cardiol. 5:357–362, February 1985   2–3

Subjective improvement has been described in children with cyanotic congenital heart disease and relative anemia (hemoglobin concentration in the low to normal range) after blood transfusion or iron therapy. However, the physiologic consequences of relative anemia in these patients have not been studied. The short-term effects of increasing hemoglobin concentration were evaluated at cardiac catheterization in seven children, aged 0.3 to 7.5 years, with a right-to-left ventricular shunt (ventricular septal defect and pulmonary stenosis) and a central venous hemoglobin concentration of less than 15 mg/100 ml. Six children had tetralogy of Fallot and one had L-transposition of the great vessels with ventricular septal defect and pulmonary stenosis. The following variables were measured before and 20 minutes after isovolumic partial exchange transfusion with 20 ml/kg packed red blood cells: hemoglobin, partial pressure of oxygen (P_{O_2}), oxygen consumption, oxygen saturation and pressure in the aorta, superior vena cava, and right and left atria.

After transfusion, hemoglobin concentration increased from 13.7 ± 0.5 to 16.4 ± 0.4 gm 100 ml ($P < .001$). In response to this, right-to-left shunting decreased by 59%, from 1.44 ± 0.29 to 0.59 ± 0.10 L/minute/sq m ($P < .01$). Effective pulmonary blood flow increased by 17%, from 2.72 ± 0.10 to 3.17 ± 0.10 L/minute/sq m ($P < .01$). Systemic arterial oxygenation from 84.3% ± 2.3% to 90.9% ± 1.3% ($P < .002$), and arterial P_{O_2} increased from 55.0 ± 3.5 to 62.0 ± 4.1 mm Hg ($P < .01$). Despite a slight increase in systemic blood flow, systemic oxygen transport increased from 658.2 ± 47.5 to 737.9 ± 45.4 ml/minute/sq m ($P < .002$). Systemic vascular resistance increased from 15.9 ± 1.1 to 20.0 ± 1.4 units ($P < .01$). A significant relation was found between the percent increase in systemic resistance and both the percent decrease in right-to-left shunt ($P < .01$) and percent increase in systemic arterial P_{O_2} ($P < .02$). Increasing the hemoglobin concentration did not affect oxygen consumption.

Increasing the hemoglobin concentration in children with right-to-left ventricular shunt and relative anemia not only augments blood oxygen-carrying capacity, but also decreases right-to-left shunting, increases effective pulmonary blood flow, and improves systemic arterial oxygen saturation. These acute hemodynamic changes appear to be related to the increase in systemic resistance after partial exchange transfusion. Therefore, hemoglobin concentration should be kept above 15 gm/100 ml in these children, and appropriate measures should be instituted if it falls below this level.

▶ The observations by the authors in an acute setting are relevant to the management of infants and children with tetralogy of Fallot physiology during a cyanotic spell, at cardiac catheterization, or during the immediate postoperative period after palliative surgery. Hemodynamic deterioration can often be avoided by maintaining hemoglobin concentration above 15 gm/100 ml. However, the observations may also be applied to the long-term ambulatory care of these patients. In children and particularly in infants with cyanotic heart disease, it is important to monitor independently the degree of hypoxemia and the accompanying hematopoietic response. Relative anemia should be assessed in relation to the severity of the hypoxemia. During office visits, measurement of hemoglobin concentration should be accompanied by a noninvasive measurement of systemic oxygen saturation (by pulse volume oximeter or ear oximeter) or oxygen tension (transcutaneous P_{O_2}). When relative anemia is present, appropriate therapy, usually iron supplementation, may be instituted.—Amnon Rosenthal, M.D.

Therapeutic Effect of Propranolol on Paradoxical Hypertension After Repair of Coarctation of the Aorta
Samuel S. Gidding, Albert P. Rocchini, Robert Beekman, Cheryl A. Szpunar, Catherine Moorehead, Douglas Behrendt, and Amnon Rosenthal (Univ. of Michigan)
N. Engl. J. Med. 312:1224–1228, May 9, 1985   2–4

Self-limited but severe systemic hypertension often develops 1 week after repair of coarctation of the aorta (paradoxical hypertension). Both the sympathetic nervous system and the renin-angiotensin system have been implicated in the genesis of paradoxical hypertension thus, a controlled trial was undertaken in 14 children to determine whether pretreatment with propranolol would prevent paradoxical hypertension. Seven patients were randomly assigned to receive 1.5 mg propranolol per kilogram body weight per day orally for 2 weeks before surgery, intravenously (0.05 mg per kg body weight/day) during the immediate postoperative period, and orally throughout the first postoperative week. Seven patients were assigned to receive standard postoperative care. Heart rate, right-arm blood pressure, plasma renin activity, and plasma catecholamine levels were measured.

During the immediate postoperative period, both groups had a similar significant increase ($P < .05$) in the plasma norepinephrine levels in response to surgery. However, when compared with the control group, children pretreated with propranolol had significantly lower systolic ($P = .004$) and diastolic ($P = .003$) blood pressures and smaller rise in plasma renin activity ($P < .01$). These differences were significant despite the treatment of 4 control patients with other antihypertensive agents. As expected, the heart rate was consistently lower in the propranolol-treated group ($P = .075$).

Prophylactic pretreatment with propranolol can prevent paradoxical hypertension after coarctation repair and should therefore become a routine part of the operative care of patients with coarctation of the aorta. The antihypertensive action of propranolol appears to be mediated by its cardiac actions (relative bradycardia) and ability to inhibit renin release.

▶ Propranolol pretreatment resulted both in a relative bradycardia and a smaller increase in plasma renin activity, suggesting that the antihypertensive effect of propranolol after repair of coarctation is mediated both by propranolol's cardiac actions and by inhibition of renin release. Whether the administration of renin just prior to, during, and after surgery will have a similar effect in eliminating paradoxical hypertension after repair is unknown. Of interest is the observation of the absence of paradoxical hypertension, decreased sympathetic response, and renin release when the coarctation is relieved by balloon angioplasty in patients with unoperated coarctation. Surgery itself, perhaps through interruption of sympathetic innervation, may alter arterial receptor mechanisms, peripheral vascular tone, or neural actions; this leads to the paradoxical hypertension.—Amnon Rosenthal, M.D.

Efficacy and Safety of Captopril in the Treatment of Severe Childhood Hypertension: Report of the International Collaborative Study Group
Bernard L. Mirkin and Thomas J. Newman (Univ. of Minnesota and Squibb Inst. for Med. Research, Princeton, N.J.)
Pediatrics 75:1091–1100, June 1985   2–5

Hypertension constitutes a significant disease process in children. The therapeutic efficacy and safety of captopril in children with severe (systolic and/or diastolic blood pressure above the 95th percentile for age and sex) and refractory hypertension were evaluated in 73 patients, aged 15 years or younger, enrolled in a collaborative international study. Most patients (90%) had hypertension attributable to renal disease or vascular abnormalities. Captopril was generally started with a single dose of 0.3 mg/kg every 8 hours. Thereafter, stepwise increments were made, not to exceed 6.0 mg/kg. Most patients received some form of antihypertensive therapy prior to captopril therapy.

Captopril was administered for periods of less than 3 months to more than 1 year. Both systolic and diastolic blood pressures were significantly reduced in 75% of patients by captopril treatment, usually in conjunction with other antihypertensive agents (most commonly diuretics and β-blockers). About 80% of those patients whose systolic and/or diastolic pressures were normalized at month 2 also had normal pressures at month 6. The average daily dosage administered at 1 week was significantly greater than the dosage used at month 3 ($P < .05$) or month 6 ($P < .01$). The response to captopril was sustained over a 12-month period.

Adverse reactions were reported in 49% of patients. However, 48% of patients had also experienced adverse effects from other antihypertensive agents prior to captopril therapy. The most frequent reactions during captopril therapy were hypotension, vomiting, postural symptoms, anemia, rash, and anorexia. Leukopenia was reported in 6 patients, all of whom had renal impairment. Two of these patients had received concomitant therapy with immunosuppressants, and 1 had systemic lupus erythematosus. Captopril was discontinued in 2 of these 6 patients. Small but statistically significant changes in serum urea nitrogen, serum potassium, and serum carbon dioxide levels were observed. Significant increases in serum creatinine levels were observed in 19 patients, including patients with renovascular hypertension or renal transplant recipients or patients with preexisting renal parenchymal disease. However, significant decreases in serum creatinine levels were also observed in 7 patients. Not all these effects could be exclusively attributed to captopril because the patients received multidrug therapy and had significant intrinsic disease.

Captopril, in conjunction with other antihypertensive agents, is an effective and safe drug for use in children wtih severe and refractory hypertension.

▶ Captopril represents the first of a new class of antihypertensive agents (angiotensin I converting enzyme inhibitors). Its initial use in children has been for the treatment of severe refractory hypertension. In this group of patients, it has proved to be a very effective and safe agent. The study of Mirkin and Newman clearly illustrates the therapeutic efficacy and safety of captopril in the treatment of children with refractory hypertension. However, the potential clinical implications of this drug in childhood are much larger than just the treatment of refractory hypertension. Captopril is already being used in adults as first-line therapy for the treatment of mild to moderate hypertension. It has the following advantages over many of the other more commonly used antihypertensive agents: It does not raise either serum cholesterol or serum uric acid levels, it does not alter glucose tolerance or produce central nervous system side effects, and it has been shown to be effective in reversing the myocardial hypertrophy associated with systemic hypertension.

In addition to its use as an antihypertensive agent, captopril has also been reported to be effective both in symptomatically treating patients with refractory congestive heart failure and in reducing proteinuria in patients with diabetic nephropathy.

Captopril is an important new pharmacologic agent that will become a key component not only in the medical treatment of children with hypertension, but also in the treatment of many other diseases, such as congestive heart failure and diabetic nephropathy.—Albert P. Rocchini, M.D.

Mucocutaneous Lymph Node Syndrome: Clinical, Hemodynamic and Angiographic Features of Coronary Obstructive Disease
Toshio Nakanishi, Atsuyoshi Takao, Makoto Nakazawa, Masahiro Endo, Koichiro Niwa, and Yoshiaki Takahashi (Heart Inst. of Japan, Tokyo)
Am. J. Cardiol. 55:662–668, March 1, 1985   2–6

The incidence of children with mucocutaneous lymph node syndrome (Kawasaki disease) presenting with significant coronary stenosis has been increasing. However, clinical and hemodynamic findings in these patients have not been described. Thirty patients with severe obstruction ($\geq$90% diameter reduction) of coronary arteries with or without a myocardial infarction (MI) pattern on ECG were evaluated to determine the clinical, hemodynamic, and angiographic features of coronary obstructive disease in Kawasaki disease.

The mean age at the onset of Kawasaki disease was 2.9 ± 1.9 years and that at cardiac catheterization was 6.3 ± 2.8 years. The male to female ratio was 4 to 1. Obstructive lesions were noted in the right coronary artery in 12 patients (group I), in the left anterior descending (LAD) artery in 6 (group II), in both right coronary artery and LAD in 10 (group III), and in the left main coronary artery in 4 (group IV). Cardiac symptoms were present in 22 patients: MI in 10, angina in 5, and chronic congestive heart failure in 8. Cardiac symptoms (64%) and an MI pattern on the ECG (81%) appeared within 1 year after the onset of Kawasaki disease. Cardiac symptoms were observed less frequently in group I (41%) than in other groups: 100% in group II, 80% in group III, and 100% in group IV ($P < .05$). Typical symptoms of MI were observed infrequently (31%). Abnormal values of left ventricular (LV) end-diastolic pressure, end-diastolic volume, and ejection fraction were observed less frequently in group I patients, 32% vs. 83% in group II, 78% in group III, and 100% in group IV ($P < .05$). Ejection fraction in patients with anterior and anteroinferior MI was significantly less than in patients with normal QRS. Mitral regurgitation was observed in about 50% of patients. The LV ejection fraction was lower in patients with mitral regurgitation than in patients without. Segmental LV wall motion was abnormal in 92% of patients with an MI pattern on the electrocardiogram and normal in all patients without an MI. The rate of bypass occlusion was rather high. There were no deaths in groups I and II, while 8 of 14 died from groups III and IV.

Coronary obstruction due to Kawasaki disease can cause depressed LV function, mitral regurgitation, and LV wall motion abnormalities in children. Clinical and hemodynamic features of isolated right coronary artery obstruction are relatively benign compared with those of left coronary obstruction, either isolated or combined with right obstruction. Since most patients are referred after they developed cardiac symptoms or an ECG abnormality, the present study may represent the patients who had survived the initial episode of coronary obstruction. Therefore, the incidence of coronary obstruction in patients with Kawasaki disease or in patients with coronary aneurysm may be understated. These are the limitations of a retrospective study.

▶ The spectrum of acute and chronic coronary artery problems in infants and children with Kawasaki disease indicates the need for long-term medical follow-up in patients with the syndrome. However, the incidence of late coronary artery disease remains low. In a group of over 200 patients with Kawasaki disease followed at our institution over the past 8 years, excluding those with documented infarction during the acute phase of the illness, none has shown late evidence of significant coronary stenosis. Noninvasive evaluation with periodic ECG and exercise treadmill testing are performed in all patients. In those who developed aneurysms or significant cardiac involvement during the acute or convalescent phase, periodic echocardiograms are also obtained. Cardiac catheterization and coronary cineangiograms may also be necessary in those patients with clinical or noninvasive evidence of coronary artery involvement. The use of streptokinase for lysis of coronary artery thrombus present during the acute and convalescent phases of the syndrome and the use of balloon angioplasty for treatment of late-appearing stenotic lesions are being explored at a number of institutions.—Dennis C. Crowley, M.D.

Probable Efficacy of High-Dose Salicylates in Reducing Coronary Involvement in Kawasaki Disease
Gideon Koren, Vera Rose, Sasson Lavi, and Richard Rowe (Univ. of Toronto, Ontario)
JAMA 254:767–769, Aug. 9, 1985   2–7

Coronary aneurysms are frequent in patients with Kawasaki disease, and fatal myocardial infarction can result. Moreover, absorption of acetylsalicylic acid is impaired in the febrile phase of the disease and requires high-dose treatment. High-dosage aspirin therapy was evaluated in a series of 54 patients with Kawasaki disease diagnosed between 1982 and 1984. Thirty-six children received acetylsalicylic acid in daily doses of 80–180 mg/kg, given in four equal portions at 6-hour intervals, starting in the febrile phase. Eighteen others were given acetaminophen or casual aspirin therapy in doses no greater than 30 mg/kg daily before Kawasaki disease was diagnosed. In study cases the dose was adjusted to produce serum salicylate levels of 20–30 mg/dl. The two groups were comparable in age, body weight, and severity of disease.

High-dose salicylate therapy was given for a mean period of 8 days during the febrile phase of disease. Only a few patients had therapeutic serum salicylate levels higher than 20 mg/dl; twofold-higher levels were achieved in the later, nonfebrile phase of disease. The prevalence of coronary involvement was 17% in the study group and 50% in the control group, as defined by dilatation of the proximal coronary arteries or aneurysms by 3 mm or more. One study patient and 7 control patients had coronary aneurysms. Two control patients with aneurysms had myocardial infarction, and 1 of them died. The duration of fever, peak erythrocyte sedimentation rate, and maximum platelet count were comparable in the two groups.

High-dose acetylsalicylic acid therapy is appropriate once Kawasaki disease is diagnosed, but the dose may have to be adjusted after fever resolves and salicylate absorption improves. High-dose treatment can prevent the coronary complications of Kawasaki disease.

▶ Salicylates remain the mainstay of therapy for patients with Kawasaki disease during the acute and convalescent phases of the illness. The authors present convincing evidence that large doses (up to 100 mg/kg/day) are required during the febrile phase to obtain therapeutic salicylate levels and to reduce the incidence of associated coronary artery disease. However, the tendency for high-dose salicylates to enhance platelet aggregation should be considered and the dose reduced to less than 30 mg/kg/day when platelet levels rise. We continue low-dose salicylate therapy for 3 months in all patients and for an indefinite period in patients with coronary artery aneurysm. Recent controlled studies on the use of gamma globulin to prevent aneurysm formation suggest that such therapy may be effective. At present we fell that gamma globulin should be administered to the severely ill and young high-risk patient with Kawasaki disease.—Dennis C. Crowley, M.D.

Rhythm and Conduction Disorders

In Utero Diagnosis and Treatment of Fetal Supraventricular Tachycardia
Charles S. Kleinman, Joshua A. Copel, Ellen M. Weinstein, Thomas V. Santulli, Jr., and John C. Hobbins (Yale Univ.)
Sem. Perinatol, 9:113–129, July 1985   2–8

Fetal echocardiography has been used to evaluate 245 fetuses with a chief complaint of "arrhythmia". Abnormal cardiac rhythm was found initially in 81% of cases. Isolated extrasystoles were present in 84% of these fetuses, and persisted postnatally in 14 of them. Sustained arrhythmias in 35 cases included supraventricular tachycardia (SVT) in 16, atrial flutter or fibrillation in 5, and atrioventricular block in 10. Two-dimensional echocardiography was performed using a segmental analysis of situs and intracardiac connection. The pulsed Doppler technique can be used to determine the hemodynamic sequelae of arrhythmias.

The 21 cases of fetal supraventricular tachyarrhythmia seen in the past 5 years are shown in Table 1. All patients had normal cardiac anatomy on echocardiography. Ventricular rates in the 16 cases of SVT ranged from 240 to 280 beats per minute. In utero treatment was with maternally administered antiarrhythmic agents (Table 2). Combined treatment with digoxin and orally administered verapamil has consistently led to conversion to sinus rhythm. All infants remained free of arrhythmia after the

TABLE 1.—Fetal Supraventricular
Tachyarrhythmias*

Supraventricular tachycardia	(n = 16)
Gestational age	19–28 wk
Hydrops fetalis	15/16 cases
In utero control	15/16 cases
Postnatal control	1/16 cases
Mortality	0
Atrial flutter	(n = 3)
Gestational age	30–38 wk
Hydrops fetalis	3/3 cases
In utero control	0/3 cases
Postnatal control	1/3 cases
Mortality	2/3 cases
Atrial fibrillation	(n = 2)
Gestational age	19–38 wk
Hydrops fetalis	0
In utero control	1/2 cases
Mortality	0

*N = 21.
(Courtesy of Kleinman, C.S., et al.: Sem. Perinatol. 9:113–129, July 1985.)

TABLE 2.—Supraventricular
Tachycardia In Utero Therapy†

*One patient, initially controlled with a regimen of digoxin and verapamil was changed to one of digoxin and propranolol because of maternal heart block following administration of verapamil.
†N = 16.
(Courtesy of Kleinman, C.S., et al.: Sem. Perinatol. 9:113–129, July 1985.)

neonatal period on prophylaxis with digoxin, alone or with propranolol or verapamil. Two fetuses with atrial flutter died, whereas 1 responded to electrical cardioversion in the delivery room. Both fetuses with atrial fibrillation survived.

The transplacental passage of various antiarrhythmic agents is shown in Table 3. In utero treatment is preferable to premature delivery, especially with an unfavorable lecithin:sphingomyelin ratio. Premature delivery is performed only if a trial on sequential drugs fails and hydrops fetalis persists or worsens. Close hemodynamic monitoring of both the mother and fetus is necessary with in utero treatment.

▶ After you read the digest, I suggest that you go to the library and obtain a copy of the full article. This report provides an excellent and comprehensive review of the pathophysiology, diagnosis, management, and prognosis of fetal supraventricular tachycardia. The day is rapidly approaching when we will witness the establishment of a new clinical program or entity within pediatric

TABLE 3.—TRANSPLACENTAL ANTIARRHYTHMIC AGENTS

	Digoxin*	Verapamil†	Propranolol‡	Procainamide§	Quinidine‖
Loading					
PO	1.0–2.5 mg				
IV	0.5–2.0 mg	5.0–10.0 mg	0.5 mg q5min	12 mg/kg	Do not give
Maintenance					
PO	0.25–0.75 mg/d	80–120 mg q6–8h	20–160 mg q6–8h	6 mg/kg q4h	250–500 mg q6h
IV	0.25 mg				Do not give
Protein bound	20%	90%	90%–95%	15%	60%–90%
Eliminating organ	Kidney	Liver	Liver	Kidney	Liver
Transplacental passage (cord/maternal serum level)	0.6–1.0	0.3–0.4	0.1–0.3	0.8–1.3	0.2–0.9
Therapeutic plasma concentration	0.5–2.0 ng/mL	50–100 ng/mL	50–1,000 ng/mL	4–14 mcg/mL	2–8 mcg/mL

*Level may increase when verapamil or quinidine is added, fetus may tolerate (? need) higher level than adult.
†Extensive first pass metabolism, may cause heart block, inotropic agent, do not give with propranolol.
‡Extensive first pass metabolism, do not give with verapamil; fetal bradycardia, hypoglycemia, growth retardation, maternal bronchospasm.
§Active metabolite, N-acetyl procainamide (NAPA), may accumulate in fetus or neonate.
‖ Do not give IV, may increase digoxin levels, neonatal thrombocytopenia, in utero deaths reported, in atrial fibrillation/flutter pretreat with digoxin or verapamil.
PO = orally, IV = intravenous.
(Courtesy of Kleinman, C.S., et al.: Sem. Perinatol. 9:113–129, July 1985.)

cardiology—fetal cardiology. When it arrives, it is likely to be initiated at Yale.—Amnon Rosenthal, M.D.

Prediction of Digoxin Treatment Failure in Infants With Supraventricular Tachycardia: Role of Transesophageal Pacing
D. Woodrow Benson, Jr., Ann Dunnigan, David G. Benditt, Theodore R. Thompson, Athi Narayan, and Stephen Boros (Univ. of Minnesota, St. Paul-Ramsey Hosp., and St. Paul Children's Hosp.)
Pediatrics 75:288–293, February 1985

2–9

Chronic digoxin therapy is a recommended prophylaxis to prevent recurrence of supraventricular tachycardia (SVT) in infants. A quantitative definition for the severity of SVT in infants is proposed. Using this definition, the effectiveness of digitalis derivatives in preventing SVT recurrences is compared to its ability to prevent the initiation of SVT by transesophageal atrial pacing in 24 infants, aged 1 to 34 days, with ECG documentation of SVT. Six infants received no treatment. Chronic oral digoxin prophylaxis (8–12 μg/kg/day) in 18 infants we based on the following criteria: SVT resulting in signs of congestive heart failure, a single SVT episode lasting more than 3 hours, three or more SVT episodes exceeding 15 minutes duration in 24 hours, or five or more SVT episodes in 24 hours. In these 18 patients, the effectiveness of digoxin therapy in preventing the initiation of tachycardia by transesophageal pacing was compared with its ability to prevent spontaneous recurrences of SVT.

Chronic oral digoxin therapy did not prevent reinitiation of SVT by transesophageal atrial pacing in 15/18 (83%) infants. In these infants, digoxin had no effect on tachycardia cycle length and atrioventricular

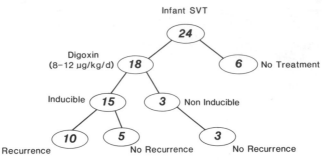

Fig 2–1.—Results in 24 infants with SVT. Eighteen infants were treated with digoxin and 10 had recurrences of SVT. The 6 untreated infants had no recurrences in 6 months of follow-up. (Courtesy of Benson Jr., D.W., et al.: Pediatrics 75:288–293, February 1985. Reproduced by permission of Pediatrics.)

interval. During 6 months of follow-up, 3 infants in whom sustained tachycardia could not be reinitiated during digoxin prophylaxis showed no spontaneous recurrences, while 10/15 (67%) infants in whom tachycardia could be reinitiated showed clinically significant spontaneous recurrences of SVT (Fig 2–1). Hence, chronic digoxin therapy was effective in preventing significant recurrences in only 8/18 (44%) infants. Six infants who received no chronic prophylactic therapy had no significant recurrences during follow-up.

Digoxin is not an effective prophylaxis for some infants with SVT. The ability to initiate SVT with transesophageal atrial pacing may be useful in determining which digoxin-treated infants are at risk for recurrence. In addition, use of the quantitative definition of severity of SVT may permit identification of some infants who do not require chronic prophylaxis during the first 6 months of life.

▶ The long-held clinical axiom that an infant with SVT should be treated with digoxin for at least 1 year is essentially empiric; it antedates the emergence of acute drug testing, transesophageal atrial pacing, and knowledge of the potential adverse response of an accessory connection to digoxin. This paper reports the application of modified acute drug testing (atrial burst pacing) delivered through the transesophageal route to the issue of chronic prophylaxis of SVT in infants by digoxin. The data demonstrate that the majority of infants are not successfully prophylaxed from either induced or spontaneous SVT by therapeutic serum levels of digoxin and that, to some extent, success or failure can be predicted by transesophageal pacing. Digoxin does not seem to do much good in these infants. Importantly, in at least the 5 patients with an antegradely conducting accessory connection (Wolff-Parkinson-White syndrome), digoxin did not do any harm either. Two caveats: First, the follow-up covered only the first 6 months after digoxin treatment; second, the digoxin serum levels, although "therapeutic," may have reached more effective concentrations at higher dosages. The authors correctly suggest that there is little rationale for a relationship between higher serum levels and successful control; on the other hand, the weight of clinical experience and practice urges that this question be addressed. For the present, it is, I think, safe to say that digoxin therapy, after conversion to sinus rhythm and in the absence of congestive heart failure, may be withheld in infants with SVT if there is little hemodynamic or symptomatic consequence; likewise, digoxin may be withdrawn earlier than after 1 year if no spontaneous or induced SVT is present.—Macdonald Dick II, M.D.

Wolff-Parkinson-White Syndrome and Supraventricular Tachycardia During Infancy: Management and Follow-up

Barbara J. Deal, John F. Keane, Paul C. Gillette, and Arthur Garson, Jr. (Harvard Univ. and Baylor Univ.)

J. Am. Coll. Cardiol. 5:130–135, January 1985   2–10

The records of all patients with the diagnosis of Wolff-Parkinson-White (WPW) syndrome observed at the Texas Children's Hospital, Houston, and the Children's Hospital, Boston, between 1951 and 1982 were reviewed. The 90 infants (57 boys and 33 girls) who had a prolonged episode of tachycardia in the first 4 months of life are the subject of this report. Structural heart disease was present in 20%, most commonly Ebstein's anomaly. All patients presented with a regular narrow QRS tachycardia, and preexcitation became evident only when normal sinus rhythm was established. Only 1 infant had atrial flutter, and none had atrial fibrillation. Type A WPW syndrome was most common (49%), with heart disease occurring in only 5% of these patients. In contrast, heart disease was identified in 45% of those with type B syndrome (table).

Initially, a normal sinus rhythm was achieved in 88% of the 66 infants treated with digoxin with no deaths. Normal sinus rhythm resumed after electric countershock in 87% of the 15 infants so treated. Maintenance digoxin therapy was used in 85 patients. The WPW pattern disappeared in 36% of the patients. Four infants died of cardiac causes during the mean follow-up period of 6.5 years. Two of these 4 infants had congenital heart disease. In the third, with a normal heart initially, ventricular fibrillation developed; she died of cardiomyopathy considered related to resuscitation. The remaining infant, with a normal heart, died suddenly at 1 month of age. All were receiving digoxin. A wide QRS tachycardia appeared in 3 patients, all with heart disease, 1 of whom died. In the initial

CLASSIFICATION OF WOLFF-PARKINSON-WHITE PATTERNS

Type	All Patients (n = 90) No. (%)	Patients With Normal Heart (n = 72) No. (%)	Patients With Heart Disease (n = 18) No. (%)
A	44(49)	42(58)	2(11)
B	29(32)	16(22)	13(72)
C	16(18)	14(20)	2(11)
A + B	1(1)	0	1(6)

(Courtesy of Deal, B.J., et al.: J. Am. Coll. Cardiol. 5:130–135, January 1985. Reprinted with permission from the American College of Cardiology.)

treatment of narrow regular QRS supraventricular tachycardia in this group of patients, digoxin was safe and effective (88%) for restoration of normal sinus rhythm; electric cardioversion was equally effective (87%) in those critically ill. After age 1 year, 33% of the infants experienced recurrent tachycardias; these were more frequent in patients with type B WPW syndrome and in those requiring more than one drug to maintain normal sinus rhythm during the initial hospitalization.

Analysis of this series of infants with WPW conduction and supraventricular tachycardia confirms the previously reported male preponderance and the incidence of congenital heart disease in approximately 20% of patients. Digoxin, administered to 66 infants in stable condition, was successful in restoring normal sinus rhythm in 58; no deaths occurred. Therefore, in the initial management of infants in stable condition with a regular narrow QRS supraventricular tachycardia, digoxin and electric cardioversion (0.5 joule/kg) were both safe and equally effective in this selective series of patients. Direct current countershock remains the treatment of choice for urgent conversion of life-threatening tachycardia. In the future, the technique of esophageal pacing may become more widely available for use in the infant and may provide an alternative to electric cardioversion. Mortality associated with the use of digoxin in this patient group may be at least 2%, and could be as high as 5%. Excessive amounts of digoxin may precipitate ventricular fibrillation in these infants. Thus, in the absence of electrophysiologically demonstrated safety of digoxin, the use of propranolol should be considered, particularly in the setting of recurrent supraventricular tachycardia.

Among those patients with significant recurrent episodes of typical supraventricular tachycardia, drugs such as propranolol, quinidine, or procainamide alone or in combination may be necessary. Verapamil, effective in older patients, may be used in older children, but experience with its use in infants is limited. In patients who manifest a wide QRS complex tachycardia or atrial fibrillation, or both, the use of digitalis is contraindicated.

▶ This paper adds to the world experience of WPW in infants. It underscores the good prognosis of most infants with this disorder, but at the same time highlights the risk in those infants with associated heart disease. Digoxin is again affirmed as a useful drug—but on an empiric basis. We would suggest adding the technique of acute drug testing through transesophageal atrial extrastimulation and pacing to the management plan presented.—Macdonald Dick II, M.D.

Surgical Management of Refractory Supraventricular Tachycardia in Infants and Children
David A. Ott, Paul C. Gillette, Arthur Garson, Jr., Denton A. Cooley, George J. Reul, and Dan G. McNamara (Texas Heart Inst., Houston)
J. Am. Coll. Cardiol. 5:124–129, January 1985   2–11

Available data are scarce concerning the diagnosis and surgical man-

LOCATION OF ACCESSORY CONDUCTION PATHWAY
(KENT BUNDLE) AND RATE OF RECURRENCE OF TACHYCARDIA
AFTER SURGERY

Location of Accessory Pathway	No.	%	Recurrence	
			No.	%
Right anterior or lateral	19	34.5	3	16
Left posterior or lateral	22	40.0	3	14
Posterior septal	10	18	1	10
Anterior septal	2	4	0	0
Both right and left	2	4	1	50
Total	55		8	14.5

(Courtesy of Ott, D.A., et al.: J. Am. Coll. Cardiol. 5:124–129, January 1985. Reprinted with permission from the American College of Cardiology.)

agement of supraventricular tachycardia caused by the presence of an accessory conduction bundle (Kent bundle) in infants and children. To obtain further information on surgical resolution of the tachycardia, 67 children aged 4 months to 18 years (mean age, 11 years) underwent attempted surgical correction of refractory supraventricular arrhythmia. The procedure combined intraoperative electrophysiologic mapping and surgical division or cryoablation of an aberrant conduction pathway or atrial ectopic focus.

Of the 55 children who underwent operative ablation of the accessory conduction bundle, 36 (65%) had classic Wolff-Parkinson-White syndrome with a delta wave of preexcitation seen on the surface electrocardiogram; 19 (35%) had only retrograde conduction across the accessory bundle and normal findings in the surface electrocardiogram during sinus rhythm. Left posterior or posterolateral Kent bundles were the most common location (40%). At a mean follow-up of 34.9 months, seven immediate failures and one late recurrence of arrhythmia were reported (table). However, increasing experience in electrophysiologic mapping and refinements in the surgical technique, including the use of cryoablation for posterior septal Kent bundles, improved the outcome, resulting in only two failures (8%) in the later 25 attempts. Of 12 patients operated on for atrial ectopic tachycardia, 7 underwent cryoablation, 1 had excision, and 4 had both excision and cryoablation. Immediate surgical ablation was achieved in 11 patients (92%) with no late recurrences, and only 1 patient had late recurrence at a mean follow-up of 16.6 months.

The results demonstrate the feasibility, predictability, and safety of electrophysiologic mapping and surgical treatment of supraventricular tachycardia, including atrial ectopic tachycardia, in infants and children. Children with refractory supraventricular tachycardia, even in the absence of preexcitation on the electrocardiogram, should undergo complete electrophysiologic evaluation to elucidate the mechanism of the tachycardia.

▶ This is one of the largest, if not the largest, series of children operated upon for Kent bundles. The techniques of diagnosis and treatment used were identical to those used in adults, and they appear to work very well in children. Thirty-five percent of the children had no delta waves, a percentage similar to that seen in adults; and of particular interest to me, only 10% had structural congenital defects. The difficulty in administering medications to children and the possible long-term side effects of antiarrhythmic drugs provide an indication for operation in children that is not present in adults. However, the bottom line in this report is that children are not much different from adults in the mode of presentation and methods of diagnosis or treatment and, therefore, that the much more extensive experience in adults can be successfully applied to children.—D. Behrendt, M.D.

Atrial Flutter in the Young: A Collaborative Study of 380 Cases
Arthur Garson, Jr., Margreet Bink-Boelkens, Peter S. Hesslein, Allan J. Hordof, John F. Keane, William H. Neches, Co-Burn J. Porter, and the Pediatric Electrophysiology Society (Houston)
J. Am. Coll. Cardiol. 6:871–878, October 1985   2–12

Atrial flutter is seen increasingly as more children with congenital heart

TABLE 1.—CARDIAC DIAGNOSIS IN 380 PATIENTS

	%
D-transposition of great arteries	20.5
Complex congenital lesions	17.8
Atrial septal defect	12.1
(80% secundum, 10% primum, 10% sinus venosus)	
Tetralogy of Fallot	7.9
Normal	6.3
Congestive cardiomyopathy	5.8
Atrioventricular canal	5.0
Total anomalous pulmonary venous return	4.7
Congenital mitral disease	4.2
Rheumatic mitral disease	3.7
Ventricular septal defect	2.6
Tricuspid atresia	2.4
Ebstein's anomaly	2.1
Wolff-Parkinson-White syndrome	1.6
Mitral valve prolapse	1.1
Aortic stenosis	0.8
Tricuspid insufficiency	0.5
L-transposition of great arteries	0.3
Pericarditis	0.3
Rhabdomyoma	0.3
Total	100

(Courtesy of Garson, A., Jr., et al.: J. Am. Coll. Cardiol. 6:871–878, October 1985. Reprinted with permission from the American College of Cardiology.)

TABLE 2.—FINAL STATUS OF 368 PATIENTS*

Cardiac Diagnosis	Alive (%)	Sudden Death (%)	Nonsudden Cardiac Death (%)
D-TGA	87	10	3
Complex	66	25	8
ASD	98	2	0
ToF	86	7	7
Normal	100	0	0
Congestive cardiomyopathy	61	13	26
TAPVR	100	0	0
TA	100	0	0

*D-TGA, D-transposition of the great arteries; ASD, atrial septal defect; ToF, tetralogy of Fallot; TAPVR, total anomalous pulmonary venous return; TA, tricuspid atresia.
(Courtesy of Garson, A., Jr., et al.: J. Am. Coll. Cardiol. 6:871–878, October 1985. Reprinted with permission from the American College of Cardiology.)

disease live into adolescence and adulthood. A multicenter study was conducted of 380 patients aged 1–25 years with atrial flutter. The cardiac diagnoses are listed in Table 1. About 60% of the patients had repaired congenital heart disease. The mean age at onset of atrial flutter was 10 years. Some 30% of the patients were asymptomatic at the first episode. Syncope was most frequent in patients with a normal heart and those with Wolff-Parkinson-White syndrome.

Drugs were used to treat atrial flutter in 91% of the patients, with an overall success rate of 58%. The most effective approach was a combination of digoxin with a type I antiarrhythmic drug, e.g., quinidine or procainamide. The most active agent overall was amiodarone, which was successful in 7 of 9 patients. Drug efficacy generally was independent of the type of underlying heart disease. Sixty-six patients had surgery after the onset of atrial flutter. In 357 patients followed for an average of 6½ years, atrial flutter lasted for 2½ years. Atrial flutter continued despite treatment in 35% of the surviving patients. The outcome is related to cardiac diagnosis in Table 2. A pacemaker was implanted in 17% of the patients. Sudden death occurred in 5% of the patients in whom atrial flutter was eliminated pharmacologically and in 20% of those without effective control.

Prophylactic digoxin therapy may be indicated in patients at high risk for the development of atrial flutter, including those operated on for transposition, patients having repair of tetralogy of Fallot with resultant tricuspid insufficiency, and patients who have congestive cardiomyopathy or an echographic left atrial dimension of more than 150% above the upper normal limit. Effective control of atrial flutter leads to lower mortality for both sudden and nonsudden cardiac death. Surgery, when indicated, is much more likely to improve atrial flutter than to worsen it.

Atrial Overdrive Pacing for Conversion of Atrial Flutter in Children

Robert M. Campbell, Macdonald Dick II, Janice M. Jenkins, Robert L. Spicer, Dennis C. Crowley, Albert P. Rocchini, A. Rebecca Snider, Aaron M. Stern, and Amnon Rosenthal (Univ. of Michigan)

Pediatrics 75:730–736, April 1985   2–13

Atrial flutter is a potentially unstable tachyarrhythmia in pediatric patients. The efficacy of rapid atrial pacing was determined in 23 consecutively seen patients with 27 separate episodes of sustained atrial flutter. Fifteen patients (group 1) with 16 episodes and a mean age of 9 years had high right atrial intracardiac pacing noted during cardiac catheterization. The conditions of 8 other patients (group 2) with 11 episodes of atrial flutter and a mean age of 10 years were managed by transesophageal atrial pacing. The most frequent diagnoses were transposition following Mustard repair and tetralogy of Fallot after intracardiac repair. Most patients were receiving digoxin at the time of the study, and most were examined within 3 months of the first episode of sustained atrial flutter.

Characteristics of atrial flutter were similar in the two treatment groups. Group 1 patients whose arrhythmia converted to baseline rhythm were younger than the others and had had surgery more recently. Ten episodes of flutter in group 1 (62.5%) were successfully converted, as compared with 73% of episodes in group 2 patients. The mean flutter cycle length for all episodes was 219 msec, and the mean successful pacing conversion cycle length was 72% of the flutter cycle length. Conversion could not be predicted by the hemodynamic or electrophysiological findings in either treatment group. No significant bradycardia or prolonged overdrive suppression followed conversion by either method.

These findings are comparable to those obtained in adults. More recent experience suggests successful results in two thirds of cases using either technique. Neither requires general anesthesia. Transesophageal pacing may be especially useful in young children where venous access is difficult, particularly after multiple surgical and catheterization procedures. Outpatient conversion by the transesophageal method is especially of interest in patients with repeated episodes of atrial flutter. Serious esophageal damage has not resulted during even prolonged pacing.

▶ Digest 2–12 represents an outstanding example of the value of the cooperative studies sponsored by the Pediatric Electrophysiology Society. Atrial flutter is not a very common disorder in the pediatric age-group. Pooling the experience of multiple institutions permits the collection of sufficient data to properly define the clinical features, to determine risk factors, and to formulate valid therapeutic recommendations. In the management of children with atrial flutter, the goal, as stated by the authors, is to eliminate all episodes of flutter rather than to allow atrial flutter to continue with a controlled ventricular rate. The treatment of choice for initial conversion of flutter to sinus rhythm is electroversion, preferably by transesophageal pacing. Maintenance of sinus rhythm is accomplished by long-term use of digoxin plus quinidine. Surgery is indicated if an underlying cardiovascular abnormality is present that is amenable to repair. Anticoagulation therapy, in order to prevent embolization, seems prudent for a month prior to cardioversion in children with long-standing atrial flutter, very dilated atriae, and/or myocardial dysfunction. An echocardiogram should be obtained prior to cardioversion to search for the presence of an atrial or ventricular thrombus. If sick sinus syndrome coexists or is suspected, a temporary transvenous pacemaker may be required prior to electrical cardioversion. Overall prognosis is poorer for the child with atrial flutter and underlying cardiac disease. No deaths occurred among patients with a normal heart.—Amnon Rosenthal, M.D.

Prevention of Sudden Death After Repair of Tetralogy of Fallot: Treatment of Ventricular Arrhythmias
Arthur Garson, Jr., David C. Randall, Paul C. Gillette, Richard T. Smith, Jeffrey P. Moak, Pat McVey, and Dan G. McNamara (Texas Children's Hosp. and Baylor Univ., Houston)
J. Am. Coll. Cardiol. 6:221–227, July 1985   2–14

Most sudden deaths after repair of tetralogy of Fallot (TOF) have been presumed to be due to ventricular arrhythmia. However, the effect of antiarrhythmic therapy on the incidence of sudden death has not been analyzed. To determine this effect, a review was undertaken of data on 488 patients followed up for more than 1 month after repair of tetralogy of Fallot. Since 1978, all patients were treated aggressively with antiarrhythmic agents (phenytoin, mexiletine, propranolol, quinidine, or amiodarone) if there were any premature ventricular complexes on a routine ECG or more than ten uniform premature ventricular complexes per hour on a 24-hour ECG. A drug was considered effective if there were fewer than ten uniform premature ventricular complexes per hour on two consecutive 24-hour ECGs.

Premature ventricular complexes were noted on routine ECG in 67

TREATMENT OF VENTRICULAR ARRHYTHMIAS IN 46
POSTOPERATIVE PATIENTS

Drug	No. of Trials*	% Success	Side Effects (%)
Phenytoin	34	88	Rash (12)
Propranolol	9	67	Lethargy (11)
Quinidine	7	14	0
Disopyramide	2	50	0
Mexiletine	9	89	Nausea (22); rash (11)
Amiodarone	5	80	0

*Since patients may have received more than one drug, the total number of trials is greater than the total number of patients.
(Courtesy of Garson, Jr., A., et al.: J. Am. Coll. Cardiol. 6:221–227, July, 1985. Reprinted with permission from the American College of Cardiology.)

(13.7%) patients, appearing from 2 months to 21 years postoperatively (mean 7.3 years). Ventricular arrhythmia was found in 71 of 97 patients (73%) who underwent a 24-hour ECG. Patients with ventricular arrhythmias had significantly higher postoperative right ventricular systolic ($P <$ .001) and end-diastolic pressures ($P <$ .05), longer duration of follow-up ($P <$ .01), older age at operation (30 years and above), and older age at follow-up. Ventricular arrhythmia occurred in 100% of patients who died suddenly compared with 12% of those who did not ($P <$ .0001). An "effective" antiarrhythmic drug was given in 44 of 46 patients at an average of 1.4 drugs per patient. Average duration of treatment was 2.3 years (range 6 months to 6.2 years). Phenytoin was used most frequently and was successful in 88% of patients (table). There were no sudden deaths among the 44 patients with successful antiarrhythmic therapy compared to 7 of 21 untreated and 2 of 2 unsuccessfully treated with antiarrhythmic therapy ($P <$ .001).

With aggressive use of antiarrhythmic drugs and adequate control of ventricular arrhythmia, the incidence of sudden death after repair of tetralogy of Fallot can be significantly reduced.

▶ The controversy over prophylaxis or no prophylaxis of ventricular ectopic activity (VEA) in the postoperative patient with tetralogy of Fallot is further fueled by this report from Texas Children's Hospital. Garson and his colleagues present persuasive data and analysis that suggest that a single ventricular premature beat on an electrocardiogram in a postoperative tetralogy of Fallot patient should be suppressed. Although we are impressed with this experience, we do not agree. The experience of several centers, including ours, suggests that this approach, as the present authors admit, may be overly aggressive and expose many patients to potentially toxic agents. With this in mind, the following approach has evolved at our institution: All patients with postoperative tetralogy of Fallot have an electrocardiogram every 1 to 2 years; if either VPBs (or symptoms of palpitations) are present, two separate 24-hour Holter tracings are obtained. Single isolated ventricular premature beats (less than 30 per hour) are not treated. If more than 30 ventricular premature beats per hour are observed, treatment is initiated with a single drug in the following sequence: dilantin, quinidine/procainamide, amiodorone. In addition, if a residual hemodynamic lesion is suspected by clinical evaluation, cardiac catheterization along with programmed ventricular extrastimulation is performed. If a residual lesion such as described by Garson and associates is found and if it is treatable, surgery is advised. To date, this approach has been successful. We join the authors in suggesting the need for a placebo-control prospective study; we would add that the study should be a collaborative, multicentered study similar to that currently being considered by the National Institutes of Health for postinfarct antiarrhythmic prophylaxis. Such an enlarged database may allow for analysis of such factors as surgical technique (which is changing even now), variability in tetralogy anatomy, right and left ventricular function, and other postoperative features. This paper presents a well-argued approach to the problem of postoperative TOF ventricular ectopic activity; it does not, however solve it.—Macdonald Dick II, M.D.

Ventricular Tachycardia in Children Without Heart Disease

David R. Fulton, Kyung J. Chung, Burton S. Tabakin, and John F. Keane (Tufts Univ., Harvard Univ., and Univ. of Vermont)
Am. J. Cardiol. 55:1328–1331, May 1, 1985   2–15

Reports on the management of ventricular tachycardia (VT) in children without heart disease have been inconclusive. The clinical course of 26 children aged 1 day to 15 years (mean, 4 years 11 months) was evaluated to assess the natural history of VT structurally normal hearts. All of the children were seen at Children's and Boston Floating Hospitals. Evaluations consisted of 24-hour Holter monitoring in 22 patients, echocardiography in 19, graded treadmill exercise testing in 16, and invasive electrophysiology in 4.

Symptoms related to the arrhythmia (e.g., palpitations, dizziness, and chest pain) were present in 8 children at some time during the course of follow-up. The arrhythmia was first identified in 12 patients during ambulatory Holter monitoring. It was evident at rest in 23 patients and only during exercise in 3. The rates of VT ranged from 120 to 230 beats/minute (median, 150), and the duration varied considerably. Exercise induced or exacerbated VT in 9 patients, but suppressed rhythm in 7. Findings on echocardiography were normal in 19 children, as were results of invasive electrophysiology in 4. There were no known deaths during a follow-up period of 1 month to 34 years (mean, 4 years 11 months). Ten patients who were never treated remained asymptomatic. Of the remaining 16 treated patients, antiarrhythmic therapy was discontinued in 10 when no significant effect was noted as determined by electrocardiography or Holter monitoring; 6 continued to receive therapy without complications.

Based on these findings and a review of the literature concerning childhood VT, symptomatic children, after undergoing complete noninvasive cardiac evaluation, should be treated and studied with invasive electrophysiology if antiarrhythmic therapy is ineffective. Asymptomatic patients do not appear to benefit from therapy, but warrant follow-up observation because rare deaths have been reported in untreated asymptomatic children with VT. Neither age at onset nor rate of VT is predictive of outcome in asymptomatic patients.

▶ The asymptomatic child with a normal heart and nonsustained ventricular tachycardia presents a number of significant dilemmas. These include the extent and type of investigations required to determine whether the heart is structurally normal, the need for restriction of physical activity, and the advisability of pharmacologic therapy to suppress the ventricular ectopy. The recommendations of the Pediatric Dysrhythmia Conference (*Ped. Cardiol.* 4:65–68, 1983) are that in children with ventricular tachycardia and a normal heart, the following in addition to "routine assessment," should be performed: exercise study, Holter monitoring, and cardiac catheterization (including hemodynamic, angiographic, and electrophysiologic studies). Treatment was also recommended by the majority of the participants in the seminar. In an effort to exclude underlying structural heart disease, we would recommend performing a resting and, if appropriate, exercise thallium nuclide study to search for abnormalities in myocardial perfusion. When this study and other noninvasive studies fail to disclose cardiac abnormalities, a cardiac catheterization should not be performed. With respect to physical activity, we follow the recommendation of the 16th Bethesda conference on recommendations regarding eligibility for competition (*J. Am Coll. Cardiol.* 6:6, 1229, 1985), which state that "patients who have no syncope or presyncope, no structural heart disease and a nonsustained ventricular tachycardia of uniform configuration that does not exceed 150 beats/minute during maximal exercise may participate in all competitive sports with caution." We would agree with Fulton et al. that pharmacologic treatment is not indicated in asymptomatic patients with nonsustained ventricular tachycardia and a normal heart.—Amnon Rosenthal, M.D.

Pacemaker Management for Acute Onset of Heart Block in Childhood
Larry T. Mahoney, William J. Marvin, Jr., Dianne L. Atkins, Edward B. Clark, and Ronald M. Lauer (Univ. of Iowa)
J. Pediatr. 107:207–211, August 1985   2–16

Myocarditis usually does not cause symptoms or significant abnormalities in children, and complete heart block is unusual. Life-threatening dysrhythmias may, however, occur without other clinical manifestations of myocarditis. The typical pattern that is seen on ECG is one of diffuse low-voltage QRS complexes, nonspecific ST changes, and a small or absent Q wave in the left precordial leads. Ventricular premature contractions are not uncommon and can lead to ventricular tachycardia or fibrillation. Conduction abnormalities usually are manifested as first- or second-degree heart block.

Three girls and one boy who were seen at University of Iowa Hospitals required pacemakers because of Stokes-Adams syndrome, which was the primary cardiac manifestation of complete heart block. All 4 had mild antecedent symptoms without signs of congestive heart failure. Complete heart block was documented along with other conduction abnormalities. Two patients required permanent pacing.

Twenty-eight cases of complete heart block secondary to myocarditis in childhood, including the present 4, have been described. Syncope was the presenting feature in 82% of cases. Only 32% of these patients had congestive failure and cardiogenic shock. Abnormalities were found at ECG study in 22 cases. Only 15 of the 28 had normal conduction on follow-up ECGs. There were 3 deaths, and complete heart block persisted in 6 children, 4 of whom required a permanent pacemaker.

Complete heart block may be more frequent in myocarditis than has been recognized. Decreased cardiac output from bradycardia carries a poor prognosis, and this makes ECG monitoring important when acute myocarditis is suspected. If complete heart block is present, conduction can be improved by giving atropine, or infusion of isoproterenol can be used to increase the heart rate of the lower focus unless premature rentricular contractions are present. Temporary transvenous pacing is indicated if the heart is slowed, especially if peripheral perfusion is reduced or heart failure is evident. A permanent pacemaker is suggested if marked bradycardia persists beyond 2 weeks.

▶ Myocarditis in childhood, in contrast to that in early infancy, is often subtle in its manifestations. It is not commonly considered in the differential diagnosis of syncope in an otherwise healthy child. However, the inflammatory process may significantly affect the conduction tissue, leading to transient or permanent complete heart block, which results in syncope. The diagnosis in the past generally has been made on clinical findings or at necropsy. The increased use and demonstrated safety of endomyocardial biopsy in children now make a definitive diagnosis possible. Indeed, not long after this report appeared, a 9-year-old girl was sent to us for a syncopal episode that developed while she was playing ball with her parent. Complete heart block was present and an endomyocardial biopsy demonstrated myocarditis with acute inflammatory process.

Insertion of a temporary pacemaker is life saving in these children. A permanent pacemaker may not be required, since approximately half of children developing complete heart block with myocarditis will then revert to normal conduction within days or a few weeks. Medical therapy with anti-inflammatory agents such as steroids or immunosuppressive drugs remains controversial.—Amnon Rosenthal, M.D.

Interpretation of Excessive Serum Concentrations of Digoxin in Children
Gideon Koren and Ruth Parker (Toronto Hosp. for Sick Children and Strong Mem. Hosp., Rochester, N.Y.)
Am. J. Cardiol. 55:1210–1214, April 15, 1985   2–17

Children are thought to be less sensitive than adults to digoxin and to require higher doses, but excessive serum levels do not necessarily indicate

MECHANISMS INVOLVED IN EXCESSIVE (≤5 NG/ML)
SERUM CONCENTRATION OF DIGOXIN IN 47
CHILDREN

	No. of Children*
High postmortem levels	10
Sampling error	15
Overdose	6
Renal insufficiency	10
Endogenous digoxin like substance	6
Digoxin-amiodarone interaction	1

*In some children, more than one mechanism could be shown (e.g., renal failure and endogenous digoxin-like substances), whereas in four cases, the high measured level of digoxin could not be explained by any of the above factors.
(Courtesy of Koren, G., and Parker, R.: Am. J. Cardiol. 55:1210–1214, Apr. 15, 1985.)

toxicity. Digoxin levels of 5ng/ml or above were recorded in 47 children aged 2 days to 16 years in a 3-year period (table).

Ten infants with inoperable congenital heart disease had postmortem digoxin levels significantly higher than antemortem levels, independent of the time elapsed after death. Sampling errors were implicated in 40.5% of living patients, when estimates were made too close to administration of a dose. None of these 15 patients had toxic manifestations. Ten patients had renal failure and a prolonged digoxin elimination half-life; 3 of them had signs of digoxin toxicity. There were 6 cases of overdose, including accidental ingestions, pharmacy error, and a suicide attempt. An endogenous digoxin-like substance contributed to the excessive serum level in 6 instances. One patient had a digoxin-amiodarone interaction. Digoxin toxicity was diagnosed in 10 living patients in all, or 63% of cases excluding sampling errors and cases with an endogenous digoxin-like substance. Nine of these patients had overdose or renal insufficiency.

An excessive serum digoxin level may not indicate toxicity. Possible explanations that should be considered include sampling error, postmortem estimation, and a circulating endogenous digoxin-like substance.

▶ The physician's response to an excessive serum digoxin level commonly is to assume that toxicity may be present, to withhold the drug temporarily, and then to repeat the assay. The authors provide convincing explanations why an excessive serum concentration may not necessarily reflect drug toxicity. Sampling error at peak levels (blood obtained minutes to 3 hours after administration) was the most common cause of an excessive serum concentration level. The simple measure of performing selective and appropriately timed blood samples may avoid needless physician and parental anxiety, repeated testing, and adverse potential medical-legal problems.—Amnon Rosenthal, M.D.

Echocardiography and Doppler Echocardiography

Accuracy of Prospective Two-Dimensional Echocardiographic Evaluation of Left Ventricular Outflow Tract in Complete Transposition of the Great Arteries
Alvin J. Chin, Scott B, Yeager, Stephen P. Sanders, Roberta G. Williams, Fredrick Z. Bierman, Bruno M. Burger, William I. Norwood, and Aldo R. Castaneda (Harvard Univ.)
Am. J. Cardiol. 55:759–764, March 1, 1985   2–18

Accurate noninvasive diagnosis of the presence and type of left ventricular (LV) outflow tract obstruction in transposition of the great arteries (TGA) is important. Thirty-two consecutive infants younger than age 2 years with TGA and ventricular septal defect underwent subxiphoid two-dimensional echocardiography. Two independent observers evaluated each echocardiogram for the presence or absence of LV outflow tract obstruction, whether outflow tract obstruction was dynamic or fixed, or both, and the precise anatomical type of fixed obstruction (Fig 2–2).

For diagnosing the presence or absence of LV outflow tract obstruction,

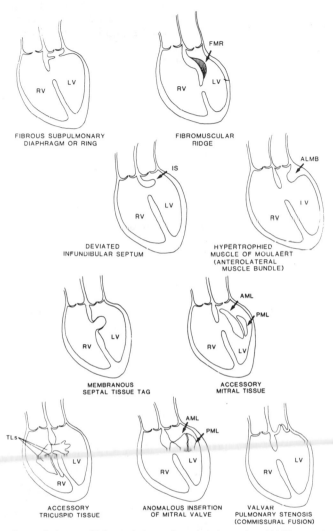

Fig 2–2.—Anatomical types of left ventricular outflow tract obstruction. ALMB, anterolateral muscle bundle; AML, anterior mitral leaflet; FMR, fibromuscular ridge; IS, infundibular septum; PML, posterior mitral leaflet; RV, right ventricle; TLs, tricuspid leaflets. (Courtesy of Chin, A.J., et al.: Am. J. Cardiol. 55:759–764, March 1, 1985.)

two-dimensional echocardiography yielded low false negative (7% to 13%) and false positive rates (0% to 6%) compared with the LV-to-pulmonary artery (PA) pressure gradient obtained at cardiac catheterization. However, the false negative cases were only minor errors, since the measured LV-PA gradients proved to be less than 25 mm Hg. In detecting LV outflow tract obstruction, which was at least partly fixed, two-dimensional echocardiography yielded no false negative results when compared with the long-axial oblique LV angiogram. Compared with autopsy and/

or surgical observations, two-dimensional echocardiography did not make any significant errors in delineating the anatomical type of fixed obstruction.

The diagnostic accuracy of two-dimensional echocardiography in detecting and characterizing LV outflow tract obstruction limits the need for "routine" cardiac catheterization before repair in infants with TGA and intact ventricular septum. With two-dimensional echocardiography it is possible to select out, as early as age 3 months, the rare patients who have early onset pulmonary vascular obstructive disease and who may need catheterization. In addition, because certain types of fixed LV outflow tract obstruction are difficult for the surgeon to visualize and alleviate, precise knowledge of the anatomical type of fixed obstruction influences the type of repair chosen—Rastelli, intraatrial baffle, or arterial switch procedures in patients with TGA and ventricular septal defect.

▶ In this article, the authors showed that two-dimensional echocardiography is a very accurate technique for the diagnosis of left ventricular outflow tract obstruction in infants with complete transposition of the great arteries. In addition, the technique was extremely useful for characterizing the exact anatomic type of fixed left ventricular outflow obstruction. The information provided should prove to be extremely helpful in eliminating the need for routine cardiac catheterization in infants with D-TGA and intact ventricular septum and in planning a surgical approach—especially in infants with D-TGA and ventricular septal defect. One would expect even more quantitative information if Doppler echocardiography were used along with the imaging techniques described in this article.—A. Rebecca Snider, M.D.

Subxiphoid Two-Dimensional Echocardiographic Identification of Tricuspid Valve Abnormalities in Transposition of the Great Arteries With Ventricular Septal Defect
Barbara J. Deal, Alvin J. Chin, Stephen P. Sanders, William I. Norwood, and Aldo R. Castaneda (Harvard Univ.)
Am. J. Cardiol. 55:1146—1151, April 15, 1985   2–19

The presence of structural abnormalities of the tricuspid valves in patients with d-transposition of the great arteries (TGA) and ventricular septal defect (VSD) may influence surgical management, particularly in patients without severe subpulmonary stenosis who undergo intra-atrial baffle repair and VSD closure. Using subxiphoid two-dimensional echocardiographic imaging, tricuspid valve morphology was examined in 39 infants with TGA and VSD (group I) aged 2 years or younger; the results were correlated with those of surgery and postoperative cardiac catheterization. Age-matched control groups consisted of 21 patients with simple TGA (group II), 30 patients with VSD and normally related greater arteries (group III), and 15 normal patients (group IV). Only 1 child (group I) had moderate tricuspid regurgitation with biventricular dysfunction as deter-

TRICUSPID VALVE ABNORMALITIES VERSUS TYPE OF
VENTRICULAR SEPTAL DEFECT (VSD)*

Type of VSD	TGA and VSD	Simple VSD
Malalignment	13/20 (65%)	5/16 (31%)
AVC	5/5 (100%)	1/3 (33%)
Membranous	5/11 (45%)	0/9 (0%)
Muscular	2/3 (66%)	0/2 (0%)
Total	25/39 (65%)	6/30 (20%)

*AVC, atrioventricular canal; TGA, transposition of the great arteries.
(Courtesy of Deal, B.J., et al.: Am. J. Cardiol. 55:1146–1151, April
15, 1985.)

mined by preoperative right ventricular angiography. Intra-atrial baffle repair was performed in 27 group I children (median age at surgery, 3.5 months) and in 19 group II children (median age, 4 months).

Tricuspid valve abnormalities were identified in 25 group I patients (64%), but in none of the patients in group II or IV, and in 6 group III patients (20%). Valve abnormalities consisted of chordal attachments to the infundibular septum or ventricular septal crest, straddling, overriding, or some combination of these defects. The incidence of tricuspid valve abnormalities was related to the type of VSD present: malalignment and atrioventricular canal-type VSDs were associated with a high incidence of abnormal tricuspid valve attachments among group I patients (table). Six of 27 group I patients and 1 in group II died early after surgery. Postoperative cardiac catheterization indicated tricuspid regurgitation in 8 of 17 group I patients (62%) but in none of 8 group II patients ($P = .01$). All patients in whom tricuspid regurgitation was not present preoperatively had abnormal chordal attachments; 3 required valve replacement. The two-dimensional echocardiographic analysis of tricuspid morphology was confirmed by autopsy findings.

Tricuspid valve abnormalities are common in patients with TGA and VSD, and the incidence appears to be higher than that previously reported. The significant incidence of postoperative tricuspid regurgitation in patients with TGA and VSD is related to the difficulties created by the abnormal chordal attachments during VSD patch placement. Preoperative two-dimensional echocardiography can identify this subset of patients who are at increased risk for tricuspid regurgitation.

▶ This article reviews the usefulness of two-dimensional echocardiography for the detection of tricuspid valve abnormalities in patients with transposition of the great arteries and ventricular septal defect. Using subcostal imaging techniques, the authors were able to detect anomalies of the tricuspid valve (chordal attachments to the infundibular septum or ventricular septal crest, overriding tricuspid annulus, straddling tricuspid valve, cleft anterior leaflet, tricuspid valve tissue protruding through the ventricular septal defect and producing left ventricular outflow obstruction) in two thirds of these infants. The information provided by two-dimensional echocardiography about the exact anatomy and chordal attachments of the tricuspid valve is very important in planning the type of surgical repair. This information often cannot be obtained by cineangiography because of the presence of a large ventricular shunt. The incidence of tricuspid valve anomalies detected in infants with D-TGA and VSD may be a factor contributing to the higher early mortality of reparative surgery and the development of postoperative tricuspid insufficiency in these infants. These patients may be better managed surgically by the arterial switch procedure because the right ventricle in this situation becomes a low-pressure chamber leading to the pulmonary circulation.—A. Rebecca Snider, M.D.

Localisation of Ventricular Septal Defects by Simultaneous Display of Superimposed Colour Doppler and Cross Sectional Echocardiographic Images
E. Ortiz, P. J. Robinson, J. E. Deanfield, R. Franklin, F. J. Macartney, and R. K. H. Wyse (Inst. of Child Health, London)
Br. Heart J. 54:53–60, July 1985   2–20

A color-coded Doppler system that superimposes flow data on conventional cross-sectional ultrasonographic images was used in an attempt to improve the diagnosis of small ventricular septal defects such as those within the trabecular septum. At the Hospital for Sick Children 23 patients who had not had an operation for ventricular septal defect and 8 who had had surgical closure were evaluated, along with 12 normal children. Eleven of the 23 had a defect that was too small to be visualized by conventional cross-sectional echocardiography.

A color-coded blood flow jet that entered the right ventricle during systole was identified in all 23 patients who had had no surgical closure. Nineteen perimembranous and 5 trabecular defects were precisely localized (1 patient had 2 defects). In 1 case the color Doppler method demonstrated flow across the defect in the presence of an elevated right ventricular peak systolic pressure. A systolic flow jet that emanated from the patch site was visualized in the right ventricle in all 5 postoperative patients with systolic murmurs but in none of the 3 without a systolic murmur. The absence of a residual defect was confirmed at cardiac catheterization in the latter cases.

Direct visualization of transseptal blood flow by the color Doppler method is a reliable means of excluding ventricular septal defects in patients with innocent murmurs and in those who have surgical closure of a defect. Defects that are otherwise invisible on cross-sectional echocardiography can be accurately localized, and the method should prove helpful in estimating the likelihood of spontaneous closure of a given defect.

▶ In this article, the authors examined the utility of color-coded Doppler echocardiography for the detection of ventricular septal defects. Of 18 unoperated patients with a perimembranous ventricular septal defect, only 9 were imaged on conventional cross-sectional echocardiography; all 18 were imaged with color Doppler echocardiography. Of 5 patients with a trabecular ventricular septal defect, 3 were imaged by cross-sectional echocardiography and all 5 were imaged with color Doppler echocardiography. The results are interesting and suggest that color Doppler echocardiography may play an ancillary role in the noninvasive diagnosis of ventricular septal defect; however, there are several factors that should be considered when one interprets these results. First, the incidence of detection of membranous ventricular septal defect with cross-sectional echocardiography alone is much lower in this study (9 of 18, 50%) than in many other reported series. Second, only 5 patients with trabecular ventricular septal defect were included in the study so that it is difficult to draw conclusions about the sensitivity and specificity of color Doppler echocardiography in the detection of trabecular ventricular septal defect. Last, because of the study design, we do not know whether the defects that were detected only by color Doppler echocardiography might have been detected with a combination of conventional pulsed Doppler and two-dimensional echocardiography.— A. Rebecca Snider, M.D.

Accuracy of Two-Dimensional Echocardiography in the Diagnosis of Congenital Heart Disease
Howard P. Gutgesell, James C. Huhta, Larry A. Latson, Doug Huffines, and Dan G. McNamara (Baylor Univ.)
Am. J. Cardiol. 55:514–518, Feb. 15, 1985   2–21

Two-dimensional echocardiography is the most commonly used noninvasive imaging technique for evaluation of children with congenital heart disease. To determine its accuracy in the diagnosis of congenital cardiac abnormalities, prospective two-dimensional echocardiograms were performed in 126 infants and children before cardiac catheterization and angiography. Segmental studies were performed from multiple imaging sites and included determinations of intracardiac, great artery, systemic venous, and pulmonary venous anatomy. Echocardiographic assessment, either by actually doing the procedure (76%) or reviewing videotapes of studies done by technicians or cardiology fellows, was performed by pediatric cardiologists with a major interest in echocardiography. The results were compared to those identified by catheterization.

Of the 259 separate cardiovascular abnormalities seen on catheterization, 226 (87%) were identified by two-dimensional echocardiography. There were 8 false positive diagnoses giving a specificity of the technique of 94%. The most common lesions and the sensitivity and specificity of echocardiography were: patent ductus arteriosus (n = 41), 83% and 100%, respectively; ventricular septal defects (n = 35), 86% and 100%; atrial septal defect (n = 26), 85% and 99%; pulmonary valve stenosis (n = 25), 77% and 97%; transposition of the great arteries (n = 16), 100% and 100%; and total anomalous pulmonary vascular connection (n = 14), 85% and 100%. In addition to identifying the less common intracardiac abnormalities such as atrioventricular canal (10 of 10 patients), tetralogy of Fallot (10 of 10), and single ventricle (4 of 4), the multiple-site imaging approach was useful in detecting extracardiac vascular abnormalities such as persistent left superior vena cava (7 of 10), right aortic

---

ERRORS IN DIAGNOSIS OF CONGENITAL HEART
DISEASE BY TWO-DIMENSIONAL ECHOCARDIOGRAPHY
IN 126 PATIENTS

	False Negative (n = 32)	False Positive (n = 8)
Personnel performing study		
Pediatric cardiologist (n = 96)	17	8
Technician or postdoctoral fellow (n = 30)	15	0
Cause of error		
Recorded data overlooked or misinterpreted	10	7
Data not recorded	5	
Technical limitation of imaging method	9	1
Undetermined	8	

(Courtesy of Gutgesell, H.P., et al.: Am. J. Cardiol. 55:514–518, Feb. 15, 1985.)

---

arch (8 of 8), coarctation of the aorta (10 of 12), interrupted aortic arch (4 of 4), and absence of the hepatic segment of the inferior vena cava with azygos continuation (2 of 3). In 33 patients (26%), the errors in echocardiographic analysis were judged to have surgical importance. Most errors were the result of overlooking or misinterpreting data that had been appropriately recorded on videotapes (table).

Most intracardiac as well as extracardiac abnormalities in congenital heart disease can be confidently diagnosed or excluded by two-dimensional echocardiography. However, this does not eliminate the need for catheterization. Pulmonary valve stenosis and patent ductus arteriosus are the lesions most likely to be misdiagnosed in ultrasound studies relying solely on two-dimensional echocardiography.

▶ Echocardiography has reduced the overall number of diagnostic cardiac catheterizations being performed in children with congenital cardiac abnormalities. However, the predictions by many that echocardiography will replace cardiac catheterization in the diagnosis of cardiac disease have not been borne out. The additional use of Doppler echocardiography, introduction of color-coded Doppler echocardiography, and the utilization of computerized quantitative analysis of cardiovascular structures and myocardial function will further replace conventional assessment, which now requires invasive procedures. In the zeal to replace cardiac catheterization, the limitations of echocardiography and Doppler echocardiography must not be overlooked. Results are highly dependent on the precise definition of the clinical problem or question, the skill of the echocardiographer (the study is often performed by a technician), and the quality of the equipment and recording. Sedation, frequently utilized for the study, may have its own complications, particularly since the patients are usually not monitored as closely as they are in the catheterization laboratory. The physician's fee for the procedure is also rapidly approaching that for cardiac catheterization. The gold standard for the definition of many anatomic lesions and most physiologic abnormalities remains cardiac catheterization and angiography. After a complete clinical evaluation, including selective noninvasive studies, has been performed, one should catheterize the patient when there is still some doubt.—Amnon Rosenthal, M.D.

Interventional Procedures

Management of Congenital Stenosis of a Branch Pulmonary Artery With Balloon Angioplasty: Report of 52 Procedures

John C. Ring, John L. Bass, William Marvin, Bradley P. Fuhrman, Thomas J. Kulik, John E. Foker, and James E. Lock (Univ. of Minnesota and Univ. of Iowa)

J. Thorac. Cardiovasc. Surg. 90:35–44, July 1985   2–22

The initial experience on the use of percutaneous balloon dilation angioplasty for the treatment of congenitally stenotic and hypoplastic pulmonary arteries was accepted with cautious enthusiasm. In an attempt to obtain a more extensive experience and to define important aspects of technique and patient selection, 24 children underwent balloon dilation angioplasty of hypoplastic or stenotic branch pulmonary arteries. Their ages ranged from 4 months to 16 years. Nine children were aged 2 years or younger. Most children had tetralogy of Fallot, with or without pulmonary atresia, or isolated peripheral pulmonary artery stenosis. All children satisfied at least two of the following requirements: congenital stenosis or hypoplasia of at least one branch of the pulmonary artery, diameter of the narrowed segment of 7 mm or less, right ventricular or main pulmonary artery-systemic artery pressure ratio of 0.50 or more, and a systolic pressure of 60 mm Hg or greater in the right ventricle or main pulmonary artery proximal to the obstruction. Fifty-two dilations were attempted, 44 in the catheterization laboratory and 8 in the operating room. Vascular access was established percutaneously in all but 2 patients.

Twenty-six (50%) angioplasties were judged successful. The average vessel diameter increased from 4.1 ± 0.3 to 7.2 ± 0.3 mm ($P < .005$) in 76% patients (Fig 2–3), the gradient across the narrowed segment decreased from 60 ± 10 to 36 ± 5 mm Hg ($P < .005$) in 92%. Pressure in the right ventricle or in the main pulmonary artery decreased from 83 ± 10 to 66 ± 6 mm Hg ($P < .005$) in 86%, and the radionuclide-determined fraction of cardiac output directed to the lung ipsilateral to the dilated pulmonary artery increased from 40 ± 4 to 51 ± 4 ($P < .005$) in 76%. Reasons for failure included inadequate technique (such as using a balloon that was too small or the inability to position the balloon or wire in 14 patients) and the refractory nature of the lesion itself in 11 patients. Technical failures were age dependent. Nondilatable lesions were more common in children older than age 2 years (10 of 25) vs. younger children (1 of 10), or with isolated peripheral pulmonary artery stenosis (5 of 7). Five of 8 stenoses near previous shunts were nondilatable. Although 1 child died from exsanguination following rupture of pulmonary artery during dilation, other complications were few. Eight dilations, followed up for an average of 6 months after initial dilation, showed angio-

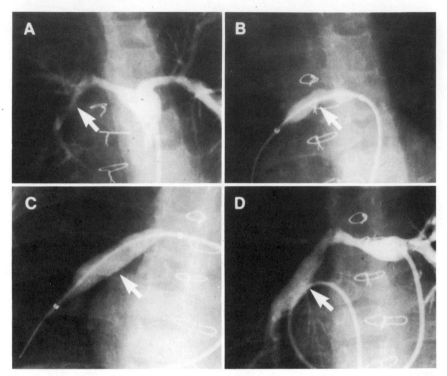

Fig 2–3.—Successful balloon dilation angioplasty from patient 2. **A,** predilation angiogram. The *arrow* denotes hypoplasia of the right lower lobe pulmonary artery. **B,** low-pressure inflation of the dilating balloon, showing a waist. **C,** high-pressure inflation of the balloon, demonstrating disappearance of the waist. **D,** postdilation angiogram. The right lower lobe pulmonary artery is considerably enlarged, with small concentrations of dye along the inferior margin denoting intimal tears. Note that the proximal right pulmonary artery stenosis near a Blalock-Taussig shunt persists. (Courtesy of Ring, J.C., et al.: J. Thorac. Cardiovasc. Surg. 90:35–44, July 1985.)

graphic persistence of improvement. Two of 4 patients were successfully redilated to a larger size a mean 8.2 months after initial dilation.

Percutaneous balloon dilation angioplasty is an effective and relatively safe procedure for the treatment of patients with congenital hypoplastic or stenotic pulmonary arteries. It should be performed before age 3 years. Optimal technique should include a balloon diameter about four times the size of the narrowed segment, careful positioning of the balloon such that the narrowed segment is centered and maintaining of that position during inflation, use of relatively high dilating pressures (5 to 7 atmospheres), and continued dilation of the stenosis until the waist disappears (usually 20 seconds).

▶ Balloon angioplasty for peripheral pulmonary stenosis or hypoplasia in patients with isolated peripheral pulmonary stenosis or in postoperative patients with tetralogy of Fallot is often the only therapy that is currently available. The results are variable and success, reported in multiple series to occur in approximately 50% of patients, is measured by the degree of improvement, not cure or complete alleviation of the obstruction. The best results appear to occur in younger patients and in those with tetralogy of Fallot complex. The poorest results are observed in stenoses at the site of a prior aortopulmonary shunt (Blalock-Taussig or Waterston). The procedure requires experience, great skill (often two skilled catheterizers), use of multiple catheters, and on the average an hour of fluoroscopy time. Therefore, I believe that its use should be restricted to major medical centers or cardiac catheterization laboratories. Long-term persistence of the dilatation seems likely, unlike the results from balloon angioplasty for pulmonary venous obstructions, which have been transient. Repeat dilatation may also be carried out after an appropriate healing period of at least a few months. Some time in the next year or so, a report should be forthcoming from the Pediatric Cardiology Interventional Registry, which has collected data from many centers around the country on nearly 1,000 interventional procedures.—Amnon Rosenthal, M.D.

Transluminal Balloon Coarctation Angioplasty: Experience With 27 Patients
Zuhdi A. Lababidi, Dimitris A. Daskalopoulos, and Harry Stoeckle, Jr. (Univ. of Missouri)
Am. J. Cardiol. 54:1288–1291, Dec. 1, 1984   2–23

Varying results have been reported with balloon angioplasty (BA) in the management of coarctation of the aorta (COA) in symptomatic infants. Twenty-seven consecutive patients with COA had BA in 1982–1984. Seven patients were infants with various cardiac defects, 7 had restenosed COA, and 13 patients had unoperated, undilated COA. The latter patients were aged 2–27 years. No. 5 F balloon catheters were used in infants, and No. 9 F catheters in older children. The inflated balloon was intended to be 1–2 mm smaller than the diameter of the descending thoracic aorta, or equal to the isthmus diameter in cases of preductal COA. The balloon was inflated up to 120 psi for 5 to 10 seconds under fluoroscopic control. Thirteen patients had follow-up cardiac catheterization 3 to 24 months after BA.

There were no deaths or serious complications from BA. Balloon rupture occurred in 5 patients, without evidence of embolization or other ill effect. No aneurysms were seen on follow-up. All patients had satisfactory immediate results (Fig 2–4). The systolic pressure gradient was significantly reduced, and the COA diameter increased, without a reduction in cardiac index. In 4 infants the gradient rose slightly at follow-up, but the infants remained markedly improved clinically.

The data indicate that BA can be safely performed in infants and in older children or adults with restenosed COA or with unoperated, undilated COA. The late results in infants can be less optimal than the immediate outcome because of the hypoplastic isthmus, but BA can be useful in critically ill neonates. Total repair may be carried out later at a lower risk following palliation by BA.

▶ A consensus exists among pediatric cardiologists and cardiovascular sur-

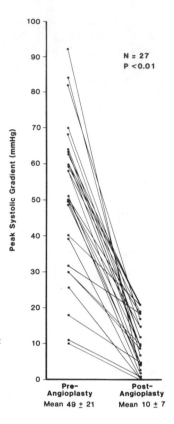

Fig 2–4.—Significant decrease in the peak systolic gradient across the coarctation immediately after balloon coarctation angioplasty. (Courtesy of Lababidi, Z.A., et al.: Am. J. Cardiol. 54:1288–1291, Dec. 1, 1984.)

geons that balloon angioplasty for restenosed coarctation of the aorta is a desirable and effective procedure. Reoperation in these patients is often more difficult than the initial procedure and may require partial bypass and repair with the use of a prosthetic patch or conduit. However, balloon angioplasty for unoperated children with coarctation of the aorta is controversial because of the reported occurrence of aneurysms at the site of dilatation. These aneurysms, however, have not been observed in all centers performing the procedure. Whether these small aneurysms, which undoubtedly result from subintimal and muscular tear, will heal spontaneously or lead to serious complications is unclear. Therefore, it seems prudent for the present to restrict balloon angioplasty in children with unoperated coarctation of the aorta to an experimental design that includes very close follow-up by angiography, digital radiography, or MRI studies. Another concern that has recently been raised has been the increased potential for paraplegia when surgical repair is undertaken following balloon angioplasty in these patients because of the diminution of aortic collaterals during the months after the procedure. As far as balloon angioplasty in neonates and young infants with complex coarctation (i.e., coarctation of the aorta that is associated with tubular hypoplasia of the arch and other cardiovascular malformations such as ventricular septal defect and aortic or mitral valve disease) is concerned, we have not performed the procedure in this group because of the nature of the anatomic defect, inherent technical problems, and the potential complications. With greater experience and improvements in techniques, it may indeed be possible to successfully palliate selected young infants with complex coarctation and postpone repair of the residual coarctation and/or associated defects until a little later in infancy.—Amnon Rosenthal, M.D.

Percutaneous Balloon Valvuloplasty for Aortic Valve Stenosis in Infancy
Gerhard Rupprath and Karl-Ludwig Neuhaus (Univ. of Goettingen, Federal Republic of Germany)
Am. J. Cardiol. 55:1655–1656, June 1, 1985   2–24

Recently, balloon valvuloplasty was reported to be effective in children and adolescents with pulmonary and aortic valve stenosis (AS). The authors report data on three infants, aged 4 to 8 weeks, with severe AS who underwent balloon aortic valvuloplasty (BAVP). All infants were in severe congestive heart failure and refractory to medical therapy. Other severe cardiac malformations (such as small aortic anulus, pulmonary hypertension, right-to-left shunt through a patent ductus, and coarctation or endocardial fibroelastosis) were present in two infants. All patients underwent percutaneous catheterization.

Left ventricular cineangiography was performed before BAVP and a Grüntzig coronary dilatation catheter (4.3 F), 2 cm long and 4.2 mm in

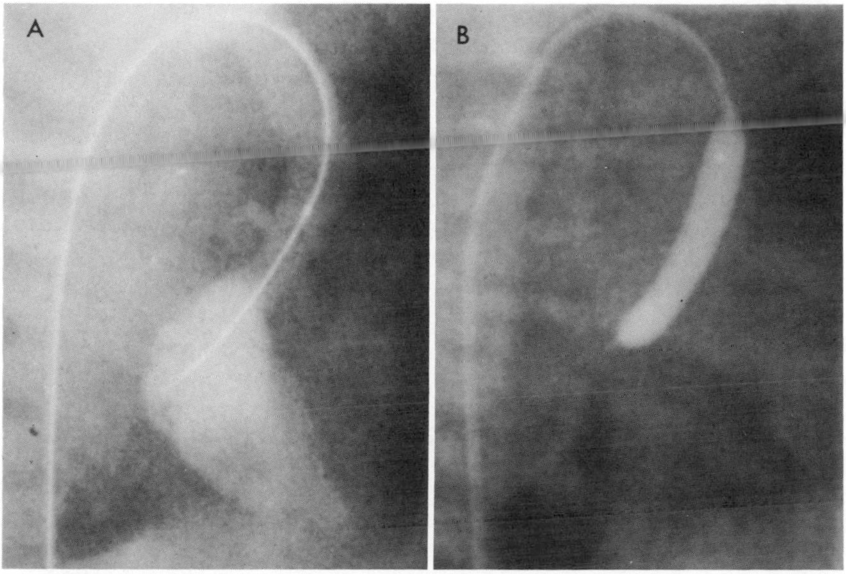

Fig 2–5.—**A,** lateral left ventricular cineangiogram of patient 1 before valvuloplasty. Aortic anulus is narrow. **B,** same patient with the balloon inflated during balloon aortic valvuloplasty. (Courtesy of Rupprath, G., and Neuhaus, K.: Am. J. Cardiol. 55:1655–1656, June 1, 1985.)

inflated diameter, was introduced. The balloon catheter was filled with 50% diluted contrast medium and inflated to pressures of 100 to 140 psi. With the catheter positioned across the aortic valve, 4 to 6 inflations were performed within 15 minutes, each lasting 6 to 12 seconds (Fig 2–5). Attention was paid to a full extension of the balloon without waisting.

No major complications resulted from BAVP. No surgical intervention was necessary. The peak systolic gradient across the stenotic valve was reduced from 73 ± 3 mm Hg to 34 ± 6 mm Hg. There was no evidence of aortic regurgitation. The morphology and movement of the thickened aortic valve remained unchanged on two-dimensional echocardiography. The right-to-left shunt was reversed after BAVP with normal oxygen saturation and pressures in the descending aorta. All infants improved clinically, with one infant still in moderate cardiac insufficiency as a result of the endocardial fibroelastosis and poor left ventricular function.

Percutaneous BAVP is an effective nonsurgical technique for reducing the obstruction and subsequently postponing operative intervention and decreasing operative mortality risk among infants with severe AS.

▶ The demonstration of successful percutaneous balloon valvuloplasty for young infants with critical aortic stenosis is a major contribution to the therapy of this disease. It follows closely a recent report of intra-operative balloon dilatation of critical aortic stenosis with a Grunzig catheter from Indiana University (*Ann. Thorac. Surg.* 39:376–378, 1985). Surgical valvulotomy carries a significant mortality (20%–50%) and is a palliative procedure. Success of percutaneous balloon angioplasty in critical aortic stenosis may be measured by a decrease in mortality, a significant reduction in the gradient, and the absence of significant aortic regurgitation. The procedure, like that for coarctation of the aorta or peripheral pulmonary stenosis, requires a great deal of skill and should, at least for the near future, be considered experimental, with its use limited to major medical centers. It should not be attempted without the availability of a standby cardiac surgical team.—Amnon Rosenthal, M.D.

Percutaneous Catheter Commissurotomy in Rheumatic Mitral Stenosis
James E. Lock, M. Khalilullah, Savitri Shrivastava, V. Bahl, and John F. Keane (Children's Hosp., Boston; G. B. Pant Hosp. and All India Inst. of Med. Sciences, New Delhi, India)
N. Engl. J. Med. 313:1515–1518, December 1985   2–25

Large-diameter balloons that are mounted on flexible catheter shafts now are available for use in closed percutaneous, blind mitral commissurotomy. Between January and April 1985 an attempt was made to dilate the rheumatic mitral valve in eight children and young adults with valve stenosis. All had exertional dyspnea or hemoptysis, or both, and classic clinical signs of moderate or severe mitral stenosis. Age range was 9 to 23 years. Hemodynamic studies confirmed significant mitral stenosis with a substantial transmitral gradient and left atrial hypertension in all cases.

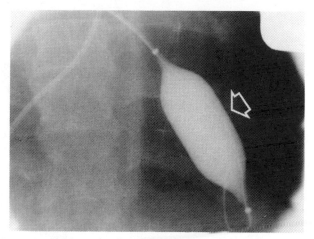

Fig 2–6.—Positioning of valvotomy catheter (25 mm) across mitral annulus. Catheter is inflated with diluted contrast material to 3 atm. *Arrow* indicates level of mitral annulus. (Courtesy of Lock, J.E., et al.: N. Engl. J. Med. 313:1515–1518, December 1985. Reprinted by permission of The New England Journal of Medicine.)

Valvuloplasty balloons 18 to 25 mm in diameter were used (Fig 2–6). Multiple dilations were used only to confirm correct balloon positioning.

Catheter commissurotomy was achieved in all eight attempts. The end-diastolic gradient fell from 21 to 10 mm Hg on average, and the cardiac index rose from 3.8 to 4.9 L/minute/sq m. Seven patients had no mitral regurgitation after the procedure; one had minimal regurgitation. Morbidity from the procedure was minimal.

All six patients who were recatheterized had a persistent increase in mitral valve area. The only patient with evidence of substantial restenosis had a minimal left-to-right shunt that was seen only on pulmonary angiography.

Balloon mitral commissurotomy appears to hold promise as an effective and safe means of treating children and young adults with rheumatic mitral stenosis, but further experience will be necessary to determine whether it can have an important role in this setting.

▶ Catheter commissurotomy for rheumatic mitral stenosis is an exciting and innovative, though not surprising, approach to the treatment of severe mitral stenosis. The increasing experience in pediatric cardiology with balloon dilatation of valvular and vascular stenoses and the accompanying development of appropriate catheters have made the procedure feasible. Much credit should go to Dr. Charles Mullins, who led the way in advocating the transseptal technique in children and developed the long transseptal sheath, which enables passage of a catheter across the interatrial septum and then through the mitral valve. Catheter commissurotomy of the mitral valve remains an experimental procedure, and although the short-term results and absence of serious complications are encouraging, the long-term relief of stenosis has not been demonstrated. Patients with mixed mitral stenosis and mitral regurgitation and those with significant mitral valve calcifications and left atrial thrombi do not appear to be suitable candidates for the procedure at this time. The technique would seem to provide the greatest benefit to countries that continue to have a high incidence of rheumatic fever. The high cost of the cardiac catheterization procedure and procedures using transseptal and balloon catheters may, however, in this situation be more costly than a noninvasive diagnosis of severe mitral stenosis and a surgical closed commissurotomy.—Amnon Rosenthal, M.D.

Findings on Endomyocardial Biopsy in Infants and Children With Dilated Cardiomyopathy
Alan B. Lewis, Harry B. Neustein, Masato Takahashi, and Paul R. Lurie (Children's Hosp. of Los Angeles and Univ. of Southern California)
Am. J. Cardiol. 55:143–145, Jan. 1, 1985   2–26

Lymphocytic myocardial infiltration has been reported in 5% to 63% of adult patients with idiopathic dilated cardiomyopathy (DC) and has been reported responsive to immunosuppressive therapy. However, because the use of immunosuppressive agents carries a considerable risk in children, 15 infants and children with DC, with a mean duration of illness of 0.9 ± 0.3 years (range, 1 month to 5 years), underwent transvascular endomyocardial biopsy to evaluate for the presence of myocardial inflammation. Both light and electron microscopic sections were examined for the presence of lymphocytes as an indicator of active myocarditis. Both ventricles were biopsied in 13 patients. In 2 patients, only right ventricle specimens were obtained. In 9 children, cardiac biopsy was performed within 6 months and in 4 patients within 2 months of the onset of congestive heart failure.

None of the 76 endomyocardial specimens revealed an inflammatory process. Interstitial fibrosis and myofiber degeneration or hypertrophy were frequently observed. Ultrastructural abnormalities of the mitochondria, T tubules or Z bands, were noted in approximately one third of patients. Antibody titers against echovirus, Coxsackie virus, Ebstein-Barr virus, and adenoviruses were negative. Two patients had a family history of cardiomyopathy, one of whom had an X-linked mode of inheritance.

Persistent active myocarditis is an uncommon cause of DC in children. The lack of inflammatory findings cannot be due to inadequacy of biopsy specimens since an average of five specimens was obtained per patient, in addition to biopsy material obtained from both ventricles. Therefore, immunosuppressive therapy should be considered only after myocardial inflammation has been documented by endomyocardial biopsy.

▶ The etiology of dilated cardiomyopathy in most afflicted infants and children remains unknown. In each case we search for etiologic factors such as antecedent myocarditis, carnitine deficiency, selenium deficiency, and systemic neuromuscular disorder. In the majority we come up emptyhanded. Endomyocardial biopsy is often unrewarding as well. However, since many of the patients undergo cardiac catheterization for assessment of myocardial function, evaluation of atrioventricular valve regurgitation, or the possible presence of a coronary artery abnormality, a myocardial biopsy may well be advisable, particularly if the etiology is unknown or myocarditis is suspected. The additional procedure carries a minimal hazard. The increasing application of cardiac transplantation to infants and children has led to the widespread use of endomyocardial biopsy for the diagnosis of rejection. We have performed more than 200 such biopsies without a single serious complication. One child, transplanted at age 2 years, died suddenly at home at age 4 years and at postmortem was shown to have had severe coronary arteriosclerotic disease. Forty right ventricular biopsies were performed in this child. At necropy the areas of biopsy were covered by endothelium and could not be grossly distinguished from normal endocardium or myocardium. We would certainly agree with the authors that given the considerable risk of chronic use of immunosuppressive agents in children (growth retardation, bone marrow suppression, and increased susceptibility to infection), a definitive diagnosis of an inflammatory disease should be made before such therapy is initiated.—Amnon Rosenthal, M.D.

Balloon Occlusion Angiography in Infancy: Methods, Uses and Limitations
John F. Keane, Richard McFaul, Kenneth Fellows, and James Lock (Harvard Univ. and Maine Med. Ctr., Portland)
Am. J. Cardiol. 56:495–497, Sept. 1, 1985   2–27

Ventriculography alone often fails to provide precise anatomical definition before corrective cardiac surgery is undertaken. Balloon occlusion angiography (BOA) via the antegrade approach prevents loss of contrast medium and enhances local anatomical definition. In a recent 5-year period, 37 infants whose median age was 5 days underwent BOA. The most frequent diagnoses were tetralogy of Fallot with pulmonary atresia, coarctation of the aorta, and interruption of the aortic arch. A 5 F Berman catheter was introduced usually through a femoral vein. Balloon inflation was with CO_2. Occlusion was in the mid-descending thoracic aorta in 33 patients. Contrast medium was injected mechanically in a median volume of 1.5 ml/kg. Balloon occlusion times did not exceed 5 seconds.

All collaterals to all lung segments were visualized in 11 of 12 infants with tetralogy of Fallot with pulmonary atresia. Filling of the central mediastinal pulmonary arteries was evident in 10 infants (Fig 2–7), and the coarctation was clearly outlined in 9 of 11 (Fig 2–8). The site of aortic arch interruption was best seen in the left oblique view. Anatomical information was inadequate in 3 instances. No complications were ascribed to BOA itself, but catheter passage through the ductus may have dislodged a thrombus in an infant with coarctation, resulting in compromise of circulation to the leg.

Balloon occlusion angiography is a useful technique, especially for visualizing central pulmonary arteries and collaterals in infants with tetralogy of Fallot with pulmonary atresia, as well as aortic arch anatomy in

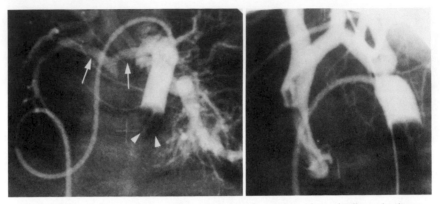

Fig 2–7 (left).—Balloon occlusion angiography in an infant with tetralogy of Fallot and pulmonary atresia in the sitting (45 degrees) position. The occluding balloon *(arrowheads)* is seen in the midthoracic aorta. The direct collaterals are seen together with retrograde filling of the central pulmonary arteries *(arrows)*.

Fig 2–8 (right).—Balloon occlusion angiography in an infant with coarctation of the aorta, long axial oblique view. The venous catheter traverses a small patent ductus arteriosus to reach the thoracic aorta. The contrast medium refluxes as far as the aortic valve and outlines the discrete coarctation of the aorta at the isthmus.

(Courtesy of Keane, J.F., et al.: Am. J. Cardiol. 56:495–497, Sept. 1, 1985.)

those with coarctation or interruption of the aortic arch. In the latter patients, left ventricular biplane angiography should be done first in the long axial oblique projection, followed by BOA if required.

▶ The paper describes a useful technique for use in neonates that obviates the need for a retrograde arterial catheterization to define the anatomy of the aortopulmonary collaterals or central pulmonary arteries in pulmonary atresia with a ventricular septal defect or the nature of the obstruction in coarctation of the aorta. While retrograde arterial catheterization in these infants is occasionally associated with complications, it nonetheless is highly desirable for monitoring pressure, systemic arterial oxygen saturation, or blood gases when the infant is critically ill, is unstable, or requires prostaglandin infusion. An umbilical arterial line is suitable, but in its absence a retrograde arterial catheter would seem to be the more conservative and safe approach. The no. 4 or 3.5 thin-walled pigtail catheter used in retrograde arterial catheterization has the ability to deliver contrast material at a much faster rate than a balloon-tipped angiographic catheter.—Amnon Rosenthal, M.D.

Surgical Management

Coarctation of the Aorta in Patients Younger Than Three Months: A Critique of the Subclavian Flap Operation
Adnan Cobanoglu, Joseph F. Teply, Gary L. Grunkemeier, Cecille O. Sunderland, and Albert Starr (Oregon Health Sciences Univ.)
J. Thorac. Cardiovasc. Surg. 89:128–135, January 1985   2–28

Little is known of the efficacy of the subclavian flap operation for coarctation of the aorta in very young infants. Review was made of 134 infants younger than age 3 months who underwent repair of coarctation of the descending thoracic aorta between 1960 and 1983. The mean age at operation was 25 days; two thirds of infants were younger than age 1 month. Most infants had intractable congestive heart failure at the time of surgery. The mean systolic pressure gradient was 38 mm Hg. All but 13% of patients had associated congenital cardiac lesions, most often patent ductus and ventricular septal defect. Repair was done on an emergency basis in 53 cases and on an urgent basis in the rest. The subclavian flap aortoplasty was used in 67 cases and end-to-end anastomosis in 55. Three patients had a bypass procedure, and 9 underwent patch aortoplasty.

The mean follow-up period was 38 months. Operative mortality was similar in the two major operative groups. Overall survival 5 years after repair was 60%; the rate was 64% after subclavian flap aortoplasty and 56% after end-to-end anastomosis. A younger age at operation was associated with both higher operative mortality and lower late survival. Most early deaths were due to low cardiac output, and most late deaths were caused by pulmonary infection and low cardiac output. Paradoxical hypertension was seen in 10% of operation survivors. Nine percent (8) of 85 survivors were hypertensive when last examined. Significantly more of the subclavian flap patients required reoperation than did those having end-to-end anastomoses. One fifth of patients were below the 5th percentile for growth at last follow-up examination.

The subclavian flap repair does not appear to be superior to resection of coarctation with end-to-end anastomosis in infants younger than age 3 months. Recurrence is more frequent after the subclavian flap operation, and it seems important to remove the coarcted aortic segment in these cases. Resection remain the procedure of choice for very young infants with coarctation of the aorta.

Coarctation of the Aorta in Infants

John L. Harlan, Donald B. Doty, Berkeley Brandt, III, and Johann L. Ehrenhaft (Univ. of Iowa)
J. Thorac. Cardiovasc. Surg. 88:1012–1019, December 1984   2–29

The cause of recurrent coarctation of the aorta developing after operative repair remains unclear. A review was made of experience gained at The University of Iowa Hospitals during a 20-year period with 47 consecutive infants less than 1 year old who were operated on for coarctation between 1962 and 1982. Eleven infants (group I) had coarctation only, 9 (group II) had an associated ventricular septal defect (VSD), and 27 (group III) had major cardiac anomalies. All of the infants had congestive failure preoperatively. At present, anastomoses are made with 7-0 or 6-0 polypropylene sutures rather than with 5-0 silk. A patch graft repair using the excised subclavian artery was done in 4 infants. Four with a VSD had simultaneous repair of the defect, and another had pulmonary artery banding. Seven infants with complex lesions had pulmonary artery banding; only 3 of the 27 had a primary 1-stage repair.

Hospital mortality was 15% in groups I and II combined and 44% in group III. Three infants required reoperation for postoperative complications. Seven of 32 infants followed up an average of 55 months after operation had significant arm-leg gradients, and 3 of them had associated hypertension. Catheterization confirmed significant gradients in these infants. Two children underwent reoperation, but 1 continued to be hypertensive after patch angioplasty and required a third operation. In 5 of these infants the anastomosis had been made with silk sutures. The 10-year actuarial survival of group III patients was 50%.

Operative mortality remains high after repair of coarctation of the aorta in infants with complex cardiac anomalies. Continued use of end-to-end anastomosis with fine polypropylene sutures is warranted in preference to angioplasty methods, which introduce prosthetic material or sacrifice the left subclavian artery. The use of absorbable monofilament suture material to create an end-to-end anastomosis while preserving the growth potential of the aorta would seem to be the optimal method from a hemodynamic viewpoint.

▶ Surgical repair of coarctation of the aorta can be lifesaving in symptomatic infants, but the long-term prognosis is less than ideal. Many such infants experience a recurrence of the coarctation that, if severe, may require reoperation. Since the middle to late 1970s, the subclavian angioplasty procedure has been promoted by many centers as the surgical procedure of choice for repair of coarctation in infancy. Theoretically, the risk of restenosis is lower than with end-to-end anastomosis because the subclavian flap operation avoids a circumferential suture line and utilizes living subclavian tissue with a potential for future growth.

Theory is fine, but well-designed clinical studies may be better! Cobanoglu and colleagues have provided the first clinical study comparing the long-term outcome following subclavian flap and end-to-end anastomosis. By the fifth postoperative year, 8% of the end-to-end patients had required reoperation compared to 25% of the subclavian flap patients, a significant difference. In the study reported by Harlan et al. a similar low incidence (9%) of recurrent coarctation was observed 10 years following resection and end-to-end anastomosis. This group feels that the risk of recurrence is decreased by the use of polypropylene suture material. Although new and innovative techniques may be attractive in concept, their advantage over old approaches can only be established with time, clinical experience, and properly designed clinical trials. These two reports suggest that the subclavian angioplasty procedure is not better, and in the authors' hands may be worse, then resection and end-to-end anastomosis in infancy.

Regardless of which operation decreases the incidence of recurrent stenosis, the risk from reoperation will undoubtedly be lower in the future with the advent of balloon angioplasty techniques. In our hands, recurrent coarctation following either type of primary repair has been successfully dilated in the majority of patients with low risk and excellent short-term results.—Robert H. Beekman, M.D.

Surgical Treatment of Subpulmonary Obstruction in Transposition of the Great Arteries by Means of a Left Ventricular-Pulmonary Arterial Conduit: Late Results and Further Considerations
Ginancarlo Crupi, Ravi Pillai, Lucio Parenzan, and Christopher Lincoln (Brompton Hosp., London, and Ospedali Riuniti, Bergamo, Italy)
J. Thorac. Cardiovasc. Surg. 89:907–913, June 1985   2–30

Surgical management of severe subvalvular left ventricular (LV) outflow tract obstruction in patients with transposition of the great arteries (TGA) with or without intact ventricular septum remains controversial. Direct relief by wedge resection or the use of a conduit between the LV and pulmonary artery (PA) are surgical alternatives in these patients.

Between January 1976 and June 1983, 16 patients with TGA and LV outflow tract obstruction underwent repair by means of a combined Mustard operation and placement of an external conduit between the LV and main pulmonary artery. Mean age and weight at operation were 5.3 years (range 1.1–11) and 19 kg (range 6–26). Ten patients had intact ventricular septum and 6 had a ventricular septal defect (VSD), which because of its size or location precluded a Rastelli repair. A fibromuscular tunnel was the most common type of subpulmonary obstruction (10 of 16, 62%). An aortic homograft conduit was used in 7 patients, a valveless woven Dacron conduit in 3, and a Hancock valved conduit in 6. Mean follow-up was 5 years (range, 7 months–6 years).

There were three early deaths and one late death. Cardiac catheterization performed at a mean interval of 45 days after operation in 10 of 13 survivors showed a significant reduction in peak systolic LV PA gradient from 66 to 8.5 mm Hg. Nine of these patients underwent repeat catheterization at a mean interval of 4 years after operation and showed continuing relief of LV outflow tract obstruction with a mean increase in peak systolic transconduit pressure gradient of only 6.4 mm Hg. In addition, angiography showed remarkably less severe obstruction in 4 patients with a subvalvular fibromuscular tunnel. One patient in whom a Hancock valve conduit was inserted showed a significant gradient due to stenosis of the porcine valve 5 years later. In contrast, none of the patients in whom a fresh antibiotic-preserved homograft or a valveless conduit was used developed a significant transconduit gradient.

Placement of an LV-PA conduit remains a good alternative to direct resection for treatment of severe fixed subpulmonary obstruction in patients with TGA and intact ventricular septum or with VSD when a Rastelli repair is precluded. The use of an oversized fresh homograft or a valveless conduit rather than a porcine valved conduit may delay reoperation.

▶ Surgical repair of the child with D-transposition of the great arteries and severe subpulmonary stenosis in the absence of a ventricular septal defect or with an uncommitted ventricular septal defect remains a challenging and difficult operation. Resection of the subpulmonary stenosis usually is not feasible, particularly when it is of a fibromuscular tunnel type; a left ventricular to pulmonary artery conduit appears to be an excellent alternative, especially when the fresh homografted or valveless conduit is used. Homografts are being used with increasing frequency in this country to establish right ventricular or left ventricular connection to the pulmonary arteries. The current limiting factor is the availability of fresh, antibiotic-sterilized aortic or pulmonary artery homografts. The excellent long-term hemodynamic results should lead to a further increase in the use of these homografts in this country. The observation that the subvalvular fibromuscular tunnel became markedly less obstructive on long-term follow-up cardiac catheterization suggests that the placement of the external conduit diminished the stimulus for progressive hypertrophy and eventually resulted in regression of the preexisting hypertrophy. In these patients, adequate pulmonary blood flow may be established through the left ventricular outflow tract, and subsequent surgical intervention for an obstructed conduit may not be necessary.—A. Rosenthal, M.D.

Staged Partitioning of Single Ventricle
Paul A. Ebert (Univ. of California, San Francisco)
J. Thorac. Cardiovasc. Surg. 88:908–913, December 1984   2–31

Partitioning of the common ventricle is an attractive approach to repairing the univentricular heart, but difficulties with the size and paradoxic motion of the patch, and with a high rate of pulmonary hypertension, have limited its use. A staged approach to partitioning of the common ventricle was attempted in 5 patients seen between 1977 and 1983, all with signs of increased pulmonary blood flow. Three had previously undergone pulmonary artery banding. No separate rudimentary outflow chamber was discerned at cardiac catheterization. No patient was thought to have elevated pulmonary vascular resistance, and the age range at the time of initial repair was 2–10 months.

The first stage of repair was carried out via a transverse right atrial incision, with either total circulatory arrest or catheterization of the individual venae cavea. A small triangular piece of Teflon felt was attached to the posterior wall of the ventricle and a second piece was sutured between the aortic and pulmonary anuli, creating together about 70% of a ventricular septum; the central section was left open. A pulmonary artery band was placed where necessary. Four patients had normal oxygen saturation values postoperatively. At the second stage, when patients were aged 6–18 months, the remaining open area was closed with another piece of Teflon. The pulmonary artery band was removed, and the area was either patched or excised. Infundibular pulmonary stenosis was identified in one child 2 years later, and a valveless conduit was inserted, with a satisfactory outcome. No patient experienced rhythm disorder.

This approach permits the apical and base patches to stiffen and heal to the endocardium, and fewer sutures are required. The final stage is analogous to closing a moderate-sized ventricular septal defect in a patient with previous pulmonary artery banding. Conduction system injury remains a possibility. Reasonable growth and development are possible with this treatment, but it remains to be seen whether early repair will reduce the risks of ventricular fibrosis or progressive ventricular enlargement.

▶ The staged approach to partitioning the single ventricle is an ingenious method used by Dr. Ebert to achieve a satisfactory ventricular repair for this challenging lesion. The major difficulties in accomplishing one-stage septation in the past have been largely due to paradoxical motion of a large, unstable patch in addition to the frequent occurrence of heart block. This new method inserts two smaller patches as a first procedure, allowing them to "stiffen" with time before the partitioning is completed. When the defect between the patches is subsequently closed at the second stage, only a small, unstable prosthetic septum results. Further, placement of the initial patches can be done with only a few sutures directly through the myocardial wall, thereby trapping less endocardium, and may well explain the lack of heart block in this small series.

It is worth emphasizing that septation procedures appear to be a reasonable option only in those cases with the aorta anterior and leftward (double inlet LV). A straight patch can then be placed to leave the tricuspid and pulmonary valves to the right and the mitral and aortic valves to the left. Most surgeons would currently favor the Fontan procedure for this anatomy using a direct atriopulmonary connection (nonvalved). The operative mortality for this approach is low, and late results are encouraging. If the staged approach to partitioning the single ventricle produces satisfactory long-term results without conduction abnormalities, it will continue to be a valuable procedure for patients with a single ventricle.—E. Bove, M.D.

Experience With the Fontan Procedure
Hillel Laks, Jeffrey C. Milliken, Joseph K. Perloff, William E. Hellenbrand, Barbara L. George, Alvin Chin, Thomas G. Di Sessa, and Roberta G. Williams (Yale Univ. and Univ. of California at Los Angeles)
J. Thorac. Cardiovasc. Surg. 88:939–951, December 1984   2–32

Since Fontan reported the first successful surgical correction of tricuspid atresia, the procedure has been modified and applied to other forms of complex congenital heart disease. The authors present the early and late results in 45 patients, aged 2 to 38 years (mean, 12.9), who underwent various modifications of the Fontan procedure from 1975 to 1984 for complex congenital heart disease. Preoperative diagnoses included tricuspid atresia in 19 patients, univentricular heart in 24, and pulmonary atresia with intact ventricular septum in 2.

The indications for operation were increasing cyanosis and progressive exercise intolerance. However, some patients underwent elective surgery during asymptomatic periods. Mean preoperative pulmonary arterial pressure was 14.6 ± 5 mm Hg, and the mean preoperative left ventricular end-diastolic pressure was 9.2 ± 3 mm Hg. Right atrial-pulmonary arterial connections were performed in 32 patients: 11 with conduits (7 with porcine valved conduit and 4 without) and 21 by direct anastomosis with patch augmentation. Right atrial-right ventricular connections were made in 13 patients, 6 with porcine valved conduit and 7 without.

Follow-up ranged from 0.1 to 9 years (mean 2.3). There were three early deaths and two late deaths, for an overall mortality of 11%. All deaths were in patients with a univentricular heart. The late deaths were related to venous hypertension. A venous assist device (intermittent abdominal compression to 45 mm Hg for 30 seconds followed by release for 15 seconds) was used in 8 patients in the immediate postoperative period and resulted in improved cardiac output and reduced fluid accumulation. Postoperative Doppler flow studies showed biphasic pulmonary artery flow in all of 15 patients studied, regardless of the type of connection or the presence of a valve. Cardiac catheterization, performed a mean 14 months postoperatively (range, 1–42 months), revealed a reduced cardiac index in 14 of 16 patients studied. Exercise testing in 8 patients demonstrated a marked rise in right atrial pressure (from 13.9 ± 1.2 to 21.4 ± 2.3 mm Hg) with only a modest elevation in cardiac index (from 2.31 ± 0.25 to 3.41 ± 0.44 L/sq m), even in those without functional limitations. Of the 37 surviving patients, 29 (78%) were in New York Heart Association class I, 6 (17%) in class II, and 2 (5%) in class III.

In carefully selected patients, the Fontan procedure is an excellent operation for tricuspid atresia and other forms of complex congenital heart disease. The need for a valve in the right atrial-right ventricular connection remains controversial and awaits further study with long-term follow-up, while its use is not required in the right atrial-pulmonary arterial connection. The venous assist device is a valuable adjunct in certain patients in the immediate postoperative period.

▶ The selection criteria for patients undergoing the Fontan procedure remain crucial in determining the mortality and morbidity from the operation. The Ten Commandments formulated by Choussat (in Anderson, R.H., and Shinebourne, E. A., (eds.): *Pediatric Cardiology 1977,* New York, Churchill Livingston Press, 1978, p. 565) nearly a decade ago as ideal selection criteria have been modified and altered by experience. At present the major incremental risk factors for hospital death include (1) repair of cardiac anomaly other than tricuspid atresia, (2) young age (less than 1 to 4 years), (3) increased pulmonary vascular resistance (greater than or equal to 4 Wood units), 4 left ventricular end-diastolic pressure greater than 14 mm Hg, (5) need for atrioventricular valve replacement, and (6) small pulmonary arteries (a ratio of greater than or equal to 2.0 for the diameter of the right plus left pulmonary artery divided by the diameter of the descending aorta at the level of the diaphragm).

The long-term results of the Fontan procedure have not been as clearly defined. The patients' reported lack of symptoms and continued well-being are rather remarkable given the low measured resting cardiac output and limited capacity to increase cardiac output during exercise (by approximately 50%–

100%). Further investigations of the compensatory mechanism during various forms of exercise may explain this apparent discrepancy.

There are two specific issues raised by the authors in the manuscript or its subsequent discussion that are worth emphasizing. First is the value, in some patients, of a venous assist device utilizing a simple cuff around the abdomen in increasing cardiac output during the immediate postoperative period. Second is the observation that patients with a Dacron conduit between the right atrium and pulmonary artery did not require reoperation for either a peel or valve obstruction for as long as 9 years postoperatively. The authors' continued administration of aspirin and dipyridamole to all these patients in the postoperative period may be the responsible factor.—Amnon Rosenthal, M.D.

Cardiac Surgery in Children of Jehovah's Witnesses
Michael J. Carmichael, Denton A. Cooley, R. Craig Kuykendall, and William E. Walker (Texas Heart Inst. and Univ. of Texas, Houston)
Tex. Heart Inst. J. 12:57–63, March 1985   2–33

Cardiac surgery has become feasible for patients of the Jehovah's Witness faith since the advent of the bloodless prime technique during cardiopulmonary bypass. A retrospective study was done of 73 consecutive Jehovah's Witness children younger than age 2 years who were operated on for lesions of the heart and major vessels. Patients were divided into three groups: (1) neonates younger than age 31 days (n = 11), (II) children between ages 31 days and 2 years (n = 47), and (III) children requiring cardiopulmonary bypass (n = 15).

Overall mortality was 12.3% (9/73). Only three of the nine deaths were complicated by blood loss and anemia. Mortality for group I was 18.2% (2 of 11). Only one death was partly attributable to anemia. The lowest hemoglobin (Hgb) level (12.4 gm/dl) and average total blood loss (TBL) (9.0 cc/kg) were tolerated. Mortality for group II was 14.9% (7 of 47). Only two deaths were complicated by anemia. The lowest Hgb level (13.0 gm/dl) and TBL (14.8 cc/kg) were well tolerated. There were no deaths in group III patients. Average TBL was 27.8 cc/kg. Hemoglobin level fell from a preoperative level of 15.7 gm/dl to 5.5 gm/dl (diluted blood) during bypass perfusion and returned postoperatively to 10.6 gm/dl. Average time on bypass was 35.6 minutes; ischemic time averaged 27.8 minutes. Bloodless prime hemodilution techniques were used in all cases, with the pump prime ranging from 500 cc to 800 cc of Ringer's lactate. The most frequent postoperative complication was postpericardiectomy syndrome.

Cardiac surgery can be performed when indicated with acceptable mortality and morbidity rates on children on Jehovah's Witnesses. The combination of rapid, meticulous performance of the operation and bloodless prime techniques allows cardiac surgery in these children while averting the complications of severe anemia.

▶ This article and a similar one (*J. Thorac. Cardiovasc. Surg.* 89:914–920, 1985) from the Texas Heart Institute report the authors' experience with cardiac surgery on a large number of children of the Jehovah's Witness faith. The low mortality and morbidity demonstrate the safety of this technique even in small children. The patients undergoing open-heart procedures constitute the most interesting group. Hemoglobin values as low as 3.5 gm/dl on cardiopulmonary bypass, often with flows considerably below generally accepted norms, were commonly encountered. All operations were done at normothermia. A number of important details are worth emphasizing, including reducing preoperative blood studies and minimizing blood loss during catheterization. Meticulous intraoperative technique is essential. The priming volume of the bypass circuit should be reduced by shortening the tubing as much as possible. A brisk diuresis as bypass is discontinued allows the return of all diluted blood back to the patient. If crystalloid cardioplegia is used, the coronary sinus effluent should be discharged to prevent further hemodilution.

With the ever-increasing concerns regarding disease transmission through blood transfusions, hemodilution techniques such as those described by the authors will become more popular for all children undergoing cardiac surgery. More complex repairs requiring deep hypothermia in neonates are less likely to fare as well due to the greater likelihood of coagulopathies.—E. Bove, M.D.

3 Heart Disease in Adults: The Myocardium, Endocardium, and Pericardium

Mitral Valve Prolapse

Mitral Valve Prolapse Associated With Other Disorders: Casual Coincidence, Common Link, or Fundamental Genetic Disturbance?
Alasdair D. Malcolm (Airedale Gen. Hosp., Keighley, England)
Br. Heart J. 53:353–362, April 1985   3–1

Mitral valve prolapse (MVP) has been linked with other clinical conditions. A review was made of these reported associations with their pathophysiologic mechanisms and awareness of the possibility of casual coincidence.

The direct but noninvasive visualization of excessive systolic bulging of the mitral leaflets by cross-sectional echocardiography is the key to diagnosis of MVP. In evaluating possible associations between MVP and various disorders, however, it should be remembered that an echocardiographically prolapsing mitral valve is not necessarily abnormal; it may represent a normal variant or a variant that appears only at a certain time of life, particularly in young women. Pathologically, the dissolution or dysgenesis of collagen in the pars fibrosa and chordae appears to be the basic mechanism responsible for ballooning of the mitral leaflets. However, disturbance of the normal balance between ventricular and valvar size may cause anatomical prolapse in the absence of any pathologic feature of mitral leaflets or chordae. This occurs when left ventricular size is sufficiently reduced, or the shape is sufficiently altered, that maintenance of normal leaflet position and contour during systole is impossible, as in hypertrophic obstructive cardiomyopathy. In patients with secundum atrial septal defect, up to half of whom have MVP, the reduced left ventricular size with distorted ventricular geometry is probably often responsible for MVP. Tricuspid valve prolapse also coexists fairly frequently with MVP. A genetically determined abnormality of atrioventricular valve development or maintenance may explain the dual valve involvement. The abnormal sequence of ventricular activation in Wolff-Parkinson-White syndrome can give rise to MVP. Distortion of the atrioventricular area and reduced left ventricular size may be responsible for MVP in patients with progressive muscular dystrophy and straight or lordotic thoracic spines. An increased chance that MVP is present occurs among patients with thoracic skeletal deformities (narrow anteroposterior chest diameter, straight back, or pectus excavatum) or hypomastia. Mitral valve prolapse is also an integral part of many inherited connective tissue disorders, e.g., Marfan and Ehlers-Danlos syndromes. A pronounced deficiency of type III collagen may be responsible for the prolapse in Ehlers-Danlos syndrome. The basis for the association between MVP and Grave's disease remains a matter of conjecture. Ischemically induced disturbance of contractile function in papillary muscles or subjacent myocardium may result in failure to maintain chordal systolic tension, resulting in prolapse; this is the most common cause of secondary MVP.

There is no doubt that anatomical prolapse of mitral leaflets is common, but in only a small proportion of patients should this be considered abnormal. In some the prolapse is evanescent. Improved cross-sectional echocardiographic instrumentation and meticulous attention to details of technique may distinguish between "normal" and pathologic forms of prolapsing mitral valves.

▶ A timely, thought-provoking discussion of this fascinating condition, mitral valve prolapse.—W. Proctor Harvey, M.D.

Complex Arrhythmias in Mitral Regurgitation With and Without Mitral Valve Prolapse: Contrast to Arrhythmias in Mitral Valve Prolapse Without Mitral Regurgitation
Paul Kligfield, Clare Hochreiter, Harvey Kramer, Richard B. Devereux, Nathaniel Niles, Randi Kramer-Fox, and Jeffrey S. Borer (New York Hosp.-Cornell Med. Ctr.)
Am. J. Cardiol. 55:1545–1549, June 1, 1985   3–2

The prevalence and significance of arrhythmias in nonischemic mitral regurgitation were examined in 31 patients with hemodynamically significant nonischemic regurgitation, 17 of whom had evidence of mitral valve prolapse (MVP), and 63 patients with MVP and no clinical or echocardiographic evidence of hemodynamically significant mitral regurgitation. No patient had evidence of ischemic heart disease. Catheterization confirmed mitral regurgitation of grades 3 + to 4 + in all 15 study patients examined. Echocardiography, radio-nuclide cineangiography, and ambulatory ECG studies were performed.

Atrial and ventricular arrhythmias were both frequent and complex in patients with mitral regurgitation. All of these patients had ventricular premature complexes. Three fourths of the patients had multiform ventricular ectopy, and one third had ventricular salvos or ventricular tachycardia. Premature complex frequency was unrelated to the presence or absence of MVP. Patients with MVP as well as mitral regurgitation had more frequent and complex atrial and ventricular arrhythmias than did those with MVP alone, whether or not digitalis or diuretics were used.

Patients with nonischemic mitral regurgitation have a high prevalence of frequent and complex atrial and ventricular arrhythmias, regardless of etiology. These arrhythmias are more closely associated with hemodynamically significant mitral regurgitation than with MVP alone. Rather than specific structural changes, the myocardial response to abnormal loading may be important in the genesis of arrhythmias in patients with mitral regurgitation.

▶ These results are not surprising from a clinical point of view and add support to the overall good prognosis of the majority of patients having mitral valve prolapse.—W. Proctor Harvey, M.D.

Diagnostic Precision of Echocardiography in Mitral Valve Prolapse
L. Samuel Wann, Charles M. Gross, Richard J. Wakefield, and John H. Kalbfleisch (Medical College of Wisconsin, Milwaukee)
Am. Heart J. 109:803–808, April 1985   3–3

Standard echocardiographic criteria for the diagnosis of mitral valve prolapse (MVP) include late systolic or pansystolic bowing of the mitral leaflets seen on M-mode echocardiography, and extension of mitral leaflet tissue through the plane of the mitral anulus into the left atrium seen on two-dimensional echocardiography. To determine the precision with which these criteria can be applied in the diagnosis of MVP, three independent observers (A, B, and C), two of whom were experienced echocardiographers and one a cardiology fellow-in-training, analyzed the separate M-mode and two-dimensional echocardiograms of 50 patients. Of these, 27 were previously identified clinically as having echocardiographic evidence of prolapse.

In interpretation of M-mode echocardiography, observer A's intraobserver repeatability was 92%, observer B's was 84%, and observer C's was 90%. For two-dimensional echocardiography, observer A's intraobserver repeatability was 98%, observer B's was 80%, and observer C's was 82%. This variability in intraobserver repeatability appeared to be related to the frequency with which individual observers identified prolapse, and probably reflected differences in the sensitivity and specificity of each observer. With M-mode echocardiography, intraobserver repeatability was 64% for observer A vs. B, 80% for observer A vs. C, and 66% for observer B vs. C. With two-dimensional echocardiography, interobserver repeatability was 54% for observer A vs. B, 70% for observer A vs. C, and 52% for observer B vs. C. There were no significant differences in intraobserver and interobserver repeatability of M-mode vs. two-dimensional echocardiography. A review of findings that were subject to considerable variation in interpretation revealed relatively subtle or mild changes that were not repeatably identifiable.

The magnitude of interobserver and intraobserver repeatability in the diagnosis of MVP is sufficiently low not to be of serious clinical concern. However, it should be emphasized that MVP is a syndrome, not an isolated echocardiographic finding. Hence, clinicians should integrate data obtained by history, physical examination, and laboratory evaluation, including an understanding of the inherent variability in echocardiographic evaluation.

▶ The last paragraph of this article is worthy of reemphasis. As part of the total evaluation, the stethoscope remains the single most valuable instrument to diagnose MVP. One must remember to listen to patients in the various positions of lying flat, turned to the left lateral position, sitting, standing, and squatting. Also, the physician should be familiar with the many variants of the auscultatory findings of MVP. It is important to remember that, in some patients, the typical findings on auscultation are heard in only one phase of respiration, either inspiration, expiration, or both. Believe your ears!—W. Proctor Harvey, M.D.

Mitral Valve Prolapse and Bacterial Endocarditis: When Is Antibiotic Prophylaxis Necessary?
Andrew J. Hickey, Stephen W. MacMahon, and David E. L. Wilcken (The Prince Henry Hosp., Little Bay, Australia)
Am. Heart J. 109:431–435, March 1985   3–4

The frequency of mitral valve prolapse (MVP) makes the question of antibiotic prophylaxis an important one. The risk of bacterial endocarditis occurring in a 1-year period was estimated from a case-control study of 56 patients with bacterial endocarditis and the incidence of this disease in adults living in New South Wales in 1980. All patients with bacterial endocarditis were at least 15 years of age and had no known antecedent cardiac lesions. Bacterial endocarditis was confirmed histologically in all 30 patients who were operated on. The series included 32 men (mean age, 51 years) and 24 women (mean age, 45 years). Controls undergoing echocardiography were matched with cases for sex and age; three controls were chosen for each case.

Mitral valve prolapse was found in 20% of the cases and in 4% of the controls. Eight cases and all of the controls had late systolic prolapse observed on M-mode echocardiography. The odds ratio for the association in men was 7.7, but the ratio of 3.0 in women was not significant. The risk of bacterial endocarditis also was increased in association with chronic hemodialysis and parenteral drug use, but exclusion of these cases did not alter the association with MVP. The estimated probability of bacterial endocarditis occurring in a person with MVP in a 1-year period was 4.7 times greater than in the general population.

An estimated 14 of every 100,000 adults with MVP will have bacterial endocarditis in a 1-year period, compared with 3 of 100,000 in the general population. Antibiotic prophylaxis is not warranted for all patients with MVP, but it might be used in patients who have systolic murmurs, those with a previous episode of bacterial endocarditis, and those at special risk for other reasons.

▶ I advise antibiotic prophylaxis for those patients with MVP who have systolic clicks as well as systolic murmurs. I have seen patients with only a click (or clicks) with infective endocarditis. Also, some patients have a transient murmur as well as clicks, sometimes heard and at other times, not heard. Murmurs can often be heard in only one position, or in only one phase of respiration, or a murmur might be brought out by physical effort. Although, statistically, infective endocarditis is uncommon in a patient with MVP who has only clicks, when it does occur, it is 100% as far as that particular patient is concerned.—W. Proctor Harvey, M.D.

Mitral Valve Prolapse and Ruptured Chordae Tendineae

Robert M. Jeresaty, Josse E. Edwards, and Surendra K. Chawla (St. Francis Hosp. and Med. Ctr., Hartford, Conn.)
Am. J. Cardiol. 55:138–142, Jan. 1, 1985   3–5

Although the association of mitral valve prolapse (MVP) and chordal rupture has been reported frequently, the etiologic link between the two entities has been debated. To determine the cause of ruptured tendineae and a suspected etiologic role for MVP, the mitral valve in 25 consecutive patients with surgically confirmed chordal rupture was examined. The diagnosis of MVP was based on the presence of redundance and marked interchordal hooding of the mitral leaflets, a large mitral anulus, and histologic changes.

Mitral valve prolapse was the underlying pathologic abnormality in 23 patients, only one of whom had infective endocarditis that was responsible for the rupture. Thus, MVP was the only underlying cause of ruptured chordae tendineae in 22 of 25 patients (88%) and endocarditis in only 2 patients (8%). In one patient the cause of chordal rupture was undetermined. Only one patient with endocarditis also had MVP. Rupture of chordae to the anterior leaflet occurred in 10 patients, to the posterior leaflet in 13, and to both in 2. Rupture of chordae of the middle scallop was most common in the posterior leaflet. The characteristic hooding was not limited to the segment of the valve attached to the ruptured chordae. A large mitral anulus was noted in 15 of 23 patients with MVP and ruptured chordae tendineae. Histologic examination revealed myxomatous changes on the mitral valve; among the chords that ruptured, the most consistent change was loss of clear, collagenous staining with the van Gieson counterstain. In four patients, MVP was documented 4–11 years (mean, 7 years) before chordal rupture, adding further support to the causal relationship. No patient had endocarditis previously. Mitral valve prolapse is probably the most common cause of so-called spontaneous chordal rupture.

▶ This study supports the strong clinical impression that spontaneous rupture of the mitral valve is a definite serious complication of MVP. Rupture of the chordae, of course, occurs as a complication of infective endocarditis. Whatever the cause, chordal rupture represents the most common and serious complication of MVP.—W. Proctor Harvey, M.D.

Primary (Spontaneous) Chordal Rupture: Relation to Myxomatous Valve Disease and Mitral Valve Prolapse
Andrew J. Hickey, David E. L. Wilcken, John S. Wright, and Bruce A. Warren (Univ. of New South Wales, Sydney)
J. Am. Coll. Cardiol. 5:1341–1346, June 1985   3–6

The causes of chordal rupture unrelated to infective endocarditis or trauma remain uncertain. Review was made of data on 152 patients who had isolated primary mitral valve replacement between 1979 and 1983. Seventy-nine patients had isolated mitral regurgitation. A floppy mitral valve was the underlying abnormality in 28% of the patients and nonrheumatic valve disease in 61%. Primary chordal rupture was found at operation in 31 patients, each of whom had a floppy valve. Chordal rupture involved the posterior leaflet in 27 patients, the anterior leaflet in 2, and both leaflets in 2. Four patients, who also had a floppy valve, had secondary chordal rupture because of endocarditis.

Myxomatous mitral valve disease was identified histologically in 39 of 42 excised floppy valves. Extensive surface fibrosis was present in 24 valves. All but 2 of the 31 patients with primary chordal rupture had myxomatous mitral valve disease. One of these had a definite history of rheumatic fever. Only one patient was hypertensive. Chordal rupture was diagnosed in 13 of 16 patients by two-dimensional echocardiography. Preexisting mitral prolapse was clearly documented in seven patients with myxomatous mitral valve disease.

The floppy mitral valve with underlying myxomatous valve disease is a major cause of severe mitral regurgitation, requiring valve surgery. More than one fourth of all isolated mitral replacement operations performed in a 4-year period at the authors' institution were done for this reason. Primary chordal rupture is the most frequent precipitant, and it almost always indicates the presence of myxomatous valve disease. There is some evidence of an association between myxomatous valve disease and mitral valve prolapse.

▶ Spontaneous chordal rupture occurs much more frequently than is generally realized. At times, one obtains a history of unusual physical exertion (e.g., lifting a heavy object, shoveling coal) that appears to be a precipitating factor. I advise against weight lifting as a type of physical conditioning of patients who have mitral valve prolapse. Certainly, clinical rupture of the chordae tendineae is the most common serious complication of this very prevalent condition.— W. Proctor Harvey, M.D.

Prevalence of Aortic Valve Prolapse With Bicuspid Aortic Valve and Its Relation to Aortic Regurgitation: A Cross-Sectional Echocardiographic Study

William J. Stewart, Mary Etta King, Linda D. Gillam, David E. Guyer, and Arthur E. Weyman (Massachusetts Gen. Hosp., Boston)
Am. J. Cardiol. 54:1277–1282, Dec. 1, 1984   3–7

Although aortic valve prolapse (AVP) has been suggested as a cause of aortic regurgitation in patients with bicuspid aortic valves, its prevalence and association with aortic regurgitation in these patients remain undefined. To determine these relationships, studies were made in 64 patients aged 2 weeks to 60 years (mean age, 20 years) with bicuspid aortic valves diagnosed by two-dimensional echocardiography. Twenty normal persons matched for age and sex were also studied to define the normal diastolic position of the aortic cusps. The presence and degree of AVP were defined using three quantitative terms: aortic valve prolapse distance (AVPD), aortic valve prolapse area (AVPA), and aortic valve prolapse volume (AVPV). Each was corrected for patient size with reference to the diameter of the aorta at the level of insertion of the valve cusps.

The mean corrected AVPD was significantly greater among patients with bicuspid valves than in the normal group [0.26 ± 0.10 (range, 0.11–0.59) vs. 0.09 ± 0.06 (range, 0–0.16), $P = .00005$]. Similarly, the mean corrected AVPA was significantly greater among patients with bicuspid valves [0.35 ± 0.17 cm (range, 0.05–0.90) vs. 0.08 ± 0.06 cm (range, 0–0.15), $P = .00005$]. When AVPD criteria were used, 81% of the bicuspid valves were abnormal; when AVPA criteria were used, 87% were abnormal. Although the presence of AVP was not related to the presence of aortic regurgitation, the degree of prolapse as defined by AVPV was significantly greater in patients with bicuspid aortic valves and clinical aortic regurgitation than in those without (mean, 0.24 ± 0.08 cm vs. 0.19 ± 0.09 cm, $P = .000$). However, because of the overlap between groups, there was no point at which the degree of AVP could be considered predictive of aortic regurgitation. There was no relationship between the degree of prolapse and either age or degree of cusp asymmetry. The degree of AVP was greater in bicuspid valves with vertical than in those with horizontal commissures. However, there was no relationship between commissure orientation and aortic regurgitation.

Aortic valve prolapse frequently occurs in patients with bicuspid aortic valves. However, neither the presence nor the degree of AVP can be used to predict clinical aortic regurgitation.

▶ It is in the recent past that interest in prolapse of the aortic valve has been documented on the basis of echocardiographic studies. This article shows no correlation between the presence of AVP and aortic regurgitation, although I would have predicted there would be a correlation. This work does reinforce the fact that prolapse is more prevalent than heretofore appreciated.—W. Proctor Harvey, M.D.

Echocardiography (Including Doppler)

Increasing Importance of Doppler Echocardiography
Harvey Feigenbaum (Indiana Univ. at Indianapolis)
J. Am. Coll. Cardiol. 6:366–368, August 1985   3–8

Hemodynamic information obtained from Doppler echocardiography, with morphological data from two-dimensional and M-mode studies, can contribute significantly to clinical cardiology. Doppler flow velocities were first used to measure blood flow and are now used to assess intracardiac pressures as well. The Bernoulli equation is used to convert blood flow velocity to a pressure fall or gradient across a stenotic valve. The technique is valuable in determining the severity of aortic stenosis. The pressure gradient across a regurgitant valve can also be determined. The gradient across an incompetent tricuspid valve provides a means of determining right ventricular systolic pressure. If there is no pulmonary outflow obstruction, the right ventricular systolic pressure should equal pulmonary artery systolic pressure. The same approach can be used to measure the pressure differential between the ventricles in a patient with ventricular septal defect.

Velocities distal to an obstructing lesion are usually high and cannot be detected by pulsed Doppler methods. A continuous-wave technique can be used, but the Doppler sample then cannot be placed at a specific distance from the transducer. The angle between the ultrasound beam and the path of the red blood cells producing the Doppler signal is an important consideration. The examination can be tedious, but it must not be hurried. Graphic recordings of Doppler studies are less readily evaluated than is the M-mode or two-dimensional echocardiogram.

▶ Doppler echocardiography is unquestionably here to stay. Harvey Feigenbaum is one of our leading experts and a pioneer in this field. Worthy of emphasis is his admonition that the technical aspects of this newer modality can be time consuming, and that knowledge of M-mode and two-dimensional echocardiograms does not ensure competency with Doppler techniques.

▶ ↓ The next paper illustrates the usefulness of this method.—W. Proctor Harvey, M.D.

Quantitative Assessment by Doppler Echocardiography of Pulmonary or Aortic Regurgitation
Stanley J. Goldberg and Hugh D. Allen (Univ. of Arizona)
Am. J. Cardiol. 56:131–135, July 1, 1985   3–9

An attempt was made to quantify semilunar valve regurgitation by Doppler measurement of flow in consecutive patients with isolated aortic or pulmonary regurgitation and no more than mild concomitant stenosis. In addition to a standard pulsed Doppler study, pulmonary artery and midascending aortic velocities were recorded. Forward and reverse flows were assessed, and reverse flow was subtracted from total forward flow to yield net flow, which in turn was compared with forward flow distal to the normal semilunar valve. Recordings were satisfactory in 18 of the 20 patients studied.

Mean net flow was not significantly different from mean flow measured in another part of the heart. The correlation coefficient for the paired measurements was 0.91. The percent regurgitation ranged from 29% to 73%. All patients with clinically severe regurgitation had a percent regurgitation exceeding 53%. The Doppler findings generally correlated well with both clinical and angiographic assessments.

Doppler echocardiography is a reasonably accurate means of evaluating patients with semilunar valve regurgitation if an internal control is included in each instance. The result obtained should be considered an estimate. The study is not simple and requires experience. Further confirmation of its usefulness is required in patients with aortic regurgitation. The method cannot be applied strictly to patients with combined stenosis and regurgitation.

▶ Note that these authors also stress what Dr. Feigenbaum (in the preceding article) stated. They also caution: "The Doppler technique is not simple and requires practice and experience in computing cardiac outputs in great vessels."—W. Proctor Harvey, M.D.

Clinical Value of Doppler Echocardiography in the Assessment of Adults With Aortic Stenosis
Iain A. Simpson, Alan B. Houston, Chris D. Sheldon, Ian Hutton, and T. D. V. Lawrie (Royal Infirmary, Glasgow)
Br. Heart J. 53:636–639, June 1985   3–10

The accuracy of continuous-wave Doppler ultrasound in predicting valve gradients was assessed in 41 adults, mean age 52 years, with clinically suspected aortic stenosis who were undergoing cardiac catheterization. Continuous-wave velocimetry was performed using a continuous-wave and pulsed-wave velocimeter with a 2-MHz transducer. Satisfactory Doppler signals were recorded in all 41 patients. The suprasternal notch was the best position in which to obtain an optimal signal, but other sites sometimes were more informative.

Thirty-three evaluable patients had a mean catheter gradient of 43 mm Hg and a mean Doppler gradient of 49 mm Hg. The overall correlation between the Doppler-derived and catheter gradients was 0.98 when the studies were done simultaneously in the sedated patient. The Doppler study indicated a surgically significant gradient, generally defined as one exceeding 50 mm Hg, in all 12 patients clinically thought to have a significant gradient; this was confirmed at catheterization. Twelve patients had inconclusive findings. The Doppler study suggested an insignificant lesion in seven patients, in agreement with the clinical impression, and this was confirmed. In two other patients with clinically insignificant lesions, the Doppler study correctly showed surgically significant lesions.

Doppler echocardiography, when combined with clinical and other non-invasive studies, can accurately predict the presence or absence of a significant gradient in patients with aortic stenosis. Surgery can be recommended in an appreciable number of patients without the need for previous cardiac catheterization.

▶ Another report attesting to the accuracy and value of this important technique.—W. Proctor Harvey, M.D.

Continuous-Wave Doppler Echocardiographic Assessment of Severity of Calcific Aortic Stenosis: A Simultaneous Doppler-Catheter Correlative Study in 100 Adult Patients
Philip J. Currie, James B. Seward, Guy S. Reeder, Ronald E. Vlietstra, Dennis R. Bresnahan, John F. Bresnahan, Hugh C. Smith, Donald J. Hagler, and A. Jamil Tajik (Mayo Clinic and Found.)
Circulation 71:1162–1169, June 1985   3–11

The accuracy of the continuous-wave Doppler echocardiographic technique in evaluating the severity of aortic valve stenosis was examined in a prospective series of consecutive patients, older than age 50 years who had suspected calcific aortic valve stenosis at the time of cardiac catheterization. The 55 men and 45 women had a mean age of 69 years. Pressure measurements were made with the dual-catheter technique in 63 patients, and in 37 by withdrawal of the catheter from the left ventricle to the ascending aorta. Forty-six patients also had an outpatient Doppler study a week or less before catheterization.

Correlation between the Doppler-determined gradient and the simultaneously measured maximal catheter valve gradient was 0.92. Correlation with the mean catheter gradient was 0.93, and with the peak-to-peak catheter gradient, it was 0.91. Correlation between nonsimultaneous Doppler-determined and peak catheter gradients was only 0.79. Correlation appeared to increase as experience increased with the Doppler method. The accuracy of the Doppler method was not influenced by the cardiac index, degree of left ventricular dysfunction, or associated coronary disease.

The continuous-wave Doppler echocardiographic study, when done by experienced practitioners, can reliably estimate peak instantaneous and mean pressure gradients in adults with aortic valve stenosis. This method should greatly aid the noninvasive assessment of patients with suspected aortic valve stenosis, in conjunction with clinical data and a complete two-dimensional echocardiographic study.

▶ This represents a significant advance in "noninvasive" technology eliminating the necessity of cardiac catheterization in many. The usefulness of the Doppler method also applies to mitral lesions. Personally observed recently was a patient with mitral regurgitation associated with mitral valve prolapse. The amount of regurgitation was of a lesser degree, as shown by Doppler techniques, than was suspected clinically. Cardiac catheterization was therefore not believed to be necessary.—W. Proctor Harvey, M.D.

Auscultatory and Echocardiographic Features of Mobile Left Atrial Thrombus
Mamdouh Warda, Jonas Garcia, Leonard Pechace, Ali Massumkhani, and Robert J. Hall (Texas Heart Inst. and Clayton Found. for Research Cardiovascular Labs., Houston)
J. Am. Coll. Cardiol. 5:379–382, February 1985   3–12

Free-floating ball thrombus of the heart is a rare disorder that usually involves the left atrium, particularly in association with mitral stenosis and atrial fibrillation. The diagnosis of mobile atrial thrombus can be suspected when auscultatory changes occur in the intensity of the murmur of mitral stenosis. Because two-dimensional echocardiography is a sensitive tool in its diagnosis, a patient was studied with simultaneous two-dimensional echocardiography and phonocardiographic recordings to clarify the relationship between movement of the ball thrombus and the auscultatory findings.

Man, 51, with rheumatic mitral stenosis, was hospitalized for evaluation of progressive exertional dyspnea and orthopnea. The patient had an irregularly irregular pulse, elevated jugular venous pressure, laterally displaced apical impulse, and a left parasternal heave. A loud, high-frequency opening snap was heard at the left precordial area, separated from the aortic closure sound by an interval of 50 msec. A grade 4/6 pandiastolic rumble was heard over the apex. Spontaneous changes, as well as occasional disappearance of the rumble, were suspected.

Both M-mode and two-dimensional echocardiography revealed a mass of echoes appearing intermittently behind the anterior mitral leaflet during mid and late systole and disappearing at the beginning of systole. Simultaneous phonocardiographic recordings revealed attenuation and disappearance of the murmur as the mobile thrombus randomly drifted into the mitral valve orifice. Reappearance of the cardiac murmur was noted as the thrombus was displaced into the large atrial cavity. Because of the random motion of the mobile ball thrombus within the atrium, two-dimensional echocardiography was superior to M-mode echocardiography. Selective coronary angiography demonstrated neovascularization in the region of the left atrial appendage. Removal of a free-floating left atrial thrombus and open commissurotomy were performed.

Echocardiography and simultaneous phonocardiographic recording permit the correlation of auscultatory events with the intracardiac movements of the left atrial thrombus. Careful auscultation of patients with mitral stenosis may be essential in recognizing the spontaneous change of the murmur caused by a mobile atrial thrombus.

▶ At a symposium at the Texas Heart Institute I have had the opportunity to listen to a tape recording of this patient and at the same time see the echocardiograms that demonstrate the free-floating left atrial thrombus. Coincident with occlusion of the mitral valve orifice with the thrombus there was temporary disappearance of the typical diastolic rumble of mitral stenosis. This was a vivid demonstration of this situation. It also showed the mechanism of dizziness, syncope, or sudden death that could result. Fortunately, for this patient, the thrombus was removed at surgery.—W. Proctor Harvey, M.D.

Primary Cardiac Tumors: Experience With 30 Consecutive Patients Since the Introduction of Two-Dimensional Echocardiography
F. Earl Fyke, III, James B. Seward, William D. Edwards, Fletcher A. Miller, Jr., Guy S. Reeder, Thomas T. Schattenberg, Clarence Shub, John A. Callahan, and A. Jamil Tajik (Mayo Clinic and Found.)
J. Am. Coll. Cardiol. 5:1465–1473, June 1985   3–13

Review was made of the two-dimensional echocardiographic findings in 30 consecutive patients studied between 1977 and 1983; they had a total of 32 primary cardiac tumors. All but two tumors were identified by echocardiography. Twenty left and three right atrial myxomas were encountered, as well as three ventricular fibromas, two papillary fibroelastomas, one myxosarcoma, and one hemangiosarcoma. The diagnostic rate of primary cardiac tumor was higher than in previous years before two-dimensional echocardiography was available.

Most of the left atrial myxomas were attached to the atrial septum. Most were deformable and jelly-like in echocardiographic appearance. Echolucent areas were seen within six myxomas, corresponding to areas of hemorrhage or necrosis. The intramyocardial fibromas were nonmobile and uniform in echographic consistency. All but 4 of 29 patients underwent surgery on the basis of the two-dimensional echocardiographic findings. Constitutional symptoms were related to tumor size in patients with left atrial myxoma. About half of these patients had symptoms of heart failure despite adequate left ventricular function. Only one of four right atrial myxomas was associated with heart failure. Six patients with left atrial myxoma had clinical evidence of embolization. Two right atrial lesions produced signs of tricuspid insufficiency and stenosis. Most of the left atrial myxomas were associated with anemia, an increased erythrocyte sedimentation rate, increased gamma globulin, or all three.

Primary cardiac tumors usually can be operated on after two-dimensional echocardiographic evaluation. No operative deaths occurred in the current series and postoperative morbidity was low.

▶ Two-dimensional echocardiography has thus provided early and accurate diagnosis of cardiac tumors. Fortunately, the great majority of tumors were myxomas that could be removed at surgery. On a personal note, within 1 week recently, two patients with left atrial myxoma were studied and the findings confirmed by echocardiography. Both had successful surgery.—W. Proctor Harvey, M.D.

Echocardiographic Diagnosis of Mobile Right Atrial Thrombus: Early Recognition and Treatment
Thomas J. Quinn, Jonathan F. Plehn, and Philip R. Liebson (Rush-Presbyterian-St. Luke's Med. Ctr., Chicago)
Am. Heart J. 108:1548–1550, December 1984   3–14

Findings in the first reported patient with the preoperative diagnosis of a right atrial thrombus made by two-dimensional echocardiography are described. Surgical removal of the thrombus was successful.

Man, 66, experienced sudden onset of tachypnea, tachycardia, and diaphoresis. His history was significant for chronic atrial fibrillation, peptic ulcer disease, and recent left carotid system cerebrovascular accident. Examination revealed jugular venous distention, a grade 1/6 systolic ejection murmur at the lower left sternal border, an intermittent early diastolic sound, and hypoxemia. The ECG indicated atrial fibrillation, and nonspecific ST changes were noted. Chest x-ray films showed cardiomegaly with slight pulmonary congestion. The ventilation-perfusion scan revealed segmental defects consistent with a massive pulmonary embolus. Treatment with heparin was started. Two-dimensional echocardiographic studies showed a rotating mass in the right atrium that wedged intermittently in the tricuspid orifice during diastole and protruded into the right ventricular cavity. Surgery disclosed no evidence of the presumed thrombus in either the right atrium or ventricle, but a large thrombus was found in the main pulmonary artery. The patient improved after surgery.

In certain cases, two-dimensional echocardiography may be an appropriate diagnostic procedure for discovering the etiology of pulmonary embolism. The differential diagnosis of a right atrial mass seen on two-dimensional echocardiography includes both tumor and thrombus. Failure to visualize the presence of an attachment to the atrial walls on multiple two-dimensional echocardiographic views, in addition to 360-degree rotation, favors the diagnosis of a free-floating thrombus.

▶ Statistically, the most common etiology of this right atrial mass would be myxoma; therefore, it is understandable that the initial clinical diagnosis in this patient was just that. If it was rheumatic in origin, concomitant mitral stenosis would have been evident. In patients in whom there is a differential diagnosis between right atrial myxoma and valvular tricuspid stenosis, if dizziness or syncope is a symptom, it is most likely myxoma. Of course, this unusual patient presented in the article above could have had dizziness or syncope, or both.—W. Proctor Harvey, M.D.

Doppler Diagnosis of Valvular Aortic Stenosis in Patients Over 60 Years of Age
Arthur S. Agatston, Mathew Chengot, Aswath Rao, Frank Hildner, and Philip Samet (Mt. Sinai Med. Ctr., Miami Beach)
Am. J. Cardiol. 56:106–109, July 1, 1985   3–15

Previous noninvasive methods have failed to quantify aortic stenosis, especially in the elderly. The relationship between Doppler-derived gradients and systolic time intervals and catheterization measurements of gradients was examined prospectively in 17 men and 8 women with suspected aortic stenosis. All were older than age 60 years; the mean age was 72 years. Doppler studies were done a mean of 5 days before cardiac catheterization, and the conditions of all patients remained clinically stable during the interval. Continuous-wave Doppler echocardiography was performed to estimate the peak and mean aortic valve gradients, for comparison with catheter-derived peak-to-peak, peak, and mean gradients. Optimal Doppler signals usually were obtained from the right sternal border with the patient in the far right lateral decubitus position.

The Doppler peak gradient correlated well with the catheter-derived peak-to-peak and peak gradients, with respective correlation coefficients of 0.80 and 0.82. The best correlation (0.89) was noted between the Doppler-derived and catheter-derived mean gradients. With a single exception, a modified time-to-peak/modified left ventricle ejection time ratio of 0.3 was used to distinguish between patients with a peak-to-peak catheter gradient below and above 50 mm Hg.

The Doppler approach can be used to evaluate the conditions of elderly patients suspected of having aortic stenosis. A Doppler-derived measure of the timing of peak aortic flow velocity distinguishes patients with aortic gradients above and below 50 mm Hg and helps to avoid overestimation and underestimation of aortic valve gradients.

▶ The use of Doppler echocardiography is rapidly increasing, as is the practical usefulness of this procedure in these patients. People are living longer today, and we are seeing more and more elderly patients with aortic stenosis whose degree of obstruction can be determined without performing cardiac catheterization.—W. Proctor Harvey, M.D.

Abnormal Systolic Sound Associated With Mobile Prosthetic Mitral Valve Vegetation

Scott W. Sharkey, Richard W. Asinger, Frank L. Mikell, and Lillian Michaud (Hennepin County Med. Ctr. and Univ. of Minnesota, Minneapolis)
Am. Heart J. 108:1565–1567, December 1984   3–16

Mobile intracardiac masses are usually seen in patients with infective endocarditis, intracardiac thrombi, foreign bodies, or tumor. They produce abnormal intracardiac sounds that may provide a bedside clue to their presence. A patient was seen with bioprosthetic mitral valve endocarditis in whom an abnormal systolic sound signaled the presence of a mobile vegetation. Simultaneous echophonocardiography provided insight into the mechanism of the production of the systolic sound.

Woman, 77, with history of mitral valve replacement with an Angell-Shiley

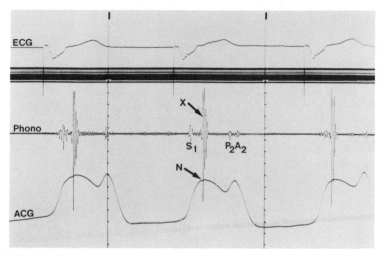

Fig 3–1.—Simultaneous phonocardiogram *(Phono)* and apexcardiogram *(ACG)* on admission. An early systolic notch *(N)* on the upstroke of the apical impulse prior to the E point was present and coincided with the high-frequency early systolic sound *(X)*. P_2 and A_2 are reversed secondary to paced rhythm. (Courtesy of Sharkey, S.W., et al.: Am. Heart J. 108:1565–1567, December 1984.)

porcine prosthesis complained of chronic fatigue and low-grade fever. Cardiac examination revealed a sustained apical impulse with a systolic notch prior to the E point (Fig 3–1) that coincided with a high-frequency sound after both tricuspid closure and aortic opening. A grade II/VI nonspecific systolic murmur was also present at the apex. Two-dimensional echocardiography revealed a large, mobile prosthetic valve vegetation that prolapsed into the left atrium during systole and into the left ventricle during diastole. Simultaneous echophonocardiography revealed the mass moving into the left ventricle to engage the prosthetic mitral orifice for about 90 msec, followed by rapid motion of the mass into the left atrium coinciding with onset of the extra heart sound. The patient refused valve replacement. Repeat echophonocardiography revealed that no abnormal cardiac sounds occurred during cycles when the valve vegetation failed to prolapse into the left atrium. The patient had clinical evidence of left femoral artery occlusion with disappearance of the mass from the mitral valve prosthesis. Emergency embolectomy was performed.

The abnormal extrasystolic sound is related to prolapse of the valve vegetation through the prosthesis into the left atrium. The early components of the sound probably result from delayed mitral valve closure, and the later component may be caused by the sudden arrest of motion of the vegetation.

▶ This sound was explained by echophonocardiography, and the subsequent clinical follow-up examination showed disappearance of this sound when the prosthetic valve vegetation dislodged and embolized to the left femoral artery. This report alerts us to the occurrence of a sound (and possible murmur) caused by vegetations. In addition, it may be more common than is generally realized.—W. Proctor Harvey, M.D.

Hypertrophic Cardiomyopathy

Life Expectancy Analysis in Patients With Chagas' Disease: Prognosis After One Decade (1973–1983)

Raúl Espinosa, Hugo A. Carrasco, Francisco Belandria, Abdel M. Fuenmayor, César Molina, Rodolfo González, and Owen Martínez (Univ. of Los Andes, Mérida, Venezuela)

Int. J. Cardiol. 8:45–56, May 1985   3–17

Knowledge about the natural history of Chagas' disease is limited. The evolution of chronic Chagas' disease was studied in 107 patients with a positive Guerreiro-Machado reaction and positive hemagglutination test results; findings were compared with those in 22 normal controls during a follow-up period of 3–10 years (mean, 4.9 years). Initial workup consisted of noninvasive evaluation and invasive studies, e.g., left and right catheterization and cineventriculography, coronary arteriography, electrophysiologic evaluation of sinoatrial node function and atrioventricular conduction, and septal endomyocardial biopsy.

Patients were classified into four groups according to the degree of myocardial damage: group IA had normal ECG findings and no evidence of heart disease, 18 patients; group IB had normal ECG findings and early left cineventriculographic signs of segmental myocardial damage, 13 patients; group II had abnormal ECG findings, advanced myocardial damage, and no signs of congestive heart failure, 42 patients; and group III had abnormal ECG findings, end-stage heart disease, and congestive heart failure, 34 patients. After reevaluation with invasive studies, one of five group IA patients (20%) progressed to group IB with signs of left ventricular apical synergy indicative of segmental damage. Four of 12 group IB patients progressed to group II (33%) with abnormal ECG findings at a mean follow-up period of 69 months. Six of 40 group II patients (15%) evolved to group III with congestive heart failure developing within a mean of 54 months. Overall, a significant decrease in life expectancy (88% for the first year, 63% after 5 years, and 40% after 10 years) was found for patients with Chagas' disease as compared with findings in controls ($P <$ .0005). Patients with normal ECG findings (groups IA and IB) had normal life expectancy during the 10-year follow-up period. In contrast, groups II and III patients had significantly decreased life expectancy (95% and 71% for the first year, 79% and 19% after 5 years, and 65% and 9% after 10 years, respectively). Overall mortality for chagasic patients was 36%; no patient in group IA or IB died. Nine in group II (23%) and 28 in group III (82%) succumbed. Main terminal events included refractory congestive heart failure, sudden death, and systemic thromboembolism. Sudden death was common in group II patients (44%), whereas refractory congestive heart failure was more frequent in group III patients (50%).

Chronic Chagas' disease follows an evolutionary course from an asymptomatic stage with normal ECG findings to arrhythmic and congestive stages. A positive Guerreiro-Machado reaction is related to decreased life expectancy in patients with abnormal ECG results or congestive heart failure.

▶ A natural history study such as this in a significant number of patients (107) is always helpful in the better understanding of the natural history of this type of cardiomyopathy as well as that of specific or idiopathic types of dilated cardiomyopathy. It remains a truism: Early suspicion, early diagnosis, early treatment.—W. Proctor Harvey, M.D.

Coronary Artery Disease in Hypertrophic Cardiomyopathy
Dennis V. Cokkinos, Zvonimir Kracjer, and Robert D. Leachman (Tzanio State Hosp., Athens, and St. Luke's Episcopal-Texas Heart Inst., Houston)
Am. J. Cardiol. 55:1437–1438, May 1, 1985   3–18

Atherosclerotic coronary artery disease (CAD) causing angina pectoris and myocardial infarction in patients with hypertrophic cardiomyopathy is being reported with increasing frequency. To determine the incidence of CAD in these patients, 85 individuals underwent hemodynamic evaluation, left ventriculography, and coronary arteriography. Significant CAD was defined as luminal diameter narrowing of more than 60%.

Sixteen patients (19%) had significant CAD in one or more coronary arteries. Overall, 94% of the patients with and 43% of those without CAD were older than 45 years ($P < .01$). Compared with patients who had no CAD, those with CAD were significantly older (mean age, 64 years vs. 42 years, $P < .001$), had more episodes of angina pectoris (81% vs. 46%, $P < .05$), and had lower left ventricular end-diastolic pressure (17 mm Hg vs. 23 mm Hg, $P < .02$). Recent worsening of symptoms was present in 5 of 13 patients with CAD and angina. After a 5-year follow-up period, all five surgically treated patients with CAD were relieved of angina. There was no operative mortality among 40 patients without CAD who underwent surgery for hypertrophic cardiomyopathy.

All patients with hypertrophic cardiomyopathy older than age 45 years, particularly those with angina pectoris, should undergo coronary arteriography in addition to hemodynamic evaluation. Patients with combined hypertrophic cardiomyopathy and CAD may benefit from corrective surgery for the former disease concomitantly with coronary artery bypass surgery; the risk of mortality is relatively low.

▶ Useful information in a significant number of patients (85) having hypertrophic cardiomyopathy.—W. Proctor Harvey, M.D.

Active Myocarditis in the Spectrum of Acute Dilated Cardiomyopathies: Clinical Features, Histologic Correlates, and Clinical Outcome
G. William Dec, Jr., Igor F. Palacios, John T. Fallon, H. Thomas Aretz, John Mills, Daniel C.-S. Lee, and Robert Arnold Johnson (Massachusetts Genl. Hosp. and Harvard Med. School)
N. Engl. J. Med. 312:885–890, April 4, 1985   3–19

Acute heart failure caused by dilated cardiomyopathy is a dramatic manifestation of acute myocarditis. The findings were reviewed in 27 patients with acute dilated cardiomyopathy who had symptoms for less than 6 months and were followed up for an average of 18 months after referral for endomyocardial biopsy. No specific cause of dilated cardiomyopathy was found other than active myocarditis in these patients. Right heart catheterization and ventriculography were done in conjunction with transvenous endomyocardial biopsy. Nine patients received immunosuppressive therapy, usually both azathioprine and prednisone.

The mean patient age was 42 years. Sixty-five percent of patients had biventricular heart failure, whereas most of the others had left heart failure. Ten patients (37%) died during the follow-up period, six of severe heart failure and four suddenly and unexpectedly. Two of the 11 patients found on monitoring to have episodic ventricular tachycardia died suddenly. Biopsy results were positive in 18 patients, but the histologic classification was not related to the outcome. Four of the nine patients given immunosuppressive therapy improved, but some patients with resolution of inflammation failed to improve clinically.

Active myocarditis can produce acute dilated cardiomyopathy, and in many patients unexplained dilated cardiomyopathy may result from myocarditis. The efficacy of immunosuppressive therapy in this setting remains to be established.

▶ This paper represents additional scientific documentation of primary myocardial involvement, such as that having a viral etiology, followed in some instances by an autoimmune response that continues the myocardial damage; in some patients this eventually results in irreversible dilated cardiomyopathy with continued decompensation.—W. Proctor Harvey, M.D.

Improved Survival With Amiodarone in Patients With Hypertrophic Cardiomyopathy and Ventricular Tachycardia
William J. McKenna, Celia M. Oakley, Dennis M. Krikler, and John F. Goodwin (Royal Postgrad. Med. School, London)
Br. Heart J. 53:412–416, April 1985   3–20

In about 25% of patients with hypertrophic cardiomyopathy, ventricular tachycardia is observed on ECG monitoring; these patients are at an increased risk of sudden death. Amiodarone treatment was evaluated in 86 patients aged at least 5 years seen between 1976 and 1979 with a diagnosis of hypertrophic cardiomyopathy. More than two consecutive ventricular extrasystoles with a mean rate exceeding 120 beats per minute were found in two of seven patients having 24-hour ECG monitoring and in 22 of 79 monitored for 48 hours. Most patients received propranolol, as well as disopyramide or quinidine in many instances. Of the seven patients who died suddenly during the 3-year follow-up period, five had continued to have ventricular tachycardia.

Ventricular tachycardia was detected by 48-hour monitoring in 21 of 82 subsequent patients with hypertrophic cardiomyopathy. They received amiodarone in daily doses of 150–400 mg, the median dose being 300 mg. Tachycardia was suppressed in all instances as determined by repeat monitoring. Two patients died suddenly during the 3-year follow-up period, but neither had received amiodarone. Treatment with amiodarone was significantly associated with improved survival and may prevent sudden death in patients with hypertrophic cardiomyopathy and ventricular tachycardia.

▶ Any drug that can prevent the dire complication of sudden death in patients having hypertrophic cardiomyopathy is a welcome and needed addition in management. A word of caution is that this treatment is not without complications resulting from the drug itself; therefore, the physician prescribing amiodarone should be familiar with these side effects and ensure that the patient has careful close follow-up.—W. Proctor Harvey, M.D.

Three Autopsy Cases of Progression to Left Ventricular Dilatation in Patients With Hypertrophic Cardiomyopathy

Chikao Yutani, Masami Imakita, Hatsue Ishibashi-Ueda, Kaoru Hatanaka, Seiki Nagata, Hiroshi Sakakibara, and Yusuharu Nimura (Natl. Cardiovascular Ctr., Osaka, Japan)
Am. Heart J. 109:545–553, March 1985   3–21

The course of hypertrophic cardiomyopathy is extremely variable. The hearts of three patients with congestive heart failure and dilated left ventricles caused by symptomatic hypertrophic cardiomyopathy were examined morphologically in an attempt to clarify the relationship between fibrosis and myocardial disarray and the development of fibrosis in patients with hypertrophic cardiomyopathy who die of congestive failure. One patient died suddenly and two died of profound chronic heart failure. Echocardiography showed an increased diastolic left ventricular (LV) internal dimension. Both disproportionate hypertrophy of the left ventricle and systolic anterior motion of the mitral valve contributed to the diagnosis.

The left ventricle was dilated in all three patients (Fig 3–2). In two hearts the interventricular septum was asymmetrically thickened. No patient had more than 25% narrowing of major coronary vessels. The mean area of LV fibrosis was 34.7% at the upper third level and 47.4% at the lower third level. It was associated with disarray in 84.4% of the patients. Fibrosis was most extensive in the lateral LV wall, followed by the posterior, anterior, and interventricular walls.

Disarray in these patients may be responsible for the fibrosis leading to dilatation of the left ventricle. The pathoetiology of myocardial disarray remains unknown. The hearts of most patients with hypertrophic cardiomyopathy do not exhibit the massive fibrosis observed in the present study.

▶ A few of these patients have been personally observed over the past years.

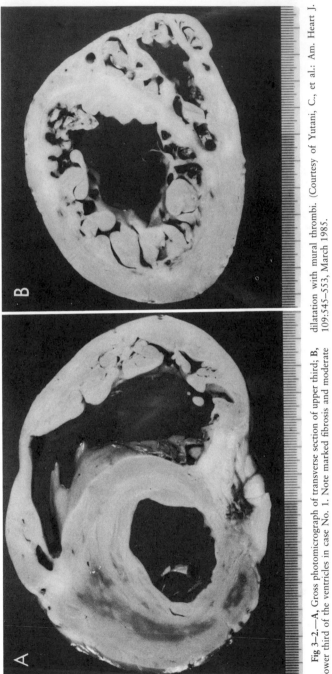

Fig 3–2.—A, Gross photomicrograph of transverse section of upper third; **B,** lower third of the ventricles in case No. 1. Note marked fibrosis and moderate dilatation with mural thrombi. (Courtesy of Yutani, C., et al.: Am. Heart J. 109:545–553, March 1985.

The possibility of this progression is a poorly recognized fact.—W. Proctor Harvey, M.D.

Apical Hypertrophic Cardiomyopathy: Evaluation by Noninvasive and Invasive Techniques in 23 Patients
Gad Keren, Bernard Belhassen, Jack Sherez, Hylton I. Miller, Rebecca Megidish, Dora Berenfeld, and Shlomo Laniado (Tel Aviv Med. Ctr. and Tel Aviv Univ.)
Circulation 71:45–56, January 1985   3–22

Japanese investigators recently described a form of nonobstructive hypertrophic cardiomyopathy characterized by disproportionate hypertrophy of the left ventricular (LV) apical region. Twenty-three patients with apical hypertrophic cardiomyopathy were seen in a 3-year period. The diagnosis was made when echocardiography showed ventricular hypertrophy virtually confined to the apical part of the left ventricle without an apparent cardiac or systemic cause. The 16 men and 7 women had a mean age of 62 years. Seven patients had a history of recurrent myocardial infarction not confirmed enzymatically. Atypical chest pain was the most frequent symptom. Seven patients had typical anginal pain. No patient used alcohol heavily, and only one was athletic.

All patients had T wave inversion in the anterolateral ECG leads. Only

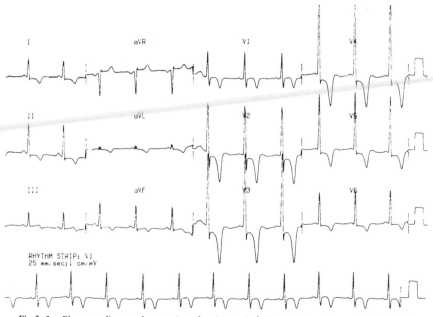

Fig 3–3.—Electrocardiogram from patient showing typical giant negative T waves and high-voltage QRS in precordial leads. (Courtesy of Keren, G., et al.: Circulation 71:45–56, January 1985; by permission of the American Heart Association, Inc.)

five had high QRS voltage with giant negative T waves (Fig 3–3). Most patients had some ST segment depression. Echocardiography showed markedly increased septal and posterior wall thicknesses toward the apex, significantly obliterating the LV cavity in the apical region. Aortic valve flow was normal on pulsed Doppler study in all cases. All but 2 of 14 patients having nuclide studies had normal LV contraction. The end-diastolic contour of the left ventricle was abnormal at cardiac catheterization in all six patients studied, but an "ace-of-spades" configuration was seen in only one. The mean ejection fraction was 72%. All patients but one had normal coronary arteries. The clinical, ECG, and echocardiographic findings were similar after a mean follow-up period of 22 months.

Apical hypertrophic cardiomyopathy appears to be a localized disturbance that does not involve the mitral apparatus. No etiologic factors were identified in the present study. A correct diagnosis is important in younger patients with chest pain and significant ECG changes. The diagnosis usually can be made noninvasively, but cardiac catheterization may be warranted in older patients with typical anginal symptoms.

▶ Obviously, this condition is not confined to Japan. The 23 patients reported were from Israel. It is now likely that similar patients throughout the world will be identified. Certainly, an ECG as shown in the above figures will serve as a reminder to us to consider this condition.—W. Proctor Harvey, M.D.

Apical Hypertrophic Cardiomyopathy in American Patients
James L. Vacek, William R. Davis, Raye L. Bellinger, and Thomas L. McKiernan (U.S. Air Force Med. Ctr., Keesler, Miss.)
Am. Heart J. 108:1501–1506, December 1984   3–23

Apical concentric hypertrophy is a subtype of nonobstructive hypertrophic cardiomyopathy described in Japanese, other Asian, and South African patients. The first three known American patients were identified recently. These patients complained of chest pain, and the ECG and ventriculographic changes described by Yamaguchi et al. were observed. No patient had a history of known heart disease or other significant systemic illness. A typical ECG is shown in Figure 3–4. Ventriculograms showed a "spadelike" configuration at end-diastole and vigorous systolic contraction. A thallium image showed increased apical isotope uptake both at rest and on exercise. A two-dimensional echocardiographic study showed concentric apical hypertrophy.

Nearly half of the described patients wtih apical hypertrophic cardiomyopathy were asymptomatic. More than 90% were male. Chest pain and exertional dyspnea were the most frequent presenting features, as in classic idiopathic hypertrophic subaortic stenosis. "Giant" negative T waves with high precordial QRS voltages were seen on the ECG, and a spadelike configuration with marked apical obliteration was seen in the right anterior oblique projection of the left ventricle in diastole. One of the present patients is the first black patient to be reported.

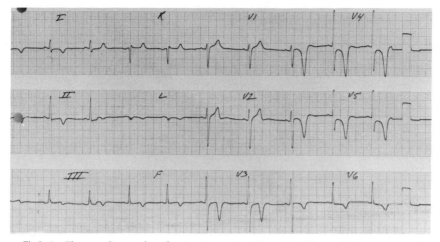

Fig 3–4.—Electrocardiogram from first American patient. Note "giant" inverted T waves in precordial leads and high precordial voltage as well as long QT$_c$. (Courtesy of Vacek, J.L., et al.: Am. Heart J. 108:1501–1506, December 1984.)

A wide racial and geographic spectrum of concentric apical hypertrophic cardiomyopathy appears to exist. The disorder may be found in Americans. The lack of left ventricular outflow tract obstruction in these patients can be ascribed to the absence of excessive septal thickness in the region of the outflow tract during systole.

▶ The ECG as shown above, in addition to the symptoms as described and the "spadelike" cavity configuration of the left ventricular angiogram, are features leading to this diagnosis. This article alerts us to look for this form of cardiomyopathy.—W. Proctor Harvey, M.D.

Progression of Hypertrophic Cardiomyopathy: A Cross-sectional Echocardiographic Study
Stefano Domenicucci, Ettore Lazzeroni, Jos Roelandt, Folkert J. ten Cate, Wim B. Vletter, A. Carntzenius, and Sunil K. Das
Br. Heart J. 53:405–411, April 1985   3–24

Because of its low sensitivity and specificity in detecting hypertrophy in patients with hypertrophic cardiomyopathy, the ECG may not be useful for studying the progression of hypertrophy. In 39 patients with hypertrophic cardiomyopathy, disease progression was monitored by cross-sectional echocardiography during a mean follow-up period of 42 months. The regional distribution of left ventricular hypertrophy as determined by cross-sectional echocardiograms was observed in the parasternal long-axis and short-axis views, the apical four-chamber view, and the apical long-axis view. Progression was defined as extension of hypertrophy to another region, from the basal to the apical region and vice versa along the left ventricular long axis, and to one or more segments of the same region along the left ventricular axis. Serial ECG was also performed in all patients.

Progression of hypertrophy was noted in four patients treated with propranolol. In two patients it affected an additional region in the left ventricular long axis plane, extending into the apical region in one and to the basal region in the other. In the other two patients it affected another segment of the same region along the left ventricular short axis extending from the septum into the free wall. Electrocardiography failed to detect the progression of hypertrophy in two of these patients: one had left bundle branch block and the other had no change. However, in the other two patients, a significant increase in QRS voltage (Sokolow-Lyon index increase of more than 10 mm) was seen on ECG, as was an increase of at least 3 points in the Romhilt-Estes score. None of the 11 patients who underwent myotomy-myectomy had progression of hypertrophy.

Serial cross-sectional echocardiographic studies accurately detect the progression of hypertrophy in affected patients. Although septal myotomy-myectomy may prevent the progression of hypertrophy and produce symptomatic improvement, this observation requires further confirmation.

▶ It appears that echocardiography is an additional method of studying progression of hypertrophic cardiomyopathy that can be added to other parameters. It is of interest that progression of hypertrophy was not seen in any of the 11 patients treated surgically with septal myotomy-myectomy; concerning this, a larger number of patients will bear watching with interest.—W. Proctor Harvey, M.D.

Dynamic Subaortic Obstruction in Hypertrophic Cardiomyopathy: Analysis by Pulsed Doppler Echocardiography
Barry J. Maron, John S. Gottdiener, Javier Arce, Douglas R. Rosing, Yvonne E. Wesley, and Stephen E. Epstein (Natl. Heart, Lung, and Blood Inst., Bethesda, Md.)
J. Am. Coll. Cardiol. 6:1–15, July 1985   3–25

It is not certain whether true obstruction to left ventricular (LV) ejection is present in patients with hypertrophic cardiomyopathy and a subaortic gradient. Pulsed Doppler echocardiography was used to estimate flow velocities and their relation to valve motion and LV dynamics in 50 patients with hypertrophic cardiomyopathy who had a markedly hypertrophied but nondilated left ventricle and no other disorder capable of producing LV hypertrophy. The mean age was 32 years. Nineteen patients were in New York Heart Association functional classes III and IV and 12 were asymptomatic. Twenty asymptomatic controls also were evaluated.

Twenty of the 50 study patients had evidence of obstructive hypertrophic cardiomyopathy. Early, rapid LV emptying was evident in these individuals. An average of 58% of forward flow velocity preceded initial mitral-septal contact, and presumably the onset of the subaortic gradient as well, whereas more than 40% followed mitral-septal contact. The LV ejection was prolonged. Most patients had a relatively small second peak in flow velocity during late systole. The 30 patients with nonobstructive hypertrophic cardiomyopathy had no evidence of impedance to LV ejection; the systolic ejection period was normal in this group.

Mechanical obstruction to forward flow does occur in some patients with hypertrophic cardiomyopathy, and a significant proportion of total LV egress is impeded by interposition of the mitral leaflets into the LV outflow tract. A greatly increased intraventricular pressure results, with the ventricle continuing to work and empty while mitral systolic anterior motion and the subaortic gradient are present. This situation can be expected to lead to excessive myocardial oxygen demand and, after chronic obstruction, to progressive hypertrophy. Abolition of the gradient and normalization of intraventricular pressures by septal myotomy-myectomy remain the rational therapeutic goals in these patients.

▶ This article and the one that follows renew the controversy of the past two decades concerning subaortic obstruction in patients with hypertrophic cardiomyopathy.—W. Proctor Harvey, M D.

Dynamic Subaortic Obstruction in Hypertrophic Cardiomyopathy: Criteria and Controversy

Robert A. Levine and Arthur E. Weyman (Massachusetts Gen. Hosp. and Harvard Univ., Boston)
J. Am. Coll. Cardiol. 6:16–18, July 1985   3–26

It has been suggested that the subaortic gradient in hypertrophic cardiomyopathy is caused by rapid, unimpeded ejection of blood from the ventricle early during systole, with contraction of the ventricular walls occurring around a virtually empty chamber after the bulk of ejection has taken place. In 1980, Murgo et al. demonstrated abnormal ejection in patients wtih hypertrophic cardiomyopathy with or without a subaortic gradient, and proposed that a gradient does not impede left ventricular (LV) outflow. In 1985, Maron et al., using both Doppler ultrasound and imaging echocardiography, found that patients with a gradient or its echographic correlate have physiologic subaortic obstruction to LV outflow, based on the criterion of flow in the presence of a gradient. Both studies indicate that, in patients with hypertrophic cardiomyopathy and a subaortic pressure gradient, most of the forward flow is ejected in the presence of a gradient.

It may be unreasonable to expect uniform physiologic findings in a disorder as pleomorphic as hypertrophic cardiomyopathy is. Further study is needed to relate flow events in the outflow tract to the onset of systolic anterior mitral valve motion. Moreover, the question remains of how mitral systolic anterior motion, if it is flow related, is maintained during late systole when aortic flow velocity is low or negligible. It also is uncertain how a second peak of aortic flow can occur while mitral-septal contact persists. The clinical features of hypertrophic cardiomyopathy reflect a complex combination of systolic, diastolic, electrical, and coronary flow abnormalities.

Relation Between Left Ventricular Gradient and Relative Stroke Volume Ejected in Early and Late Systole in Hypertrophic Cardiomyopathy: Assessment With Radionuclide Cineangiography

Declan D. Sugrue, William J. McKenna, Shaughan Dickie, Melvyn J. Myers, J. Peter Lavender, Celia M. Oakley, and John F. Goodwin (Royal Postgrad. Med. School, London)
Br. Heart J. 52:602–609, December 1984   3–27

Hypertrophic cardiomyopathy is characterized by hyperkinetic left ventricular (LV) function, but the effect of an outflow tract gradient on the hemodynamics of ejection remains controversial. Using high temporal resolution time activity curves from technetium-99m gated equilibrium radionuclide angiography, the proportion of stroke volume ejected during early and late systole was measured in 57 patients with hypertrophic cardiomyopathy with (n = 26) and without (n = 31) LV gradients to determine the functional importance of these gradients. Eighteen normal persons served as controls.

In patients with hypertrophic cardiomyopathy, the mean LV ejection fraction and peak LV ejection rate were significantly higher, and the time to peak ejection was shorter. The proportion of stroke volume ejected during the initial third, the initial 50%, and the initial 80% of systole was greater than in controls, but it was identical in patients with or without LV gradients. The duration systole was similar in all groups, together with diastolic and systolic blood pressures and end-diastolic volumes.

The findings suggest that an LV outflow gradient does not represent true obstruction. Therefore, its clinical relevance, particularly with regard to the effect of combined myotomy and myectomy, remains questionable. These findings are also consistent with those of previous reports suggesting that clinical features and prognostic indicators do not relate to gradients in hypertrophic cardiomyopathy.

▶ The authors add more fuel to the controversy and give support to the concept that the ventricular outflow gradient does not represent true obstruction.—W. Proctor Harvey, M.D.

Miscellaneous Topics

Cardiac Involvement in Coxsackie Virus Infection
N. R. Krishnan, J. Rai, M. M. Ghosh, H. L. Kher, and G. Kuppuswamy (Armed Forces Med. College, India)
Indian Heart J. 37:13–17, January–February 1985   3–28

Coxsackieviruses have been implicated in cardiac infection. When a review was made of data on 171 patients seen in 1977–1979 in Pune, India, with acute viral infection, 58 (34%) were found to have evidence of cardiac involvement. Results of virologic tests were positive in 20 patients. There were no clinical or ECG differences between the 20 patients with coxsackievirus heart disease and the others. The course of illness was similar in these groups during a follow-up period of 6–24 months.

Coxsackieviruses can cause a wide range of illnesses. The six group B subtypes are chiefly responsible for producing myocarditis. The main findings are a pericardial or pleuropericardial rub, tachycardia, and arrhythmias. A pericardial rub was heard in about half of the present patients, and five had pericardial effusion of the serous type. No patient had evidence of constrictive pericarditis on follow-up study. Three patients had moderate heart failure. There may be ECG findings of pericarditis, myocarditis, or both. Arrhythmias have been attributed to viral involvement of the atrioventricular node. The only evidence of infection in patients seen late in the course may be a high neutralizing antibody titer.

The patients in this study received symptomatic treatment only. Adequate rest, good oxygenation, and good nutrition are important. Acutely ill patients may require intensive care. Patients with myocarditis have a low threshold for digitalis toxicity. Corticosteroid treatment is best withheld early in the course, but may be highly effective in acute viral pericarditis. Administration of interferon or an interferon inducer may help to prevent viral myocarditis. The average duration of illness was about 8–12 weeks; there were no sequelae.

▶ Clinically, there appears to be no question that virus infection is the culprit causing myocarditis or pericarditis and is associated with the subsequent development of features of dilated cardiomyopathy. This report supplies evidence of viral infection of the heart. A word of caution in such patients: Look carefully and specifically for subtle signs of heart involvement [mild pulsus alternans, atrial (S_4) and ventricular diastolic (S_3) gallops] before concluding that there are no sequelae. If these findings are present, more prolonged periods of reduced activity are indicated before it can be assumed that the patient has recovered.

Although postulated by "armchair" analysis several decades ago, there was little definite proof that viruses played an important role in the etiology of dilated cardiomyopathy. Another factor, also postulated by "armchair" deduction, is that of the presence of autoimmune reactions to explain the clinical picture of progressive and irreversible dilated cardiomyopathy. This next article gives scientific support to this theory.—W. Proctor Harvey, M.D.

Autoimmune Myocarditis Induced by *Trypanosoma cruzi*
Alberto M. Acosta and Charles A. Santos-Buch (Cornell Univ.)
Circulation 71:1255–1261, June 1985   3–29

Chagas' disease, or American trypanosomiasis, is the most common cause of congestive heart failure and sudden death worldwide. An estimated 20 million persons in the western hemisphere are affected. Severe cardiac involvement can occur in the absence of intracellular *Trypanosoma cruzi* forms in the heart, and the pathogenesis of the disease is uncertain.

Antiheart immune reactions have been described in both human and experimental Chagas' disease. Autoimmunity was investigated in BALB/c mice infected with a small inoculum of the Colombia strain of *T. cruzi*. Studies were done at intervals up to 150 days after intraperitoneal inoculation of 50 trypomastigotes.

No antiheart lymphocyte cytotoxicity was evident up to 120 days after infection. No lesions or pseudocysts of *T. cruzi* amastigotes were found in the heart, skeletal muscle, or colon. Mice infected for 150 days showed specific lysis of syngeneic heart cells and also focal, but widely distributed, mononuclear cell myocarditis with myocardial cell necrosis. Intracellular pseudocysts of *T. cruzi* were not seen. The ganglioneurons of the heart were unaltered. Parasitemia was demonstrated throughout the course of infection. Mice immunized with a cross-reacting antigen from a syngeneic or heterogeneic source had splenic lymphocyte cytotoxicity to normal syngeneic heart cells as well as mononuclear cell myocarditis with focal necrosis.

Long-term infection of mice with a small inoculum of *T. cruzi* produced autoimmune antiheart lymphocyte cytotoxicity in vitro in this study. These autoimmune antiheart reactions may involve cross-reacting antigens shared by *T. cruzi* and heart muscle. Long-term infection may sensitize the host immune system to shared muscle antigen, which may trigger the development of the cell-mediated autoimmune reactions that give rise to mononuclear myocarditis and cardiac damage.

The Heart in Polyarteritis Nodosa: A Clinicopathologic Study
Margaret L. Schrader, Judith S. Hochman, and Bernardine Healy Bulkley (Johns Hopkins Univ.)
Am. Heart J. 109:1353–1359, June 1985   3–30

Previous studies found that the heart is often involved in polyarteritis nodosa, a necrotizing vasculitis affecting arteries of small and medium size. The clinical and pathologic findings in 36 autopsied patients with polyarteritis nodosa were studied to characterize cardiac involvement in this disease.

Of 18 (50%) patients with evidence of coronary arteritis, the disease was classified as healed in six, mild in five, and active in seven. Patients with active disease had short survivals (3.2 months) and concomitant mild diffuse interstitial myocarditis (43%). Those with healed disease had the longest mean survival (36 months) and the heaviest mean heart weight at autopsy (616 gm). Patients were also categorized according to the chronology of their disease (before or after 1952). The 22 patients who had onset of disease after 1952 were subgrouped into those who received steroids (13) and those who had not received them (9). A decrease in coronary arteritis was noted in the post-1952 group. The incidence of active arteritis was highest among patients whose disease had its onset before 1952 (29%) and lowest in the steroid-treated group (8%). There were no significant differences in the frequency of hypertension, congestive failure, degree of renal impairment, or cardiomegaly between those with disease onset before 1952 and the steroid-treated group. Mean survival increased in those with disease onset after 1952 (11.2 vs. 25.5 months), but was only slightly increased in the steroid-treated group.

Cardiac involvement in polyarteritis nodosa may be owing largely to the secondary effects of hypertension, renal failure, and steroid therapy. Although arteritis is present in 50% of the patients, it is healed or trivial in most.

▶ It is unusual to have a carefully documented report of 36 patients with polyarteritis among a total of 200 who had some form of arteritis. It is useful information to be remembered.—W. Proctor Harvey, M.D.

Cardiac Lesions in Acquired Immune Deficiency Syndrome (AIDS)
Carmine Cammarosano and William Lewis (Univ. of California at Los Angeles)
J. Am. Coll. Cardiol. 5:703–706, March 1985   3–31

Cardiac manifestations of the acquired immunodeficiency syndrome (AIDS) may be clinically significant, but they are not helpful in making the diagnosis. The findings in 41 patients with AIDS autopsied in 1981–1984 were reviewed. Ten patients had cardiovascular involvement. The mean age was 36 years. All ten patients were males; eight were homosexual and one was bisexual; the one heterosexual was a Haitian.

Four patients had Kaposi's sarcoma involving the heart; two had myocardial involvement. Three patients had nonbacterial thrombotic endocarditis, and two of them had systemic embolization with cerebral infarcts. The cardiac vegetations exhibited a fibrin mesh with few chronic inflammatory cells. Fibrinous pericarditis was seen in three hearts, two of which had acute diffuse fibrinous changes of the epicardium. In one patient systemic *Cryptococcus neoformans* infection involved all organs, including the heart.

Primary angiosarcoma of the heart is rare, but Kaposi's sarcoma involved the heart in several patients in this series. Nonbacterial thrombotic endocarditis is associated with various chronic wasting illnesses and malignancies. Other cardiac lesions associated with AIDS include fibrinous pericarditis and cryptococcal myocarditis. Cardiac manifestations of AIDS appear to be prevalent. They may be relatively quiescent clinically, but lead to death in some instances.

▶ One is not surprised to learn of this report documenting cardiac lesions of the dread AIDS. Certainly to be expected are increasing numbers of such patients who will be seen and reported in the medical literature. —W. Proctor Harvey, M.D.

Ocular and Pericardial Involvement in Legionnaires' Disease

Lance Friedland, David R. Snydman, Alan S. Weingarden, Thomas R. Hedges, III, Richard Brown, and Michael Busky (Tufts Univ., Boston; Bay-state Med. Ctr., Springfield, Mass.; and Holyoke Hosp., Holyoke, Mass.

Am. J. Med. 77:1105–1107, December 1984   3–32

Pericardial involvement was recently reported in certain patients with Legionnaires' disease, occurring concomitantly with pneumonia in all instances. The patient described herein with *Legionella* infection was previously healthy and was seen with pericarditis as the initial manifestation of infection.

Man, 28, experienced pleuritic chest pain as well as a nonproductive cough, dyspnea, myalgias, and watery diarrhea. The temperature was 102 F, and a pericardial friction rub was noted. The white blood cell count was 24,500/cu mm with a polymorphonuclear leukocyte value of 79% and a sedimentation rate of 71 mm/ hour. A moderate pericardial effusion was observed on M-mode echocardiography, and the ECG showed diffuse T wave inversions. Bilateral pleural effusions were found subsequently when the dyspnea worsened; thoracentesis yielded serosanguinous fluid with a polymorphonuclear leukocyte count of 28%. The patient's condition worsened despite treatment with chloramphenicol and nafcillin. Roth's spots, cotton wool patches, and hemorrhages appeared in the posterior poles of both retinas. Pulsus paradoxus of 5 mm Hg was present. Symptoms improved somewhat with erythromycin therapy alone, and the pericardial effusion diminished. A diagnostic rise in antibody to *Legionella pneumophila* was noted. The response to intravenously administered erythromycin was good. Pericarditis recurred after 7 months without serologic evidence of recrudescent *Legionella* infection. The ocular abnormalities resolved completely. Indomethacin was given, and the patient did well.

Pericardial involvement is a rare complication of Legionnaires' disease. Both acute pericarditis and Roth's spots are potential manifestations of *L. pneumophila* infection. An absence of cross reactivity to other antigens (e.g., *Mycoplasma*) supported the specificity of serodiagnosis in this case.

▶ This report alerts us to another complication of Legionnaires' disease. It is a possibility that, in some patients with pericarditis, an associated myocarditis could be present.—W. Proctor Harvey, M.D.

Long-Term Follow-Up of Asymptomatic Healthy Subjects With Frequent and Complex Ventricular Ectopy

Harold L. Kennedy, James A. Whitlock, Michael K. Sprague, Lisa J. Kennedy, Thomas A. Buckingham, and Robert J. Goldberg (St. Louis Univ. Med. Ctr.)

N. Engl. J. Med. 312:193–197, Jan. 24, 1984   3–33

Frequent and complex ventricular ectopy in patients with known ischemic heart disease or myocardial disease is associated with increased risk of death and sudden death. However, its role in patients without apparent heart disease remains uncertain. From 1973 to 1983, 73 asymptomatic healthy persons (mean age, 46 years), who were discovered to have frequent and complex ventricular ectopy, were followed for 1 year to 9.5 years (mean, 6.5 years) to determine the long-term prognosis of asymptomatic ventricular ectopy. Asymptomatic healthy status was confirmed by noninvasive cardiologic examination. However, cardiac catheterization in a subsample of 31 patients disclosed serious coronary artery disease in 19%. Hypertension, found in 23 patients (32%) was treated with thiazides or β blockers.

Ventricular ectopy, as measured by 24-hour ambulatory ECG, showed a mean frequency of 566 beats per hour (range, 78–1,994). Ventricular ectopy occurred as multiforms in 63% of the patients, ventricular couplets in 60%, ventricular tachycardia in 26%, and R and T phenomena in 4%. Ventricular ectopy occurred in bigeminy in 96% of the patients and in repetitive patterns in 60%. Follow-up studies in 70 patients (96%) who were initially asymptomatic showed that 15 experienced bothersome palpitations, and another 15 reported some form of chest pain, discomfort, or angina pectoris. There was one sudden death and another death caused by cancer. The standardized mortality ratio (Monson's United States death rate data, eighth revision) for 448 person-years of follow-up observation predicted 7.4 deaths. However, only two deaths occurred (standardized mortality ratio = 27; $P < .05$). The survival experience of these asymptomatic patients with ventricular ectopy was similar to that of patients with no coronary artery disease or with mild narrowing of the coronary arteries, and was increased as compared with that of patients with moderate coronary artery disease or unrecognized myocardial infarction.

The data show that asymptomatic healthy patients with frequent and complex ventricular ectopy have a relatively good long-term prognosis, even some of those who have asymptomatic serious coronary artery disease. The prognosis is comparable to that of the healthy United States population, suggesting no increased risk of death. The present study is limited by the absence of concurrent controls and the small sample size. Furthermore, β-blockade therapy for hypertension or coronary artery disease may have influenced the survival of the study cohort.

▶ Ventricular ectopy in asymptomatic persons is a common problem confronting the practicing physician. This report is both timely and reassuring to the patient as well as to the physician.—W. Proctor Harvey, M.D.

The Arrhythmogenicity of Antiarrhythmic Agents
Vilma Torres, David Flowers, and J. C. Somberg (Albert Einstein College of Medicine)
Am. Heart J. 109:1090–1097, May 1985 3–34

Cardiac arrhythmias sometimes are worsened or facilitated by treatment with antiarrhythmic agents. The findings were reviewed concerning 181 patients referred for programmed electrical stimulation because of ventricular arrhythmias. The 121 men and 60 women had a mean age of 60 years. Arteriosclerotic heart disease was present in most of them, but 30 patients had no evidence of heart disease. Thirty-nine patients had out-of-hospital cardiac arrest, and 62 had hemodynamically symptomatic ventricular tachycardia. Treatment with an average of two drugs had failed clinically before electrophysiologic evaluation. Three fourths of the patients had evidence of heart failure. The antiarrhythmic agents given during programmed electrical stimulation included lidocaine, quinidine, procainamide, cibenzoline, bethanidine, lorcainide, flecainide, bepridil, and ethmozine.

In all, 478 drug tests were carried out. In 23% of patients, induction of ventricular arrhythmia was facilitated by treatment with at least one drug. Facilitation was observed in 13% of all drug tests. Sustained ventricular tachycardia developed during five tests. New sustained hemodynamically significant ventricular tachycardia developed in 11 tests, requiring cardioversion. More than one type of arrhythmogenic response occurred in a number of patients. Serum drug levels in the therapeutic range were found in patients with arrhythmogenic responses. A few patients had subtherapeutic drug levels. There were no significant prolongations in PR, QRS, or QT_c intervals associated with the arrhythmogenic responses for the group as a whole.

Nearly one fourth of these patients had worsening of the induced arrhythmia by treatment with antiarrhythmic agents during programmed electrical stimulation. This approach can rapidly identify drugs that may facilitate arrhythmias in a given patient and also can determine the extent of arrhythmogenicity of various drugs.

▶ This article is a reminder to us that the drugs we use to control arrhythmias can also cause them. It is, of course, important that the possibility of this adverse, sometimes very serious, effect be looked for. This is currently apropos, because many newer drugs are being introduced and advocated for treatment of arrhythmias.—W. Proctor Harvey, M.D.

Constrictive Pericarditis: Assessment of Current Diagnostic Procedures
Rick A. Nishimura, Daniel C. Connolly, Thomas W. Parkin, and Anthony W. Stanson (Mayo Clinic and Found.)
Mayo Clin. Proc. 60:397–401, June 1985   3–35

Constrictive pericarditis poses a diagnostic challenge because of its varied manifestations. However, accurate diagnosis is essential as surgical decortication yields excellent clinical results. Although the use of noninvasive procedures has helped in the diagnosis of constrictive pericarditis, the initial clinical suspicion of this diagnosis must be high for appropriate interpretation of these tests.

Man, 81, was referred for fatigue and dyspnea that worsened despite treatment for "heart failure." Physical findings included dullness to percussion and decreased breath sounds at both lung bases, elevated jugular venous pressure, quiet precordium, and moderate pitting edema. Chest x-ray films showed mild cardiomegaly with no evidence of pericardial calcifications. Small pleural effusions were present bilaterally. The differential diagnosis included dilated cardiomyopathy, restrictive cardiomyopathy, and constrictive pericarditis. Two-dimensional echocardiography disclosed normal size and systolic function of the left ventricle, mildly increased left ventricular wall thickness, mild left and right atrial enlargement, abnormal septal motion, and a dilated inferior vena cava; there was no pericardial abnormality. These features were consistent with restrictive cardiomyopathy or constrictive pericarditis. Computed tomography showed moderate thickening of the pericardium suggestive of constrictive pericarditis. Catheterization of the right side of the heart demonstrated end-diastolic equalization of pressures in the right atrium, right ventricle, and pulmonary artery, and a right ventricular pressure waveform having a dip-and-plateau configuration (square root sign); these findings were suggestive of a constrictive or a restrictive process. Thoracotomy revealed a diffusely adherent and densely fibrotic parietal pericardium and epicardium, which were widely resected. The patient improved.

Constrictive pericarditis should be considered in the differential diagnosis when patients complain of fatigue and dyspnea, and clinical findings include predominantly right-sided heart failure. Echocardiography is useful primarily for distinguishing other cardiac abnormalities simulating constrictive pericarditis, e.g., dilated cardiomyopathy and restrictive cardiomyopathy. Computed tomography is a valuable tool for assessment of pericardial thickening. In addition, evaluation of early diastolic filling by computerized digitization in conjunction with echocardiography, angiography, and invasive hemodynamics shows promise as a diagnostic tool. Despite all of these evaluations, the distinction between constrictive pericarditis and restrictive cardiomyopathy still may be difficult and in some cases may necessitate surgical exploration.

▶ We define a "cardiac pearl" as a clinical fact or finding that either makes the diagnosis or provides a clue that leads to it. The "cardiac pearl" is not changed with the passage of time. An excellent "cardiac pearl" of constrictive pericarditis may be described as (1) the detection of a sound in early diastole that at first might be confused with an opening snap of mitral stenosis (occurring, however, slightly later); this is termed the pericardial knock; and (2) abnormal distention of neck veins.

These two findings may immediately suggest the accurate diagnosis of constrictive pericarditis. In the case report presented, the patient did have jugular vein distention. The pericardial knock was not heard. However, if carefully sought, it will probably be heard in more than 90% of patients.—W. Proctor Harvey, M.D.

Right Ventricular Outflow Obstruction Caused by Constrictive Pericardial Disease

Rick A. Nishimura, Francis J. Kazmier, Hugh C. Smith, and Gordon K. Danielson (Mayo Clinic and Found.)
Am. J. Cardiol. 55:1447–1448, May 1, 1985   3–36

The classic clinical triad of chronic constrictive pericarditis includes increased venous pressure, ascites, and a small quiet heart. A patient was seen with chronic constrictive pericarditis and right ventricular obstruction caused by a pericardial band in the atrioventricular groove, simulating pulmonic stenosis.

Woman, 53, had recurrent peripheral edema and fatigue. Since age 15 she had undergone pericardial resection on several occasions because of recurrent constrictive pericarditis secondary to calcium deposition. Examination revealed jugular venous distention, right parasternal lift, a grade 3/6 systolic ejection murmur at the left sternal border followed by a grade 2/6 mitral valve diastolic rumble, and 2 + peripheral edema. Cardiac catheterization showed the following pressures (mm Hg): right atrium, 11; right ventricle, 80/11; pulmonary artery, 30/16; pulmonary wedge, 14; and left ventricle, 120/8. Selective coronary angiography revealed a prominent collar of calcium in the atrioventricular groove, a thickened pericardium that narrowed the right ventricular outflow tract below the pulmonary valve, and a systolic pressure gradient of 50 mm Hg. Surgery revealed a thick ring of calcium at the atrioventricular groove and over the right ventricular outflow tract. Mitral stenosis, presumably from a rheumatic cause, was relieved by valvotomy. The right ventricular outflow gradient was relieved after resection of the calcified pericardium and pericardial patch enlargement. The patient remained asymptomatic at 12 months postoperatively.

Chronic constrictive pericarditis may occasionally simulate other cardiac abnormalities, in this case pulmonic stenosis. The unusual feature was pronounced right-sided hypertrophy in association with a right-sided outflow murmur.

▶ From a similar mechanism in patients with constrictive pericarditis personally observed has been obstruction between the right atrium and ventricle producing a diastolic rumble that simulates tricuspid stenosis; also, in another patient, similar findings on the left side—obstruction in the left atrioventricular groove producing a diastolic rumble simulating mitral stenosis. Of course, these patients are unusual, but their records illustrate some of the uncommon clinical findings in patients with constrictive pericarditis.—W. Proctor Harvey, M.D.

Myxoid Degeneration of the Aortic Valve and Isolated Severe Aortic Regurgitation

Warren M. Allen, Jack M. Matloff, and Michael C. Fishbein (Cedars-Sinai Med. Ctr., Los Angeles)
Am. J. Cardiol. 55:439–444, Feb. 1, 1985   3–37

Findings were reviewed in 55 patients who had aortic valve replacement for pure aortic regurgitation in 1976–1982, with and without coronary bypass grafting. Seventeen control aortic valves from patients dying of noncardiac causes with no history of valve disease also were examined.

Rheumatic heart disease was established in 11 study patients, and 13 others had a history of endocarditis not associated with rheumatic disease. The diagnosis of Marfan's syndrome and congenital bicuspid aortic valve was made in two patients each. Thirteen of 21 valves from patients in

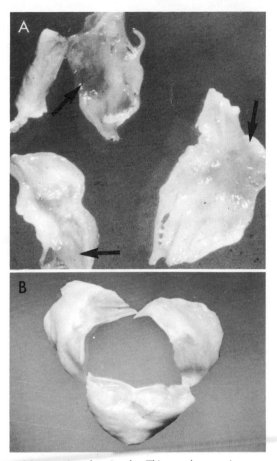

Fig 3–5 A, myxoid degeneration of aortic valve. Thin, translucent regions are present in each leaflet *(arrows)*. **B**, control aortic valve, which does not show this change. (Courtesy of Allen, W.M., et al.: Am. J. Cardiol. 55:439–444, Feb. 1, 1985.)

whom no definite cause of aortic regurgitation was found had pathologic evidence of pure myxoid degeneration (Fig 3–5). All but one of these patients were aged 50 years or older, and all but two were male. Ten of the 13 patients had long-standing systemic hypertension. A widened pulse pressure with low diastolic pressure was a frequent finding. The valves usually were thinned, with extensive cystic change and myxoid degeneration. Significant destruction of the fibrosa was a constant finding. Many of the valves also had nodular thickening, with large "pools" of myxoid material intermixed with fibrosis. Findings in the other patients in whom the cause of valvular insufficiency was unknown included long-standing hypertension and severe coronary artery disease. The valves exhibited fibrosis, focal calcification, and increased amounts of acid mucopolysaccharides.

Myxoid degeneration of the aortic valve was a frequent concomitant of isolated severe aortic regurgitation in this series. In many instances it may be secondary to long-standing systemic hypertension. Myxoid degeneration may be one of the most frequent pathologic entities associated with severe aortic regurgitation. The pathologic process may carry over into the postoperative period.

► This is useful information that is not well known. Remember, also, that in a patient who has diastolic hypertension and in whom aortic regurgitation develops (particularly if the murmur is "right-sided," i.e., heard better along third and fourth right sternal border as compared with the third and fourth left) we should think of aneurysm or dissection, or both, of the first portion of the ascending aorta.—W. Proctor Harvey, M.D.

Aortic Regurgitation in Giant Cell Arteritis
Alice V. Klinkhoff, Graham D. Reid, and Michael Moscovich (Univ. of British Columbia)
Arthritis Rheum. 28:582–585, May 1985   3–38

Giant cell arteritis (GCA) affects large arteries diffusely; it may cause claudication, aneurysmal dilatation, and aortic aneurysmal dissection and rupture. Progressive aortic dilatation and aortic regurgitation developed in a patient with confirmed GCA during a course of low-dose steroid therapy.

Woman, 65, experienced severe temporal headaches with scalp tenderness and had temporal artery biopsy findings of GCA. Prednisone was used in an initial dose of 20 mg daily and then in lower doses down to 2.5 mg daily during a 7-year period. The erythrocyte sedimentation rate fell below 35 mm/hour, and exertional dyspnea developed without chest pain or orthopnea. Clinical findings of aortic regurgitation were present. A review of chest roentgenograms showed progressive widening of the mediastinum with cardiomegaly and aneurysmal dilatation of the aorta. Arteriography confirmed a large aneurysm of the ascending aorta with dilatation of the aortic ring and gross regurgitation of contrast medium into the left ventricle. The aorta and its branch vessels also were dilated. Coronary artery disease was present, and the patient had evidence of old anterior infarction. Prednisone was given in a daily dose of 60 mg, and a daily dose of 20 mg was used 6 months later. Polymyalgic symptoms resolved, but the cardiac status remained unchanged. Chest roentgenograms showed no further increase in aortic dilatation.

This patient, with proved GCA, experienced symptomatic aortic regurgitation as well as polymyalgic symptoms during several years of low-dose prednisone therapy. Six previous reports of aortic regurgitation secondary to GCA have been published; all but one of the seven patients received steroid treatment for GCA. Two patients died of complications of giant cell aortitis. The long-term outlook for these patients is not known, but surgery probably should not be considered until an adequate course of steroid therapy has been given.

▶ This is an unusual etiology for this condition and one to remember. The diastolic murmur was a "right-sided aortic diastolic murmur," a clinical pearl that immediately affords the physician a clue to look for rightward displacement of the first portion of the ascending aorta (resulting from aneurysm or dissection, or another cause) that produces a murmur heard best along the right sternal border as compared with its counterpart on the left. This patient's murmur was described as best heard at the second right interspace. As a rule, this "right-sided murmur" is best detected at the third or fourth right interspace as compared with the left. One wonders if another factor contributing to this patient's aortic aneurysm was hypertension; the blood pressure was 180/90, even though aortic regurgitation was present.—W. Proctor Harvey, M.D.

Rupture of the Myocardium: Occurrence and Risk Factors
Mikael Dellborg, Peter Held, Karl Swedberg, and Anders Vedin (Östra Hosp., Göteborg, Sweden)
Br. Heart J. 54:11–16, July 1985   3–39

Myocardial rupture is the most important cause of hospital death after pump failure that follows AMI. Risk factors were examined in 1,746 consecutive patients hospitalized with AMI. Myocardial rupture was defined as a pathologic passage through either the free left ventricular wall or the septum found at operation or at autopsy. Five patients with isolated papillary muscle rupture were excluded. Autopsy was performed on 75% of patients who died.

Total hospital mortality was 19%. Rupture through the free wall was found at autopsy in 46 patients and through the septum in 5. Another five patients had rupture at operation. Rupture occurred in 3% of all patients and in 17% of operative deaths. Women younger than age 70 years had the highest incidence of rupture. Nearly one third of the ruptures occurred within 24 hours of onset of initial symptoms. Sustained hypertension in the coronary care unit was more frequent in patients with rupture. About 80% of study patients received no corticosteroids. Severe heart failure and antiarrhythmia therapy were relatively infrequent in rupture patients, but more analgesics were used than by controls.

Females with myocardial infarction and patients with sustained chest pain may be at an increased risk of myocardial rupture. Many ruptures may be subacute, allowing time for diagnosis and surgical treatment. The risk appears to be greatest for women younger than age 70 years with sustained pain who are having their first myocardial infarction.

▶ Rupture of the interventricular septum after AMI is probably ten times more common than rupture of the myocardium is. The diagnosis of septal perforation can be made by the history of sudden onset of a loud systolic murmur accompanied by a palpable systolic thrill felt along the left sternal border rather than at the apex. Early recognition of septal perforation or rupture of the myocardium can be life saving because of improved surgical techniques.—W. Proctor Harvey, M.D.

Surgical Pathology of Pure Aortic Insufficiency: A Study of 225 Cases
Lyle J. Olson, Ramiah Subramanian, and William D. Edwards (Mayo Grad. School of Medicine)
Mayo Clin. Proc. 59:835–841, December 1984   3–40

Few studies describe the pathologic features of incompetent aortic valves that have been excised. To determine the incidence and changes in the relative incidence of each form of aortic insufficiency observed in the surgical population during the past two decades, the gross surgical pathologic features of the aortic valve were reviewed in 225 patients. All had clinically pure aortic insufficiency and underwent aortic valve replacement during the years 1965, 1970, 1975, and 1980.

The four most common causes of pure aortic insufficiency were postinflammatory disease (46%), aortic root dilatation (21%), incomplete closure of a congenitally bicuspid aortic valve (20%), and infective endocarditis (9%). Other causes of aortic incompetence included ventricular septal defects (2%) and quadricuspid aortic valves (1%). The cause was indeterminate in 1%. The mean age of the patients at the time of valve replacement for all causes was 50 years, except for those with a ventricular septal defect. All forms of aortic incompetence were much more common in male patients, except for the postinflammatory and indeterminate types, which occurred approximately equally in both sexes. Incompetent aortic valves were either free of calcification or were only minimally involved in 86% of the patients. The incidence of postinflammatory disease and aortic root dilatation changed appreciably during the two decades reviewed. The incidence of postinflammatory disease decreased from 51% before 1980 to 29% in 1980 ($P < .006$), whereas that of aortic root dilatation increased from 17% to 37% ($P < .003$).

Aortic root dilatation is now the most common cause of pure aortic insufficiency in the surgical population. The decreased incidence of postinflammatory disease may be a result of the decreasing incidence of acute rheumatic fever reported in western countries.

► Fortunately, rheumatic heart disease is rapidly decreasing in the United States. In fact, most of our medical students today have never seen a patient with rheumatic fever. We can therefore expect that there will be a continuing decrease in aortic insufficiency resulting from inflammatory disease. Not well appreciated is that a congenital bicuspid valve can result in pure advanced aortic insufficiency and not represent the result of infective endocarditis.—W. Proctor Harvey, M.D.

Tricuspid Stenosis: Atrial Systolic Murmur, Tricuspid Opening Snap, and Right Atrial Pressure Pulse
Charles F. Wooley, Mary E. Fontana, James W. Kilman, and Joseph M. Ryan (Ohio State Univ.)
Am. J. Med. 78:375–384, March 1985   3–41

The crescendo-decrescendo atrial systolic murmur is the most important auscultatory sign of tricuspid stenosis in the presence of sinus rhythm. To investigate the atrial systolic murmur, the tricuspid opening snap, and the right atrial pressure pulse of tricuspid stenosis, right atrial and right ventricular intracardiac manometer sound and pressure recordings were obtained from five patients with hemodynamically significant tricuspid stenosis.

The right atrial pressure pulse of tricuspid stenosis differed from the normal as follows: (1) elevation of right atrial pressure; (2) different morphological features (tall, spiky A wave complete before C; small V wave with an interruption, the tricuspid snap opening notch at termination of the gradual Y descent; and a diastolic plateau, the relatively flat diastolic segment of the right atrial pressure pulse after the tricuspid opening snap notch prior to the next A wave); and (3) a relative lack of right atrial pressure and right atrial pressure pulse response with normal respiration.

The atrial systolic murmur, recorded in the right ventricular outflow tract, was complete by S_1 (Fig 3–6). The crescendo-decrescendo atrial systolic murmur configuration paralleled the right ventricular-right atrial

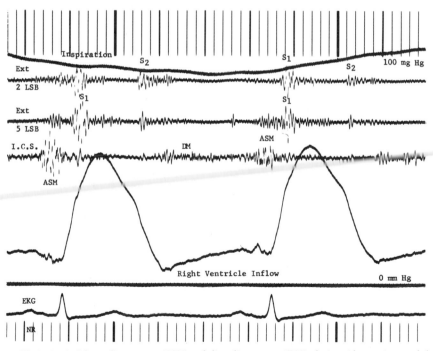

Fig 3–6.—Atrial systolic murmur *(ASM)* and diastolic murmur *(DM)* of tricuspid stenosis recorded in right ventricular inflow tract. *Top to bottom:* respirometer recording, external *(Ext)* phonocardiogram second intercostal space, left sternal border *(LSB)*; external phonocardiogram, fifth intercostal space, left sternal border; intracardiac sound *(I.C.S.)* recording, right ventricular inflow tract; right ventricular pressure pulse, electrocardiogram *(EKG)*. Scale 0 to 100 mm Hg, time lines 40 msec. *NR*, patient 2; S_1, first heart sound; S_2 second heart sound. (Courtesy of Wooley, C.F., et al. Am. J. Med. 78:375–384, March 1985.)

diastolic pressure gradient at the time of the atrial A wave. The right atrial contraction-relaxation process, as reflected by the right atrial A wave ascent and descent, was complete at the onset of ventricular systole with P-R intervals of 170–200 msec. Hence, the configuration and timing of the atrial systolic murmur of tricuspid stenosis reflected the timing and completion of the right atrial contraction-relaxation process prior to onset of right ventricular systole and the configuration of the tricuspid diastolic pressure gradient.

The tricuspid opening snap, recorded in the right ventricular inflow tract, occurred at the time of a notch at the termination of the Y descent of the right atrial pressure pulse V wave, whereas right atrial pressure exceeded right ventricular pressure. The sound-pressure events paralleled the angiographic and echocardiographic documentation of doming, ballooning, or movement of the mobile, stenosed tricuspid valve structure into the right ventricle during the Y descent of the right atrial pressure pulse. The tricuspid opening snap occurred at the time of termination of the diastolic movement of the fused tricuspid valve complex into the right ventricle.

These observations, together with historical and sequential observations, may be viewed as a continuum, with each stage of clinical awareness or technologic development contributing to a more coherent pathophysiologic basis for the observed clinical manifestations in tricuspid stenosis.

▶ The crescendo-decrescendo diastolic murmur in presystole is produced by atrial contraction, and it generally ends before the first heart sound. It does not sound like the typical presystolic murmur of mitral stenosis, which crescendos up to an accentuated first sound. It also may increase strikingly with inspiration.—W. Proctor Harvey, M.D.

Clinical Characteristics of Patients Younger Than 60 Years With Mitral Anular Calcium: Comparison With Age- and Sex-Matched Control Subjects
Chandra K. Nair, Chris Sudhakaran, Wilbert S. Aronow, Wade Thomson, Mark P. Woodruff, and Michael H. Sketch (Creighton Univ.)
Am. J. Cardiol. 54:1286–1287, Dec. 1, 1984   3–42

Mitral anular calcium (MAC) is a degenerative process commonly seen in elderly patients, but it can also occur at younger ages. The clinical features of 107 patients with MAC who were younger than age 60 were compared with those of age-matched and sex-matched controls. The study group included 55 men and 52 women whose mean age was 51 years. They were identified from echocardiographic records obtained in 1978–1982. In patients with MAC, cardiomegaly was more often seen on chest radiography, and left atrial and ventricular enlargement more often observed on echocardiography; also, precordial murmurs were more frequent. They also more often had diabetes and systemic hypertension, and conduction defects were seen more frequently on surface ECG recording. The mean serum phosphorus and calcium-phosphorus values were higher in the study group.

The prevalence of MAC increases linearly with advancing age, but other factors may accelerate its development. Conditions that elevate left ventricular systolic pressure, and thereby increase stress on the mitral apparatus, have been implicated in the accelerated development of MAC. Systemic hypertension was associated with MAC in the present study, but valvular aortic stenosis and hypertrophic cardiomyopathy were not. Patients with MAC had a higher rate of diabetes mellitus, and a higher level of serum phosphorus and product of serum calcium and phosphorus, compared with controls.

▶ One would expect that patients with diabetes mellitus would have a higher incidence of mitral anular calcification, because calcification is increased in arteries throughout the body in diabetic patients. From clinical observations also, diabetes predisposes to calcification of the mitral anulus in patients with mitral valve prolapse. Further, calcium in aortic valves appears more likely in diabetics. Atrial fibrillation is also more frequent in those who have mitral anular calcification.—W. Proctor Harvey, M.D.

Recurring Cardiac Myxoma
Ian R. Gray and W. G. Williams (Walsgrave Hosp., Coventry, England)
Br. Heart J. 53:645–649, June 1985   3–43

Myxoma is the only primary cardiac tumor seen with any frequency. A small number of recurrences have been reported. Two patients with repeated recurrence of myxoma were encountered among 15 who had atrial myxoma, 14 of whom were operated on successfully. Both patients had two further separate operations for recurrent lesions. The intervals before the second recurrences were nearly 11 years and 4½ years. Neither patient had histologic evidence of malignant change. Reported cases of recurrent myxoma are listed in the table. Most known patients have been male, in contrast to findings in primary myxoma. Recurrences were nearly always in the left atrium, as were the original myxomas. Six patients had more than one tumor each. Most recurrences developed within 4 years of initial operation. Five of the six patients with a second recurrence had more than one tumor present.

Incomplete removal of myxoma may explain some recurrences. It also is possible that recurrences are distinct from the original myxoma and represent multiple foci of neoplastic change. Myxoma generally is considered a benign tumor, but tumor emboli behaving in a malignant manner have been described. Malignant histology was reported in only one instance. A second recurrence may be found in about 25% of patients with a first recurrent atrial myxoma. The difference in sex distribution between primary and recurrent myxomas remains to be explained.

▶ Although successful removal of a left atrial myxoma is usually unassociated with recurrence, this article demonstrates that it does happen.
A patient with left atrial myxoma was personally evaluated recently. He had

REPORTED CASES OF RECURRING CARDIAC MYXOMA*

Authors	Age (yr)/sex	Site of primary myxoma	Time of recurrence	Site of recurrence
Gerbode et al (1967)	—	LA	4 yr	LA
Bahl et al (1969)	34/F	LA	6 yr 5 mnth	LA
Walton et al (1972)	—	LA	1 yr 10 mnth	LA, RA
Kelly and Bhagwat et al (1972)	—	LA	7 mnth	LA
Kabbani and Cooley (1973)	19/F	LA	1 yr 5mnth	LA (4)
Mussini-Montpellier et al (1973)	5/M	LA	2 yr	LA
Puel et al (1973)	15/M	LA	1yr 2 mnth	LA (2)
Chassignolle et al (1973)	—	LA	14 yr	LA
Maranhao et al (1973)	—	LA	3 yr 8 mnth	Mitral valve
Read et al (1974)	39/M	LA	7 mnth	LA
Hardin et al (1974)	59/M	LA	1 yr 3mnth	LA
Zackai et al (1974)	47/M	LA	2 yr 6 mnth	LA
Jugdutt et al (1975)	46/M	LA	1 yr 7mnth	LA (2)
Dang and Hurley (1976)	22/M	LA	2 yr 6 mnth	RV
Sasaki et al (1977)	—	LA	3 yr 7 mnth	LA (multiple)
O'Neil et al (1979)	18/M	LA	8 mnth	Tricuspid valve
Attar et al (1980)	—	LA	4 yr	LA
St John Sutton et al (1980)	—	LA	<3 yr	LA
			<3 yr	LA
			<4 yr	LA
Cleveland et al (1983)	—	LA		
Present series (1985)				
Case 1	19/F	LA	11 yr 11 mnth	LA, RA
Case 2	32/M	LA	1 yr 3 mnth	LA

*LA, left atrium; RA, right atrium; RV, right ventricle.
(Courtesy of Gray, I.R., and Williams, W.G.: Br. Heart J. 53:645–649. June 1985.)

no history of heart disease. He occasionally noted "stars" in his vision when he changed position from sitting or lying to standing. The ECG showed notched P waves and left atrial enlargement, and the x-ray film also demonstrated left atrial enlargement. A tumor sound ("plop" as described by Dr. Woofin Cobb) was heard in early diastole at the apex when the patient was lying flat or in the left lateral position; it was absent in the sitting or standing position. This "tumor plop" sound is a valuable bedside clue that was not described in the above report.—W. Proctor Harvey, M.D.

***Streptococcus bovis* Bacteraemia Requires Rigorous Exclusion of Colonic Neoplasia and Endocarditis**
N. J. Beeching, T. I. Christmas, R. B. Ellis-Pegler, and G. I. Nicholson (Auckland Hosp., New Zealand)
Q. J. Med. New Series 56:439–450, August 1985   3–44

Streptococcus bovis is recognized as an important cause of endocarditis that is associated with a better prognosis than enterococcal endocarditis is. *Streptococcus bovis* bacteremia has also been associated with gastrointestinal tract neoplasms. Twelve patients with *S. bovis* bacteremia were seen in Auckland between 1979 and 1984. They included the first known patient with right-sided endocarditis caused by this organism.

All 12 patients were adults, with a mean age of 66 years. Five had definite and five had probable endocarditis; two had septicemia alone. All of the patients with endocarditis had symptoms for at least 3 weeks. Two patients had dense hemiplegia. Both patients with infected homograft valves were operated on for valve destruction and progressive heart failure. Five patients received benzylpenicillin only; six were also given an aminoglycoside. One patient who was treated inappropriately died of septicemia complicating immunosuppression. In no case was there evidence of recent dental sepsis or treatment, or recent genitourinary tract surgery. Three patients had malignant large bowel neoplasms, and five had premalignant changes. Only one of the nine patients studied had no colorectal tumor. One of the three patients with colorectal villous adenoma was an alcoholic with cirrhotic liver failure. Three of the patients with neoplasms had normal radiologic findings.

Bacteremia caused by *S. bovis* should lead to studies excluding both endocarditis and large bowel neoplasia. It is important to distinguish between *S. bovis* and other causes of endocarditis because of prognostic differences. Colonoscopy is more reliable than radiologic studies are in detecting colonic neoplasms in these patients.

▶ This report describes an interesting association, the cause of which is unknown; however, the authors cite the following reference by Klein, R. S., et al: *Streptococcus bovis* septicemia and carcinoma of the colon. *Ann. Intern. Med.* 91:560–562, 1979. These authors found *S. bovis* in 50% of patients with colon adenocarcinoma compared with 28% of those with inflammatory bowel disease and 10% of the controls.—W. Proctor Harvey, M.D.

***Staphylococcus aureus* Tricuspid Valve Endocarditis in Young Women After Gynaecological Events: A Report of 3 Cases**
P. J. Swift (Cecilia Makiwane Hosp., Mdantsane, Ciskei, South Africa)
S. Afr. Med. J. 66:891–893, Dec. 8, 1984   3–45

Isolated tricuspid valve endocarditis caused by *Staphylococcus aureus* is usually associated with intravenous narcotic abuse. In three patients with *S. aureus* tricuspid valve endocarditis, the infection was preceded by a gynecologic event. Two patients had no overt pelvic sepsis or history of operative or instrumental intervention, but tricuspid valve endocarditis may have resulted from a silent genital source. The third patient had pelvic inflammatory disease.

The patients had fever, cough, and dyspnea. Laboratory examinations revealed anemia, neutrophil leukocytosis, elevated erythrocyte sedimentation rates, and blood culture results positive for *S. aureus*. Chest radiographs in all three revealed bilateral pulmonary infiltrates and abscess formation. The diagnosis of tricuspid valve endocarditis was in doubt in one patient despite the presence of a grade 1/6 systolic murmur at the tricuspid area and positive blood culture results for *S. aureus* until a C-V wave appeared in the jugular venous pulse. In another patient the significance of pelvic inflammation, bilateral pneumonia, and staphylococcal septicemia was not appreciated despite the presence of a C-V wave, because of absence of a cardiac murmur. Follow-up examination revealed a grade 1/6 systolic murmur at the tricuspid area accentuated by inspiration. All three patients improved when standard antibiotic therapy was given.

Bacterial endocarditis should be considered in any young woman who has a serious respiratory infection with bilateral infiltrates seen on chest radiography after a recent obstetric or gynecologic event, with or without overt sepsis.

▶ These are case reports to remember. Worthy of emphasis is that "we *find* what we look for" and, in addition, "we should *know* what we are looking for." With early tricuspid valve endocarditis, a systolic murmur may be present only on inspiration. An atrial sound (S_4), louder on inspiration, may also be present. These auscultatory findings may correlate with the "C-V" wave and an "A" wave. Early recognition of tricuspid valve endocarditis can lead to prompt, successful treatment, and in some patients it can be lifesaving.—W. Proctor Harvey, M.D.

Pacemakers and Cardiac Pacing

Update of Infections Involving Permanent Pacemakers: Characterization and Management
Anthony B. Lewis, David L. Hayes, David R. Holmes, Jr., Ronald E. Vlietstra, James R. Pluth, and Michael J. Osborn (Mayo Clinic and Found.)
J. Thorac. Cardiol. Surg. 89:758–763, May 1985   3–46

Infections related to permanent pacemakers remain a difficult diagnostic and management problem. Data were reviewed concerning 75 patients successfully treated for infections related to permanent pacemakers during a 10-year period. Demographic characterization, mode of presentation, types of infecting organisms, potential predisposing factors, significance of a retained infected pacemaker lead, and various medical and surgical treatment methods were analyzed.

The most common site of involvement was the generator pocket itself

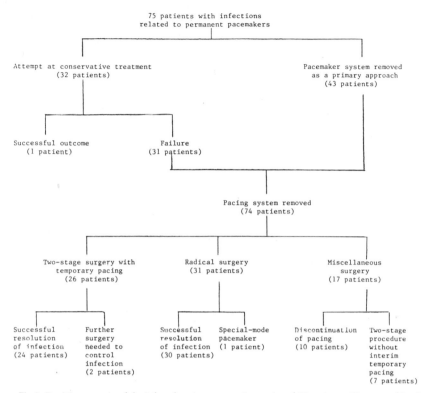

Fig 3–7.—Management of the infected pacing systems in a series of 75 patients. (Courtesy of Lewis, A.B., et al.: J. Thorac. Cardiol. Surg. 89:758–863, May 1985.)

(57 patients, 76%). The most common infecting organism was *Staphylococcus epidermidis*, which was usually detected late after implantation. Eighteen of 19 mixed microbial infections were localized at the implantation site. Seventeen of these patients had at least two pacemaker procedures at the infected site of implantation. Eight of 11 patients with early-onset infections had pure *Staphylococcus aureus* infections. Seven of these patients had generator pocket abscess associated with sepsis. Diabetes mellitus, a need for urgent lead repositioning, and treatment with steroids were associated with an increased number of infections. In addition, dermatologic diseases accounted for a significant number of secondary infections. Conservative therapy failed in 31 of 32 patients. Removal of the entire infected pacing system successfully eradicated infections in 74 patients (Fig 3–7). In one patient conservative treatment was successful. There was no difference in complications or incidence of reinfection between the 31 patients whose infected pacing system was removed at the same time that the new system was implanted and in the 26 having a two-stage procedure that included a period of temporary pacing between explantation of the old system and implantation of the new. The average duration of hospitalization was 18 days and 28 days, respectively, for these two groups.

The likely infecting organism depends on the mode of presentation and the time of infection. Optimal treatment for most patients requires removal of the entire infected pacing system. The one-stage procedure remains safe and effective, obviating the need for temporary pacing and reducing the duration of hospitalization.

▶ This report is a good update, particularly in view of the fact that increasing numbers of pacemakers are implanted each year.—W. Proctor Harvey, M.D.

Survival in Second Degree Atrioventricular Block
David B. Shaw, Christopher A. Kekwick, Dan Veale, Jim Gowers, and Tony Whistance (Royal Devon and Exeter Hosp., Exeter, England)
Br. Heart J. 53:587–593, June 1985   3–47

A 14-year prospective study was carried out to compare the outcome of patients having second-degree Mobitz type I (atrioventricular nodal) block with that of patients with Mobitz type II (distal) block, both with and without pacemakers. Between 1968 and 1982, follow-up study was made of 214 patients with chronic second-degree heart block. Seventy-seven patients had Mobitz type I block, 86 had Mobitz type II block, and 51 had 2:1 or 3:1 block. The respective mean ages were 69 years, 74 years, and 75 years. A general preponderance of males was noted. Few patients changed from Mobitz type I block to Mobitz type II block, or vice versa, during the study.

Twenty patients sustained Stokes-Adams attacks during the study, and six had other major cardiac symptoms. The overall survival at 5 years was similar in all groups, ranging from 53% to 61%. The presence or absence of bundle-branch block did not influence the outcome significantly. Pacemakers were used in 103 patients, most often in those with Mobitz type II block. Significantly more paced than unpaced patients survived in all groups. The overall 5-year survival was 78% for paced patients and 41% for unpaced patients. A difference persisted after controlling for age.

Pacing is indicated in patients with heart block chiefly to improve the chance of survival and to prevent significant symptoms, particularly Stokes-Adams attacks. In the present study, all groups of patients with chronic second-degree heart block did better when paced. Patients with chronic Mobitz type II second-degree heart block should be paced unless special considerations are present. A similar approach should be taken in those with chronic Mobitz type I second-degree block.

▶ This is a good, practical, clinical study of a significant number of patients followed for 14 years. It presents convincing evidence for advising the use of pacemakers in patients with second-degree heart block.—W. Proctor Harvey, M.D.

Complications of Permanent Transvenous Pacing
Brendan Phibbs and Henry J. L. Marriott (Univ. of Arizona and Rogers Heart

Found., St. Petersburg, Fla.)
N. Engl. J. Med. 312:1428–1432, May 30, 1985   3–48

Permanent transvenous cardiac pacing, although an important cardiologic advance, is not without complications. Medical complications fall into three major categories: thrombosis and embolism, infection, and, more rarely, pacemaker-generated arrhythmias, myocardial perforation, and tamponade. The risk of thrombotic or embolic complications is about 2%. This complication may range from a relatively benign thrombosis of the veins of the upper arm to the more serious superior vena cava syndrome, cerebral venous thrombosis, thrombosis of the external jugular vein, and large right atrial thrombus. Pulmonary embolism, often fatal, can arise from mural thrombi attached to a pacing wire in the right atrium or right ventricle. Infection may be manifest as septicemia or endocarditis, and may occur in 1% to 7% of patients. The pacemaker pocket is usually the site of entry, with the pacing wire involved frequently. The infected pacing apparatus must be removed, at times necessitating thoracotomy when pacemakers are permanently entrapped. More rare complications include constrictive pericarditis, formation of painful contractile fibroblasts around the pacemaker pocket, and tricuspid valve insufficiency.

In addition to medical complications, socioeconomic and psychological problems are common. Insurability is difficult, and the presence of a permanent pacemaker is a serious handicap in the job market. Psychological problems including anxiety and depression arise. The psyches of some patients may not tolerate a situation in which the device is permanent, frequent checkups are required, and battery or wire failure may occur. A more distressing problem is the patient who has a needlessly implanted pacemaker. As many as 75% of pacemaker implantations have been found unjustifiable. Errors in diagnosis and prognosis (e.g., predictably transient abnormalities, misinterpretation of the ECG, presence of hypothyroidism, and drug effects) account for the presence of these unnecessary pacemakers. The entire apparatus should be removed if the cardiologist is satisfied that there is no abnormality of impulse generation or conduction and no reason to suppose that any will develop. Further, about 50% of the older type of electrodes and all of the newer long-tined electrodes will become permanently entrapped and may cause infection. Their removal creates another problem, perhaps requiring cardiopulmonary bypass with major morbidity and possible death.

▶ Thanks. We needed that!—W. Proctor Harvey, M.D.

Clinical Significance of Ventricular Fibrillation-Flutter Induced by Ventricular Programmed Stimulation

Lorenzo A. DiCarlo, Jr., Fred Morady, Alan B. Schwartz, Edward N. Shen, Jeffrey M. Baerman, Ryszard B. Krol, Melvin M. Scheinman, and Ruey J. Sung (Univ. of California at San Francisco and Univ. of Michigan)
Am. Heart J. 109:959–963, May 1985   3–49

There are few data concerning the prognosis in patients in whom sustained ventricular fibrillation-flutter (VF) is initiated during electrophysiologic testing. To determine the significance of induced VF, 224 consecutive patients underwent ventricular programmed stimulation without prior documentation of the clinical occurrence of sustained ventricular tachycardia or VF. Using one, two, and three extrastimuli, programmed stimulation was performed at one-drive or two-drive cycle lengths (500 msec, or 500 and 400 msec) until ventricular tachycardia or VF having a duration of at least 30 seconds or circulatory collapse was initiated, or until nonsustained, polymorphous ventricular tachycardia with a cycle length of 210 msec or less and a duration of at least 10 seconds was initiated at least twice. Indications for programmed stimulation included palpitations or nonsustained ventricular tachycardia during ambulatory monitoring in 85 patients, unexplained syncope in 112, presyncope in 25, and family history of sudden death in 2.

Sustained VF requiring transthoracic defibrillation was induced by ventricular programmed stimulation in 18 patients (8.0%). Four patients received chronic antiarrhythmic treatment based on electropharmacologic testing, five were treated empirically, and nine received no therapy. Ten patients had heart disease. None had cardiac arrest or sudden death during a mean follow-up period of 25.2 ± 13.8 months. Ventricular fibrillation-flutter was initiated by two extrastimuli in 3 patients and by three extrastimuli in 15. The incidence of VF was similar in patients with and without heart disease (7.1% vs. 9.6%) or previous syncope/presyncope (8.8% vs. 6.9%). It was significantly higher when programmed stimulation at three ventricular sites with a current strength of 5 mA (pulse width, 2 msec) was compared with programmed stimulation of two ventricular sites using a current twice diastolic threshold (pulse width, 2 msec) (15.2% vs. 3.0%, $P < .05$).

Ventricular fibrillation-flutter initiated by VPS appears to be a nonspecific finding in patients without a documented history of sustained ventricular tachycardia or VF and does not mandate the use of antiarrhythmic therapy.

▶ This is useful information. However, I continue to be somewhat amazed at the apparent lack of apprehension of obviously confident and skilled physicians who administer and supervise ventricular programmed stimulation. I realize that this is an accepted procedure today, but I am happy not to do it as I would be concerned that defibrillation of the ventricular fibrillation might not always be accomplished.—W. Proctor Harvey, M.D.

Unilateral Neck Pulsations in a Patient With a Permanent Pacemaker
Neil L. Coplan, John A. Ambrose, and Johnathan L. Halperin (Mt. Sinai Med. Center, New York)
Chest 87:548–550, April 1985   3–50

Internal jugular vein occlusion, especially in combination with tricuspid regurgitation, may result in asymmetric neck pulsations. An asymptomatic patient who had a permanent pacemaker was seen with unilateral accentuated neck pulsations.

Man, 66, described pulsations in the right side of the neck. A permanent ventricular demand (VVI mode) pacemaker was installed previously via the left subclavian vein because of persistent high-grade atrioventricular block after an inferior wall myocardial infarction. Pertinent physical findings included a strong systolic wave palpated beneath the right sternocleidomastoid muscle with the right carotid pulse indistinguishable from the diffuse pulsation. Auscultation revealed a grade 2/6 coarse left parasternal systolic murmur without radiation that intensified with inspiration, and a grade 1/6 short high-pitched left parasternal decrescendo diastolic murmur. The left side of the neck was normal. The external jugular veins were distended bilaterally. The abdomen showed faint hepatic pulsations and minimal hepatomegaly. The venous pressure was elevated in both upper extremities, without a distended collateral venous pattern over the thorax, abdomen, or legs. Edema was absent. Chest x-ray films showed mild cardiomegaly with prominence of the right atrial border and right ventricle. The ECG revealed a predominant ventricular paced rhythm, without evidence of ventriculoatrial activation. Contrast-enhanced digital subtraction angiography revealed normal carotid arteries bilaterally but with lateral displacement of the right carotid artery; there was no evidence of an arteriovenous fistula. The right internal jugular vein was markedly dilated, but the left internal jugular vein was not opacified. Two-dimensional echocardiography revealed right atrial and right ventricular dilatation with paradoxic motion of the interventricular septum. Tricuspid regurgitation was suggested by Doppler ultrasound examination and confirmed by angiography. Right-sided catheterization showed systemic venous hypertension with ventricularization of the right atrial pressure waveform (right atrial pressure was 20 mm Hg; V wave, 30 mm Hg).

Internal jugular vein occlusion, in combination with tricuspid regurgitation, should be considered in the differential diagnosis of asymmetric neck pulsations in patients with permanent pacemakers. Severe tricuspid regurgitation causes exaggerated pulsatile venous waves and signs of volume overload of the right side of the heart, whereas the concomitant left internal jugular occlusion leads to diminished pulsations on the side of occlusion and increased pulsations on the right side of the neck.

▶ Of course, the key to the problem in such a patient having a permanent pacemaker is that the venous pulse abnormality was present only in the right neck. We can now add the above observations to the clinical information that can be derived from observation of the jugular venous pulse.—W. Proctor Harvey, M.D.

Transcutaneous Temporary Pacing in the Operating Room
David Berliner, Marc Okun, Robert W. Peters, Nathan H. Carliner, Gary D. Plotnick, and Michael L. Fisher (Univ. of Maryland)
JAMA 254:84–86, July 5, 1985   3–51

Unexpected bradyarrhythmia occurring during surgery may cause considerable morbidity and mortality, and emergency insertion of a temporary transvenous pacemaker is often difficult. Experience with transcutaneous pacing in 21 men (mean age, 55 years) having elective surgery under general anesthesia was reviewed. Ten patients had evidence of organic heart disease. General surgical and otolaryngologic procedures were done most frequently. Asynchronous pacing was initiated at a rate of about ten beats per minute above the spontaneous rate, using the shortest pulse duration (10 msec) and lowest current output (50 mamp). All patients were paced from anterior and posterior electrodes.

Complete capture was achieved in all cases. In ten patients an output of 200 mamp was necessary for consistent capture. A pulse width of 10 msec was adequate in 19 patients. The pacing threshold was unrelated to body surface area or the presence of organic heart disease, but there was a trend toward lower thresholds in younger patients, those with smaller hearts, and those with a smaller transverse chest diameter. No arrhythmias were induced by transcutaneous pacing.

Transcutaneous pacing is a rapid, safe, and effective means of initiating temporary pacing in the operating room when unexpected bradyarrhythmia develops during surgery. Its availability for standby use may reduce cardiac morbidity and mortality during surgery.

▶ This form of temporary pacing makes good sense. If larger numbers of patients such as those described in this report have similar benefit, this uncomplicated simpler form of pacing will have its place in the operating room. Because there are increasing numbers of 1-day outpatient procedures being done in our hospitals today, it is likely that more temporary pacemakers will be used as a safety precaution.—W. Proctor Harvey, M.D.

4 Coronary Arteries and Heart Disease

Asymptomatic or Minimally Symptomatic Coronary Artery Disease

▶ ↓ The following six articles were chosen as examples of heightened interest in and investigation of silent or minimally symptomatic coronary artery disease. Although absence of symptoms in the presence of myocardial ischemia is not a new concept, what has emerged over the last three decades has been the demonstration that myocardial ischemia comes about through many mechanisms of which but one is the presence of fixed atherosclerotic lesions within the coronary artery wall. The supply of coronary arterial blood may be curtailed by acute and phasic vasoconstriction either at the site of an arteriosclerotic plaque or more widespread to affect greater lengths of the coronary arteries and even the intramyocardial arteries. Furthermore, the role of platelets aggregating at the site of arteriosclerotic lesions to release potent vasoactive compounds may be yet an added factor.

What now emerges is the fact that there may be little relationship between the frequency and severity of myocardial ischemia and the presence or absence of symptoms. Even the extent of coronary atherosclerosis may be little related to the severity and frequency of symptoms (Quyyumi et al.: *Br. Heart J.* 54:362, 1985). Unfortunately, the absence of symptoms does not confer an absence of risk. Retrospective studies of silent ischemia have demonstrated a 30% incidence of a cardiac event occurring within a few years of the diagnosis having been made. It is estimated, again from retrospective studies that about 3% of middle-aged males may be prone to episodes of silent ischemia. Clearly, strategies for determining the presence of silent ischemia, the risk the patient is running, and the effects of such episodes on segmental and total left ventricular function need to be established.

The risk of future cardiac events in the presence of silent ischemia seems higher when coronary risk factors and a family history of coronary artery disease are present. In such individuals, seeking evidence of myocardial ischemia, even when they are shown to be asymptomatic by exercise ECG, and long-term ambulatory ECG monitoring may be wise. If exercise ECG suggests that ischemia is present, myocardial scintigraphy or radionuclear angiography can be used to confirm that this is so and serve as a guide to the severity of the ischemia. If severe, it may be necessary to proceed to coronary arteriography and ventriculography to determine the nature and extent of the arteriosclerotic lesions and their effects on the myocardium. This, in turn, will permit decisions about therapy to be made: medical (calcium channel blockers, β-adrenergic-blocking drugs, nitrates, aspirin), percutaneous transluminal coronary angioplasty, or aortocoronary bypass graft surgery.

Subsets of patients with silent ischemia who are at higher risk are now being recognized, including patients with unstable angina pectoris who, although made asymptomatic by medical therapy, nevertheless continue with episodes of myocardial ischemia (Gottlieb et al.: *Circulation* 72 (Suppl. III):III–163, 1985), or individuals who on exercise fail to achieve their maximum predicted heart rates (Reisman et al.: *Circulation* 72(Suppl. III):III–445, 1985). We require urgently the results of carefully conducted, randomized trials of therapy for silent ischemia, investigations to determine the sensitivity and specificity of diagnostic methods, and more basic investigations of the nature and causes of phasic ischemia of the myocardium that at times is silent and at other times symptomatic.—Leon Resnekov, M.D.

FREQUENCY OF PAINFUL AND PAINLESS EPISODES OF S-T SEGMENT CHANGE IN PATIENTS WITH CORONARY ARTERY DISEASE OF VARYING SEVERITY

Coronary artery disease	No of patients	% Of painful episodes	Number of patients:		
			With painful and painless episodes	*With painful episodes only*	*With painless episodes only*
Normal	5	8	1	0	4
Spasm only	1	39	1	0	0
No of vessels affected:					
1	11	31	5	4	2
2	17	48	5	4	8
3	24	29	14	6	4
Left main stem stenosis*	7	36	6	0	1

*These patients also included in figures for two- and three-vessel disease.
(Courtesy of Quyyumi, A.A., et al.: Br. Heart J. 54:22–26, July 1985.)

How Important Is a History of Chest Pain in Determining the Degree of Ischaemia in Patients With Angina Pectoris?

Arshed A. Quyyumi, Christine M. Wright, Lorna J. Mockus, and Kim M. Fox (Natl. Heart Hosp., London)
Br. Heart J. 54:22–26, July 1985   4–1

Treatment decisions in patients with angina are usually based on the reported frequency of pain, but ST segment changes may not be accompanied by angina in patients with or without obstructive coronary artery disease. The relationship between the reported frequency of chest pain and the objective evidence of myocardial ischemia during usual activity was examined in 100 consecutive patients undergoing coronary arteriography for chest pain. The 74 men and 26 women had a mean age of 53 years. Twenty-seven patients had evidence of old transmural myocardial infarction. Ambulatory ST segment monitoring was continued for 48 hours, during which time the patients kept an angina diary.

Seventy-four patients had coronary artery disease. All patients but nine reported typical angina. The frequency of rest or exertional angina could not be related to the coronary anatomy. About two thirds of patients with coronary disease had transient ST segment depression during monitoring. One patient had both ST depression and ST elevation. The frequency of angina was unrelated to that of observed daytime or nocturnal ST segment changes. About a third of all ST segment changes were associated with pain in patients with coronary disease. Only one such episode was accompanied by pain in patients with normal coronary arteries (table). About one fourth of patients with coronary disease had only pain-free episodes of ST segment change. Considerable variation was seen in time of onset of ST segment change in relation to perceived chest pain.

The frequency of angina is a poor indicator of the frequency of significant myocardial ischemia. Personal differences in pain perception may be an important factor. Long-term studies are needed to determine the clinical significance of asymptomatic myocardial ischemia.

Morphology of Ambulatory ST Segment Changes in Patients With Varying Severity of Coronary Artery Disease: Investigation of the Frequency of Nocturnal Ischaemia and Coronary Spasm

Arshed A. Quyyumi, Lorna Mockus, Christine Wright, and Kim M. Fox (Natl. Heart Hosp., London)
Br. Heart J. 53:186–193, February 1985   4–2

The frequency and magnitude of objectively determined myocardial ischemia during normal daily activities of patients with varying severity of coronary artery disease are unknown, as are incidence of nocturnal resting myocardial ischemia and frequency of coronary spasm in patients with normal coronary arteries and chest pain. One hundred consecutive patients with chest pain were referred for coronary angiography; exercise testing and ambulatory ST segment monitoring were also carried out. The series included 74 men and 26 women whose mean age was 53.2 years.

Overall, 52 of 74 patients with significant coronary artery disease and 6 of 26 with no significant coronary narrowing had episodes of ST segment change during 48 hours of ambulatory monitoring. One patient with normal coronary arteries and localized spasm and another with three-vessel disease had episodes of ST segment elevation. All of the other patients had episodes of ST segment depression. The frequency, duration, and magnitude of ST segment changes were greater in patients with more severe types of coronary artery disease. Thus, more than six episodes of ST segment changes per day occurred in patients with two-vessel or three-vessel disease or with left main stem stenosis and in the only patient with coronary artery spasm and normal coronary arteries. Nocturnal ischemia occurred in 15% of patients with coronary artery disease and was almost an invariable indicator of two-vessel or three-vessel coronary artery disease or left main stem stenosis. Episodes of ST segment change occurred most commonly during morning hours and least commonly during the night. The heart rate at the onset of ST segment change tended to be lower in patients with coronary artery disease than in those with normal coronary arteries.

The duration of exercise to ST segment depression tended to be shorter in patients with more severe disease, but it could not predict which patients would experience nocturnal myocardial ischemia, left main stem stenosis, or coronary spasm. Ambulatory ST segment monitoring was able to identify most of these patients.

Transient ST-Segment Depression as a Marker of Myocardial Ischemia During Daily Life
John E. Deanfield, Michael Shea, Paulo Ribiero, Christian M. de Landsheere, Richard A. Wilson, Peter Horlock, and Andrew P. Selwyn (Hammersmith Hosp., London)
Am. J. Cardiol. 54:1195–1200, Dec. 1, 1984   4–3

Asymptomatic, transient ST segment depression often occurs during ordinary life in patients with angina and coronary artery disease (CAD). To determine whether this sign is a reliable marker of myocardial ischemia, 30 patients aged 37–75 years with chronic stable angina, confirmed CAD, and a positive treadmill exercise test response underwent positron tomography with rubidium-82 (^{82}Rb). The regional myocardial uptake of ^{82}Rb, presence or absence of angina, ST segment changes, heart rate, and systolic blood pressure were recorded before, during, and after exercise tests, cold pressor test, and unprovoked episodes of ST segment depression. Sixteen normal healthy persons served as controls.

ST depression occurred during 58 of 59 technically satisfactory exercise tests, 15 of 35 cold pressor tests, and on 22 occasions without provocation. Most exercise tests were accompanied by chest pain (53 of 58), but most cold pressor tests with ST depression (12 of 15) and unprovoked episodes (13 of 22) were painless. Tomographic evidence of ischemia was found in 63 (97%) of the total 65 episodes of ST depression with angina and in all 30 episodes of painless ST depression. Perfusion abnormalities consisting of inhomogeneity, an absolute regional decrease in ^{82}Rb uptake, or both, were significantly different from those in normal individuals ($P < .01$). In each patient, perfusion defects occurred in the same abnormal myocardial segment during painful and painless ST depression. In addition, responses were reproducible in patients whose tests were repeated. The heart rate was significantly lower after unprovoked or cold pressor-induced ST depression than after exercise ($P < .01$).

ST segment depression is a reliable marker of myocardial ischemia in patients with typical chronic stable angina, CAD, and a positive exercise test response. These findings support a much wider picture of CAD activity as revealed by ambulatory monitoring with more frequent episodes of silent myocardial ischemia than of angina pectoris.

▶ The two preceding articles document the use of ambulatory ECG monitoring to determine episodes of ischemia, whether silent or symptomatic. Note the wide variation in the number of episodes that occur during daily life. Why some episodes are symptomatic (angina pectoris, fatigue, breathlessness) and others occur with no symptoms is uncertain. The number of episodes of ischemia, however, is a more accurate assessment of the patient's risk than is the number of episodes of angina.

With regard to using ambulatory ECG monitoring for determining episodes of ischemia, it is important to recognize that there are many states other than myocardial ischemia that can cause ST-T ECG deviations including heart diseases other than coronary arterial, physiologic change (e.g., vagotonia), and the effects on the myocardium of abnormalities of rhythm and conduction as well as changes brought about by various medications. In addition, variations in amplitude of R waves as occur normally throughout the 24 hours may influence ST segment shift and have nothing to do with myocardial ischemia (Hollenberg et al.: *Am. J. Cardiol.* 56:13, 1985). Meticulous attention to detail is needed to ensure satisfactory recordings of the ST segments over the long term. An apparatus capable of achieving accurate recordings at the low frequencies needed, and ensuring an absence of playback artifact, is necessary to record ST segments reliably throughout the 24 hours.—Leon Resnekov, M.D.

Analysis of ST-Segment Changes in Normal Subjects: Implications for Ambulatory Monitoring in Angina Pectoris
John E. Deanfield, Paulo Ribiero, Katherine Oakley, Shirley Krikler, and Andrew P. Selwyn (Hammersmith Hosp., London)
Am. J. Cardiol. 54:1321–1325, Dec. 1, 1984   4–4

Continuous ambulatory monitoring of the ECG in patients with angina pectoris and coronary artery disease has shown frequent episodes of depression of the ST segment, which suggest silent myocardial ischemia during normal daily life. To determine the reliability of these changes as a marker of myocardial ischemia in normal persons out of hospital, frequency-modulated ambulatory ECG recordings were performed in 80 asymptomatic normal volunteers (20 from each decade between 20 and 50 years and 20 who were older than age 50 years) and 20 patients with noncardiac chest pain, negative results on exercise and provocative tests, and angiographically normal coronary arteries.

Treadmill exercise tests were performed in all persons older than age 40 years. Significant depression of the ST segment was defined as a horizontal or downsloping shift of 0.1 mV or more that occurred for 80 msec or longer; elevation of the segment was defined as upward J-point displacement of 0.1 mV or greater. These shifts had to last at least 30 seconds to be considered significant.

Changes in T waves during normal activity were present in 53 individuals. Transient elevation of the ST segment was present in five men younger than age 40 years (Fig 4–1) and occurred at slow heart rates (mean, 65 beats per minute) usually at night and lasted a mean of 193 minutes. In three patients the elevation could be controlled by postural changes. Significant planar depression of the ST segment was found in only two persons, both older than age 40 years: One had risk factors for coronary disease and a positive exercise test response. These episodes occurred during tachycardia (mean, 128 beats per minute) and lasted for a mean of 13 minutes. No patient with normal findings on a coronary angiogram had episodes of depression of the ST segment. Upsloping, nonsustained depression of the ST segment with tachycardia was significantly more common

Fig 4–1.—Ambulatory recordings of transient changes in T wave and elevation of ST segment during normal daily life; T wave remained upright during episodes of elevation of ST segment, all of which occurred at slow heart rates. There was no significant relation between heart rate and changes in T wave. (Courtesy of Deanfield, J.E., et al.: Am. J. Cardiol. 54:1321–1325, Dec. 1, 1984.)

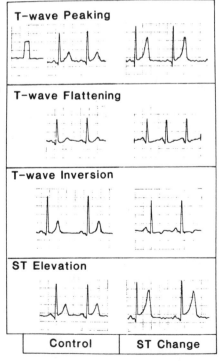

in younger patients. In five persons isolated single complexes with depression of the ST segment were seen during baseline instability.

With frequency-modulated recordings and strict criteria for interpretation of changes in the ST segment, planar depression of the ST segment is rare in a normal population. The findings lend support to the use of transient depression of the ST segment in following the activity of myocardial ischemia out of the hospital in patients who have typical angina and coronary artery disease.

Silent Myocardial Ischemia: Hemodynamic Changes During Dynamic Exercise in Patients With Proven Coronary Artery Disease Despite Absence of Angina Pectoris
Heinz O. Hirzel, Ruth Leutwyler, and Hans P. Krayenbuehl (Univ. of Zurich)
J. Am. Coll. Cardiol. 6:275–284, August 1985   4 5

Angina is considered to be a sensitive indicator of myocardial ischemia, but it may occur silently, in ways that remain to be clarified. Hemodynamic changes during exercise were examined in 36 of 258 consecutive patients with proved coronary disease who tolerated bicycle stress testing without symptoms developing. Twenty-six patients had previous myocardial infarction. Thirty-six other patients whose tests were limited by angina also were evaluated. All patients exercised to the same point. All were men, aged 26–63 years. The two groups had similar coronary status and mean vascularization indices.

The left ventricular end-diastolic pressure increased with exercise in all groups, and the left ventricular ejection fraction decreased. The changes from rest to exercise were highly significant in each group, but no significant differences were seen between corresponding groups. Regional hypokinesia developed with exercise in all patients without and in most of those with past infarction. Changes in regional contraction also were similar in all groups.

Comparable stress-induced hemodynamic changes indicating myocardial ischemia are seen in patients with significant coronary disease, with or without previous myocardial infarction, regardless of the occurrence or absence of angina. Angina, therefore, cannot be taken as a prerequisite for the development of hemodynamically significant myocardial ischemia on exertion. Silent ischemic attacks can be accompanied by hemodynamic changes as severe as those occurring in patients who experience angina.

Comparison of Preoperative, Operative, and Postoperative Variables in Asymptomatic or Minimally Symptomatic Patients to Severely Symptomatic Patients Three Years After Coronary Artery Bypass Grafting: Analysis of 423 Patients
Pim J. de Feyter, Patrick W. Serruys, Ronald W. Brower, Marcel van den Brand, Harald J. ten Katen, Paul G. Hugenholtz, and Egbert Bos (Erasmus Univ. and Interuniversity Cardiology Inst., Rotterdam, The Netherlands)
Am. J. Cardiol. 55:362–366, Feb. 1, 1985   4–6

A consecutive series of 637 patients underwent coronary artery bypass grafting (CABG) between January 1976 and December 1979. Follow-up studies were made in 423 of these patients, 79 of whom became severely symptomatic within 3 years postoperatively. All patients were seen every 6 months.

The incidence of severely symptomatic patients in New York Heart Association (NYHA) class III or IV was 19% (79 of 423 patients). The predictive value of approximately 80 clinical, angiographic, and perioperative variables was too low to be of clinical value. An adverse clinical outcome was associated with a high closure rate of the grafts. Overall, 46% of the patients could not undergo reoperation because of unsuitable coronary anatomy. With intensive medical therapy, half of these patients improved to NYHA functional class I or II, whereas 32% of those who were reoperable improved to class I or II with intensive pharmacologic treatment rather than reoperation. The nonresponders underwent reoperation, which usually resulted in improvement of symptoms to NYHA functional class I or II (83% of patients).

Coronary Vasomotor Responses

Regional Coronary Hemodynamic Responses During the Cold Pressor Test: Lack of Effect of Nitroglycerin

Robert L. Feldman, James A. Hill, C. Richard Conti, and Carl J. Pepine (Univ. of Florida and VA Med. Ctr., Gainesville)
J. Am. Coll. Cardiol. 5:1319–1325, June 1985   4–7

Immersion of a hand and forearm in ice water for 1 minute (cold pressor test) induces a diffuse reduction in the diameter of the coronary conductance vessel and may account for increased coronary resistance among patients with severe coronary artery disease. To verify this hypothesis, regional coronary blood flow and aortic and left ventricular pressures were continuously monitored in 17 patients before and during two cold pressor tests. Each test was performed before and after administration of nitroglycerin either sublingually (0.4 mg) or directly into a coronary artery (0.01 mg). Fourteen patients were taking propranolol at the time of the study. Angiography showed that 13 patients had severe coronary artery disease; 4 had normal coronary angiograms.

During the initial cold pressor test, heart rate and coronary pressures increased in all patients; however, total and regional coronary resistance usually increased before nitroglycerin was given to patients with severe coronary artery disease and usually decreased in patients with normal coronary angiograms. Sublingual administration of nitroglycerin induced variable systemic or coronary hemodynamic changes, but intracoronary administration did not. Both, however, induced persistent dilation of coronary arteries that was seen at angiography. Regardless of the route of administration, directional responses in regional coronary resistance during the cold pressor test were usually similar before and after administration of nitroglycerin.

Coronary hemodynamic responses during a cold pressor test are not altered by sublingual or intracoronary administration of nitroglycerin, indicating that changes in tone of the large coronary arteries are not important in producing the cardiac responses observed during a cold pressor test.

▶ The cold pressor test was introduced during the mid-1930s as a provocative test for the presence of systemic hypertension. Its effect is to precipitate vasoconstriction by an adrenergic mechanism. The effects, however, are widespread, involving many arterial beds and intramyocardial circulation. Since the peripheral vascular circulation is also affected and the test may result in local pain as the arm is kept in very cold water, interpretation of the results needs to be done with great care. This study and similar investigations by others point out the importance of differentiating the vasomotor effects of epicardial and intramyocardial coronary arteries. It is the role of the intramyocardial arteries as resistance vessels to control the amount of arterial blood delivered to the myocardial cells.—Leon Resnekov, M.D.

Attenuation of Coronary Vascular Resistance by Selective Alpha₁-Adrenergic Blockade in Patients With Coronary Artery Disease

Morton J. Kern, John D. Horowitz, Peter Ganz, Jorge Gaspar, Wilson S. Colucci, Beverly H. Lorell, William H. Barry, and Gilbert H. Mudge, Jr. (Brigham and Women's Hosp., Boston, and Harvard Univ.)
J. Am. Coll. Cardiol. 5:840–846, April 1985   4–8

Alpha-adrenergic-mediated coronary vasoconstriction during stress such as cold pressor testing may contribute to myocardial ischemia by increasing coronary vascular resistance in patients with severe coronary artery disease. Although nonselective α-adrenergic antagonists (e.g., phentolamine) abolish both peripheral and coronary vasoconstriction during cold pressor testing, they increase myocardial oxygen consumption because of increased inotropy and reflex tachycardia. To determine the role of selective α-receptor blockade, the changes in coronary vascular resistance during cold pressor testing were measured in 18 patients with coronary artery disease before and after intravenous administration of 100 mg of trimazosin. Cold pressor testing was performed at a constant paced subanginal heart rate of 95 ± 5 beats per minute. Plasma norepinephrine levels were also measured.

Before trimazosin, cold pressor testing increased mean arterial pressure by 9% ± 4% (102 ± 14 mm Hg to 111 ± 14 mm Hg, $P < .001$), with no change in coronary sinus blood flow ($P = $ NS). However, it significantly increased coronary vascular resistance by 14% ± 0.9% (1.02 ± 0.46 units to 1.16 ± 0.57 units, $P < .02$). Five minutes after administration of trimazosin, cold pressor testing increased the mean arterial pressure by 6% ± 5% (95 ± 9 mm Hg to 101 ± 10 mm Hg, $P < .001$) with no change in coronary sinus blood flow ($P = $ NS) or coronary vascular resistance. The increase in coronary vascular resistance during cold pressor testing was attenuated from 14% ± 4% to 6% ± 3% after trimazosin administration ($P < .02$). There were no significant increases in heart rate, arterial norepinephrine levels, or heart rate-pressure product (as an index of myocardial oxygen demand).

Selective α-adrenergic blockade with trimazosin attenuates the reflex coronary vasoconstriction during the adrenergic stimulus of cold pressor testing in patients with coronary artery disease. It has a potential advantage over nonselective α_1-adrenergic blockade in that the release of norepinephrine is also attenuated. Thus, potentially there would be less augmentation of heart rate and myocardial oxygen demand.

Coronary Hemodynamic and Metabolic Effects of Nifedipine in Patients With Coronary Artery Disease Treated With Beta-Blocking Drugs
Peter Schanzenbächer, Gerhard Göttfert, Gerhart Liebau, and Kurt Kochsiek (Univ. of Würzburg)
Am. J. Cardiol. 55:33–36, Jan. 1, 1985   4–9

In man, the direct cardiac action of nifedipine after systemic administration is modified by reflex sympathetic nerve activation and results in a positive chronotropic and inotropic response. To determine the acute coronary hemodynamic and metabolic effects of nifedipine after β-blockade by propranolol, coronary sinus blood flow (CSBF), myocardial oxygen consumption (MVO_2), heart rate, and aortic pressure were determined before, during, and after intravenous administration of propranolol, 0.1 mg/kg, followed by 1 mg of nifedipine in 12 patients with angiographically documented coronary artery disease.

Propranolol produced a decrease in heart rate (from 73 ± 14 to 66 ± 9, $P < .025$), CSBF (from 117 ± 27 ml minute to 104 ± 26 ml/minute), and MVO_2 (from 15.7 ± 2.6 ml O_2/minute to 14.0 ± 2.8 ml O_2/minute, $P < .001$), and an increase in coronary vascular resistance (CVR) (from 1.01 ± 0.22 mm Hg/ml/minute to 1.17 ± 0.28 mm Hg/ml/minute, $P < .001$) and the coronary arteriovenous oxygen difference (from 13.2 ± 1.9 vol % to 13.5 ± 1.8 vol %, $P < .01$). The mean aortic pressure did not change significantly. The subsequent administration of nifedipine caused a transient increase in CSBF (up to 148 ± 30 ml/minute, $P < .001$) and a reduction in CVR (0.66 ± 0.07 mm Hg/ml/minute, $P < .001$) and in the arteriovenous oxygen difference (8.7 ± 1.7 vol%, $P < .001$). Nifedipine administration also caused a sustained decrease in mean aortic pressure (from 116 ± 19 mm Hg to 97 ± 20 mm Hg, $P < .005$) and MVO_2 (12.9 ± 3.0 ml/O_2/minute, $P < .005$) without significant changes in heart rate.

In the presence of acute β-receptor blockade by propranolol, the positive chronotropic response to nifedipine is attenuated and nifedipine treatment reduces MVO_2 significantly. The vasodilatory effect of nifedipine is maintained, and a probable propranolol-induced inappropriate vasoconstriction may be reversed. The combination of nifedipine and β-receptor blocking agents may be useful in the treatment of patients with both effort-induced angina and angina related to changes in coronary vasomotor tone.

▶ Since nifedipine is an active smooth muscle dilator, one would predict that it would have an important role in preventing and treating coronary vasoconstriction. The combination of β-adrenergic blocking drugs with a powerful coronary artery vasodilator (e.g., nifedipine) might therefore be the most beneficial form of combined therapy to administer to the patient who has symptomatic or silent myocardial ischemia. This combination may, in fact, obviate the need for chronic nitrate therapy, which is less effective in dilating the intramyocardial circulation and suffers from the effects of tachyphylaxis. In addition, as demonstrated by Manyari et al. (*Am. J. Cardiol.:* 55:927, 1985) cross tolerance between chronic isosorbide dinitrate therapy and sublingual nitroglycerin occurs; thus, the effect of acute nitrate responses may be blunted in a patient maintained with chronic nitrate therapy.—Leon Resnekov, M.D.

Regional Coronary Vasoconstriction After Combined Beta-Adrenergic and Calcium Channel Blockade in Patients With Coronary Artery Disease
Morton J. Kern, Michael A. Petru, David R. Ferry, Steven D. Eilen, W. Kent Barr, Charles B. Porter, and Robert A. O'Rourke (Univ. of Texas at San Antonio and Audie L. Murphy VA Hosp.)
J. Am. Coll. Cardiol. 5:1438–1450, June 1985   4–10

Although β-adrenergic and calcium channel-blocking drugs are efficacious in the treatment of angina pectoris when used individually or in combination, previous studies of these agents showed opposing effects on coronary artery vasomotion. β-Adrenergic blockade potentiates, and calcium channel blockade reverses, coronary vasoconstriction during adrenergic cold stimulation in patients with coronary artery disease. To assess the coronary hemodynamic effects of combined therapy, thermodilution coronary sinus and great cardiac vein flow and mean arterial pressure were measured during serial cold pressor testing, both before and after 0.1 mg/kg of propranolol intravenously and again after the addition of 10 mg of nifedipine sublingually in 21 patients (group A); the reverse protocol (nifedipine followed by propranolol) was used in 15 patients (group B). The patients were subdivided into groups A1 (9 patients) and B1 (6 patients) who had insignificant stenoses of the left anterior descending coronary artery and groups A2 (12 patients) and B2 (9 patients) who had narrowing of the same artery of at least 50%.

During cold pressor testing, mean arterial pressures increased significantly in all groups ($P < .01$), but coronary sinus resistance responses after administration of propranolol and nifedipine were not statistically significant for any group. However, regional coronary resistance responses differed between patients with and without left anterior descending coronary artery stenosis. In group A1, great cardiac vein resistance was unchanged after treatment with propranolol and nifedipine. In contrast, in group A2, great cardiac vein flow decreased significantly after treatment with propranolol plus nifedipine ($8\% \pm 17\%$ to $-4\% \pm 12\%$, $P < .01$ vs. control) and great cardiac vein resistance increased from $4\% \pm 21\%$ to $15\% \pm 19\%$ ($P < .01$ vs. control). The same significant responses were observed in groups B1 and B2.

After administration of combined β-adrenergic and calcium channel-blocking drugs, increased adrenergic stimulation may cause regional coronary vasoconstriction in a subset of patients with significant left anterior descending coronary artery stenosis. Combined therapy modified regional coronary responses to adrenergic stimulation with an inhomogeneous distribution of blood flow to potentially ischemic regions without affecting total coronary blood flow. The beneficial effects of combined drug therapy may result primarily from a reduction in myocardial oxygen demand caused by decreased myocardial contractility, diminished left ventricular wall stress, or reduced intramyocardial resistance rather than from increased myocardial oxygen supply.

Efficacy of Calcium Channel Blocker Therapy for Angina Pectoris Resulting From Small-Vessel Coronary Artery Disease and Abnormal Vasodilator Reserve
Richard O. Cannon, III, Rita M. Watson, Douglas R. Rosing, and Stephen E. Epstein (Natl. Heart, Lung, and Blood Inst., Bethesda, Md.)
Am. J. Cardiol. 56:242–246, Aug. 1, 1985   4–11

Patients with angina but angiographically normal coronary arteries may have abnormal vasodilator reserve of the coronary microcirculation, demonstrated by pacing. Calcium channel blockade was evaluated in a double-blind, placebo-controlled study of 26 outpatients seen between 1982 and 1984 with chest pain syndromes and angiographically normal coronary arteries. Typical angina occurred during rapid atrial pacing, before or after ergonovine administration. Most patients initially received verapamil, starting with 80 mg four times daily. Six treatment-refractory patients and three who experienced side effects received nifedipine; this drug was also used initially in four others. The initial dosage was 10 mg four times daily, and the maximum was 40 mg four times daily.

Less chest pain and less nitroglycerin consumption were found in the drug phase of the study than in the placebo phase. All but 1 of 23 patients expressing a preference specified the study drug rather than placebo. The systolic pressure-heart rate product was no different in the placebo and drug phases at rest or at peak exercise. Chest pain was more frequent as an end point to exercise testing in the placebo phase than in the drug phase of the study.

Dynamic fluctuations in microvascular coronary tone may be favorably affected by calcium channel blockers, helping explain their beneficial effect in patients with abnormal vasodilator reserve. Further studies are needed to identify other mechanisms involved, especially in patients resistant to calcium channel blockade.

▶ The coronary vasodilator reserve is an important mechanism by which additional arterial blood may be delivered to the myocardium. Unfortunately, in the presence of significant coronary arteriosclerosis, the need for additional vasodilation soon exceeds the capacity of the coronary circulation to do so. Calcium channel blocking drugs can favorably affect the requirement and are more active in this regard than nitrates are.—Leon Resnekov, M.D.

Coronary Hemodynamic Responses During Spontaneous Angina in Patients With and Patients Without Coronary Artery Spasm
Robert G. MacDonald, Robert L. Feldman, James A. Hill, C. Richard Conti, and Carl J. Pepine (VA Med. Ctr. and Univ. of Florida, Gainesville)
Am. J. Cardiol. 56:41–46, July 1, 1985   4–12

Coronary hemodynamic changes have been reported to occur during spontaneous angina (angina developing without provocation at rest) in patients with variant angina. To define other possible mechanisms for spontaneous angina, data on 13 men with spontaneous angina during cardiac catheterization were evaluated. Left ventricular and systemic hemodynamics and coronary venous flows were studied; ECGs and coronary angiograms were obtained before and during an episode of spontaneous angina.

Angiography during spontaneous angina showed five patients with coronary spasm (group I) and eight without (group II). Group II was characterized by a prevalence of multivessel coronary artery disease. In group I, four patients had transient elevation of the ST segment and one had new T wave peaking during spontaneous angina. All patients in group II had transient depression of the ST segment during episodes of angina. Left ventricular end-diastolic pressure increased in all patients in both groups during these episodes. Among the five patients in group I, coronary sinus flow decreased in four, and regional blood flow declined in all five during spontaneous angina. In addition, coronary resistance and ratio of double product to coronary sinus flow increased in all patients.

Among the eight patients in group II coronary venous flow during spontaneous angina varied, coronary sinus flow decreased in five and increased in three, but regional blood flow decreased in two and increased in six. Although total coronary resistance and the ratio of double product to coronary sinus flow increased during spontaneous angina for the group as a whole, there was considerable variation in individual patient responses.

Patients with severe coronary artery disease can have spontaneous angina without angiographic evidence of coronary spasm. There appears to be no apparent uniform mechanism for spontaneous angina among patients without coronary spasm. The study also confirms a previous finding that spontaneous ischemia in patients with variant angina results from decreased coronary blood flow secondary to coronary spasm.

Aspirin, Prostacyclin, Prostaglandins, and Apolipoproteins

▶ The first three articles that follow are concerned with the effects of prostacyclin, prostaglandins, and aspirin. Since it is known that prostacyclin is not only a vasodilator but prevents abnormal aggregation of platelets, administering it to patients with AMI might indeed bring benefit, as demonstrated by the study reported by Henricksson and his colleagues. The number of patients studied, however, was small and more detailed patient investigations are needed. It is known that, following myocardial infarction, prostaglandin levels remain elevated for at least 7 days (see abstract of the article by Friedrich et al.); as a result, dangerous ventricular rhythm disturbances might emerge.

It is not clear what the best dosage regimen of aspirin is to prevent platelet aggregation and the release of adverse vasoactive compounds. It remains uncertain whether, under all circumstances, a dosage as low as 20 mg/24 hours will suffice. It seems apparent, however, that doses of aspirin in excess of 325 mg/24 hours are not needed and indeed may be detrimental, because inhibition of prostacyclin at these higher doses may emerge. Further investigation is needed, however, before the protective dosage of aspirin under a variety of circumstances and needs is known. It should be recollected that, in addition to the cyclo-oxygenase arachidonic acid pathway, there is also the lipo-oxygenase pathway from which substances such as the leukotrienes and breakdown products of eicosotetraenoeic acids are formed. These compounds may also be vasoactive, and their effects require study.—Leon Resnekov, M.D.

Prostacyclin Infusion in Patients With Acute Myocardial Infarction

P. Henriksson, O. Edhag, and A. Wennmalm (Karolinska Inst., Huddinge, Sweden)
Br. Heart J. 53:173–179, February 1985   4–13

The vasodilatory and platelet antiaggregatory effects of prostacyclin prompted researchers to suggest its use in treating AMI. Vascular formation of prostacyclin is reduced in atherosclerosis. The effects of prostacyclin therapy were examined in a double-blind study of 30 patients aged 18–75 years who were initially seen with typical chest pain and confirmatory ECG or plasma enzyme findings, or both. All were seen within 16 hours of onset of symptoms. The 15 patients in each group were clinically comparable, and similar proportions in each group received β-blocking drugs. Prostacyclin was infused in study patients at rates of 1–5 ng/kg/minute during a 72-hour period, with tapering of the dose in the last 4 hours. Glycine buffer was used for the placebo infusions.

Twelve study patients were able to receive the maximum dose of prostacyclin. Only in the placebo-treated group did the number of patients requiring treatment for heart failure increase during the study period. Four patients given placebo had evidence of infarct extension during infusion, and one of them died of ventricular rupture on the second day. No prostacyclin-treated patient had signs of infarct extension. There were no significant ECG differences between the two groups, although creatine kinase MB activity and lactate dehydrogenase activity increased less in those seen within 6 hours of onset of chest pain.

These findings suggest that prostacyclin infusion has a beneficial effect in patients with AMI. Moreover, a myocardium-sparing effect is possible in those treated within 6 hours of onset of symptoms. Myocardial risk might persist after prostacyclin infusion, and some postinfusion measure (e.g., aspirin administration) might be indicated to counteract platelet aggregation and thromboxane A_2 formation.

Follow-up of Prostaglandin Plasma Levels After Acute Myocardial Infarction

Tilman Friedrich, Jürgen Lichey, Santosh Nigam, Michael Priesnitz, and Karl Wegscheider (Free Univ. of Berlin)
Am. Heart J. 109:218–222, February 1985   4–14

Results of animal experiments suggested a role of prostaglandin in the pathogenesis of AMI. To investigate the time course of prostaglandins in transmural AMI and their association with cardiac arrhythmias, the plasma levels of 6-keto-prostaglandin $F_{1\alpha}$ (6-keto-$PGF_{1\alpha}$) and thromboxane B_2 (TXB_2), metabolites of prostacyclin and thromboxane, respectively, were measured in the venous blood of 32 patients with AMI on the first, third, and seventh days after the event.

Plasma levels of TXB_2 and 6-keto-$PGF_{1\alpha}$ in patients with AMI (up to 117 ± 237 pg/ml and 96 ± 105 pg/ml, mean $\pm$ SD, respectively) differed significantly from levels in normal controls (10 ± 12 pg/ml and 4 ± 7 pg/ml, mean $\pm$ SD, respectively) ($P < .01$). Prostaglandin values remained elevated on all 3 sample days. In most patients, 6-keto-$PGF_{1\alpha}$ levels prevailed over those of TXB_2. However, in eight patients with cardiac arrhythmias, the ratio of 6-keto-$PGF_{1\alpha}$/TXB_2 was inverse.

The study indicates that prostaglandin generation is increased for at least 7 days after myocardial infarction. An inverse ratio of 6-keto-$PGF_{1\alpha}$/TXB_2 may be associated with cardiac arrhythmias in myocardial infarction.

Cumulative Inhibitory Effect of Low-Dose Aspirin on Vascular Prostacyclin and Platelet Thromboxane Production in Patients With Atherosclerosis

Babette B. Weksler, Karen Tack-Goldman, Valvanur A. Subramanian, and William A. Gay, Jr. (New York Hosp.-Cornell Med. Center)
Circulation 71:332–340, February 1985   4–15

The best dosage of aspirin to use to prevent thrombosis is uncertain, as is the relationship between the antithrombotic efficacy of aspirin and its antiplatelet effects. This was assessed in 40 men with documented coronary artery disease scheduled for coronary bypass grafting. Twenty of the 40 men who were not taking aspirin served as controls. The 20 others took a 20-mg capsule of aspirin each morning in the week before scheduled operation. The groups were similar in age, severity of atherosclerosis, and laboratory values. Operative factors also were similar.

Platelet aggregation responses to arachidonic acid, collagen, adenosine diphosphate, and epinephrine were inhibited by aspirin use. Serum thromboxane B_2 concentrations were significantly lower in those taking aspirin than in controls. Aortic fragments from aspirin-treated patients produced less 6-keto-prostaglandin $F_{1\alpha}$ than those from controls did when incubated with sodium arachidonate. Template bleeding times were longer in aspirin-treated patients, but perioperative blood losses were similar in the two groups, as were transfusion requirements.

Low-dosage aspirin administration for 1 week before coronary bypass grafting can markedly inhibit platelet aggregation and thromboxane synthesis in patients with coronary artery disease and partially suppress vascular prostacyclin production. Hemostasis does not appear to be impaired by a daily aspirin dose of 20 mg. Cumulative inhibitory effects of aspirin on vascular and other tissues require investigation.

Lipoprotein and Apolipoprotein Levels in Angiographically Defined Coronary Atherosclerosis
Stanley B. Schmidt, Alan G. Wasserman, Richard A. Muesing, Sarah E. Schlesselman, John C. Larosa, and Allan M. Ross (George Washington Univ.)
Am. J. Cardiol. 55:1459–1462, June 1, 1985   4–16

Recent studies suggest that apolipoproteins and subfractions of high-density lipoprotein (HDL) cholesterol may be better predictors of atherosclerotic coronary artery disease (CAD) than levels of plasma cholesterol and total HDL cholesterol are. To examine this hypothesis, levels of plasma cholesterol and triglyceride, cholesterol of low-density lipoprotein (LDL), HDL and its subfractions 2 and 3, apolipoprotein A-1 (Apo-AI), apolipoprotein B (Apo-B) of LDL, and the ratio of apolipoprotein E_{II} to E_{III}, as well as ratios of several of these variables, were measured in 83 men and 43 women who underwent coronary angiography for suspected CAD.

Ninety-nine patients were found to have significant CAD; 27 had either normal coronary arteries or no significant CAD (controls). Significant CAD was defined as 50% or greater narrowing of the luminal diameter of one or more major coronary arteries. Men with CAD had significantly higher mean levels of plasma cholesterol and triglyceride, LDL cholesterol, and LDL-Apo-B than controls had, as well as lower mean levels of HDL cholesterol and ratios of HDL cholesterol-total cholesterol, HDL cholesterol-LDL cholesterol, and Apo-AI-LDL-Apo-B. After adjustment for age, use of β-blockers, and diuretic drugs, only the difference in mean level of HDL cholesterol was significant.

The ratio of HDL cholesterol to total plasma cholesterol was the only significant independent predictor of CAD. The ratio tended to be lower in men with CAD (mean, 0.17 mg/dl) than in male controls (mean, 0.23 mg/dl), and in all men with ratios of less than 0.15 mg/dl (Fig 4–2). None of the variables was a significant univariate or multivariate predictor of CAD in women, probably because of the small size of the groups, and none was a significant predictor of the extent of disease in either sex.

The ratio of HDL cholesterol to plasma cholesterol may be superior to many of the more recently described lipoprotein and apolipoprotein-derived predictors of CAD. However, because of the relatively small group of highly selected patients, the question of the value of these newer assays

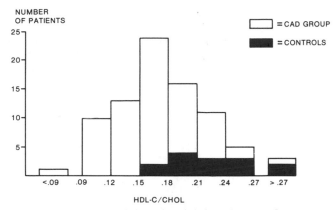

Fig 4–2.—High-density lipoprotein cholesterol-total cholesterol (HDL-C/CHOL) ratios in men with coronary artery disease and in control subjects. (Courtesy of Schmidt, S.B., et al.: Am. J. Cardiol. 55:1459–1462, June 1, 1985.)

in predicting coronary disease must be considered unanswered until large prospective studies are performed.

▶ We now have a far better understanding of processes that result in arteriosclerosis. Although much remains to be elucidated, recent information about the role of receptors in lipid metabolism and its control, and the ability to fractionate the lipoproteins, have combined to provide the clinician with a far better understanding of the effects of abnormalities of lipid metabolism. Of particular importance clinically are fractionating high-density and low-density lipoproteins and determining levels of the various apolipoproteins.—Leon Resnekov, M.D.

Coronary Artery Disease: Investigations and Diagnostic Methods

Alternative Diagnostic Strategies for Coronary Artery Disease in Women: Demonstration of the Usefulness and Efficiency of Probability Analysis
Jacques A. Melin, William Wijns, Roland J. Vanbutsele, Annie Robert, Patrick De Coster, Lucien A. Brasseur, Christian Beckers, and Jean-Marie R. Detry (Univ. of Louvain, Brussels)
Circulation 71:535–542, March 1985   4–17

The value of noninvasive testing for coronary artery disease in symptomatic women without previous myocardial infarction is unclear. Avoidance of unnecessary scintigraphy and coronary angiography would improve the quality of care and reduce costs. Diagnostic accuracy was assessed for strategies using tests on a probabilistic mode and for those based on blanket-testing decision rules in consecutive groups of women who had stress ECG and thallium scintigraphic studies within 2 weeks before coronary angiography. The series included 135 patients. The prevalences of coronary disease were 26% in 93 infarct-free women with chest pain and 48% in a prospective group of 42 consecutive female patients.

Pretest and posttest probabilities of coronary disease were derived from a computerized bayesian algorithm.

The best strategies for predicting the presence or absence of coronary disease in both groups were one considering the history and stress ECG and stress scintigraphic findings, and one in which the scintigraphic findings were considered only if the poststress probability of coronary disease was 10% to 90%. With the latter strategy, more than one-third of the scintigraphic studies could have been avoided without loss of accuracy. The proportions of patients with a probability estimate of coronary disease of 10% or lower was 29% in the prospective series and 58% in the initial group.

A probabilistic approach to diagnosis of coronary artery disease can be as accurate as blanket testing all patients, and certain unnecessary coronary angiographic studies can be avoided. Costs are thus reduced and patient discomfort minimized.

▶ It is indeed unfortunate that in women there is a higher incidence of false negative exercise ECG results for diagnosing coronary artery disease. In consequence, different strategies for investigating women for the presence of coronary atherosclerosis and myocardial ischemia are needed. Application of the principles of the Bayes theorem to clinical diagnosis demonstrates the importance of considering the probability of a particular disease being present in the individual being studied. Such considerations may well obviate the need for unnecessary testing, reduce the cost of diagnosis, and provide more accurate clinical information.—Leon Resnekov, M.D.

Symptomatic Coronary Artery Disease in Patients Aged 21 to 30 Years
Donald A. Underwood, William L. Proudfit, Juan Lim, and Julie P. MacMillan (Cleveland Clinic Found.)
Am. J. Cardiol. 55:631–634, March 1, 1985   4–18

Eighty-eight men and 13 women, aged 30 or younger, with arteriographically proved obstructive coronary artery disease (CAD) were identified and reviewed for risk factor prevalence. Findings in the men were compared with those in age-matched and date-of-catheterization matched controls who were arteriographically normal.

Significant risk factors were cigarette smoking ($P = .001$), familial CAD ($P = .002$), and familial CAD manifested by age 50 or younger ($P = .005$). Serum cholesterol values were significantly higher in the CAD group ($P = .0001$), but in most patients (54%) these values were still less than 250 mg/dl. Arteriography showed a spectrum of CAD: one-vessel in 57 patients, two-vessel in 21, and three-vessel in 22. One patient had significant left main CAD. Follow-up study was possible in all 94 Americans in the series. The 1-year mortality was 3% and the 5-year mortality, 20%. Causes of death were predominantly cardiac including myocardial infarction in ten patients, congestive heart failure in two, and sudden death in six (three patients died of noncardiac causes).

In this study, the young men with CAD had a higher prevalence of family history of CAD, premature familial CAD, and cigarette smoking than found in similarly aged patients without disease. Young men, and probably young women also, with family histories of CAD, especially premature CAD, should avoid smoking cigarettes and should have serum lipid levels measured. The use of oral contraceptives probably should be avoided by young women with positive family histories of CAD.

▶ Note the importance of smoking and a poor family history of CAD.—Leon Resnekov, M.D.

Different Recovery Process of ST Depression on Postexercise Electrocardiograms in Women in Standing and Supine Positions
Masahiro Murayama, Kiyoshi Kawakubo, Toshiaki Nakajima, Shizuo Sakamoto, Shōichi Ōno, Tsutomu Itai, and Norihisa Kato (Kanto-Teishin Hosp., Tokyo)
Am. J. Cardiol. 55:1474–1477, June 1, 1985   4–19

A false positive response to an exercise test is often observed in women. Because postexercise depression of the ST segment may be exaggerated in the standing position, the recovery process in the standing and supine positions was compared in 26 women with nonischemic depression of the ST segment and in 14 patients with typical angina pectoris to differentiate a false positive from a true positive response to testing. Exercise tests were performed twice, and the magnitude of depression of the ST segment during the immediate postexercise period was measured while the patient was standing in the first test and while in the supine position during the second test.

A typical pattern of recovery was observed among patients with false positive responses: (1) maximal depression of the ST segment occurred immediately after exercise and improved rapidly in the early recovery phase; (2) depression of the ST segment was maintained or further increased in the late recovery phase as long as the patients remained standing, in contrast to the rapid recovery that occurred when the supine position was assumed, and (3) maximal depression of the ST segment was consistently observed in lead aVF. In contrast, the recovery process of ischemic depression of the ST segment did not vary in either position.

Although the sensitivity of this procedure for diagnosing a false positive response is low (47% at 7 minutes), changing posture during postexercise ECG recording may be helpful in differentiating a false-positive from a true positive response.

▶ Vagotonic processes are but one mechanism by which ST segment change, particularly in young women, may come about and confuse the diagnosis, coronary artery disease being erroneously considered as the cause.—Leon Resnekov, M.D.

Different Susceptibility to Myocardial Ischemia Provoked by Hyperventilation and Cold Pressor Test in Exertional and Variant Angina Pectoris

Filippo Crea, Graham Davies, Sergio Chierchia, Franco Romeo, Raffaele Bugiardini, Juan Carlos Kaski, Ben Freedman, and Attilio Maseri (Hammersmith Hosp., London)

Am. J. Cardiol. 56:18–22, July 1, 1985   4–20

It has been suggested that coronary constriction at the site of atherosclerotic stenoses has an important role in modulating the frequency of symptoms in patients with exertional angina. Patients with either exertional or variant angina were subjected to hyperventilation and cold pressor tests to assess the relative susceptibility to different nonpharmacologic vasoconstrictor stimuli. Findings in 20 patients with exertional angina (mean age, 56 years), positive results of exercise tests, and coronary artery disease (CAD) were compared with those in 14 patients with variant angina (mean age, 51 years) and elevation of the ST segment during an ergonovine test. All results were considered positive when there was more than 0.1 mV of downsloping or rectilinear depression of the ST segment or more than 0.1 mV of elevation of the segment in leads without pathologic Q waves.

In patients with exertional angina, the cold pressor test produced depression of the ST segment in six patients (30%) at a peak rate-pressure product much lower than that during the exercise test; all patients had low effort tolerance and severe CAD. However, the pattern of peak rate-pressure product was also similar in four patients who had a positive result on a low-threshold exercise test but a negative response to the cold pressor test. Ergonovine produced an ischemic response in all six patients who had positive responses to the cold pressor test. In only one patient with exertional angina did depression in the ST segment develop with hyperventilation. In contrast, in patients with variant angina, hyperventilation produced elevation of the ST segment in 11 (78%), but the cold pressor test produced elevation in only 2 (14%). In six patients hyperventilation-induced ischemia occurred within a mean of 3.2 minutes after discontinuing hyperventilation.

Coronary constriction can provoke myocardial ischemia not only in patients with variant angina but also in some patients with exertional angina. A different individual susceptibility to coronary stenoses in response to vasoactive stimuli may explain the presence or absence of myocardial ischemia among patients with similar exercise tolerance and similar severity of CAD.

▶ This is an important study that differentiates the effects of hyperventilation and cold temperature both in patients with variant angina and those with more stable forms of exertional angina. It should be recollected that the important information sought is the presence of myocardial ischemia and not whether it is necessarily symptomatic.—Leon Resnekov, M.D.

Value of Lead V₄R in Exercise Testing To Predict Proximal Stenosis of the Right Coronary Artery

Simon H. Braat, J. Herre Kingma, Pedro Brugada, and Hein J. J. Wellens (Univ. of Limburg, Maastricht, The Netherlands)
J. Am. Coll. Cardiol. 5:1308–1311, June 1985   4–21

The finding of ST segment elevation in lead V_4R in acute inferior wall myocardial infarction is a sensitive and specific sign of right ventricular involvement. To determine the value of changes in lead V_4R during exercise stress testing for predicting proximal stenosis of the right coronary artery, 107 consecutive patients underwent a Bruce exercise test with simultaneous recordings of leads I, II, V_4R, V_1, V_4, and V_6 followed by coronary angiography. Along with ST segment changes in the conventional leads, ischemia in lead V_4R was defined as ST segment deviation (elevation/depression) of 1 mm or more lasting for at least 80 msec after the J point. Seventy-nine patients were evaluated for inadequate control of angina pectoris and 21 were evaluated for severe rhythm disturbances. Seven patients had myocardial infarction before age 40 years. In 46 patients who had previous myocardial infarction, the infarct location was inferior in 28 patients and anterior in 18.

Twenty-one patients had ST deviation of 1 mm or more in lead V_4R, including 7 of 14 patients with significant stenosis in the right coronary artery without inferior myocardial infarction; ST deviation was also present in 11 of 18 patients with previous inferior myocardial infarction with proximal occlusion of the right coronary artery. None of the 53 patients without significant stenosis in the right coronary artery had ST segment deviation of 1 mm or more in lead V_4R. Determination of exercise-related ST segment deviation in lead V_4R had a sensitivity of 56%, a specificity of 96%, and a predictive accuracy of 84%. Also, three patients with coronary artery disease but without ST segment elevation in the conventional leads had ST segment elevation in lead V_4R; two of these had proximal stenosis in the right coronary artery and the third had double-vessel disease with distal stenosis in the right coronary artery.

These findings suggest that lead V_4R changes during exercise testing are of value in predicting or excluding proximal stenosis in the right coronary artery.

Positive Exercise Thallium-201 Test Responses in Patients With Less Than 50% Maximal Coronary Stenosis: Angiographic and Clinical Predictors

Kenneth A. Brown, Mary Osbakken, Charles A. Boucher, H. William Strauss, Gerald M. Pohost, and Robert D. Okada (Massachusetts Gen. Hosp., Boston)
Am. J. Cardiol. 55:54–57, Jan. 1, 1985   4–22

In a group of patients, definite abnormalities were observed in thallium-201 (^{201}Tl) scans in the absence of angiographically critical coronary stenoses. To determine the incidence and causes of abnormal ^{201}Tl myocardial perfusion findings in the absence of significant coronary artery disease, data were studied on 100 consecutive patients undergoing both coronary angiography and exercise ^{201}Tl myocardial imaging for evaluation of chest pain; all had a maximal coronary artery diameter narrowing of less than 50%. Maximal coronary artery stenosis ranged from 0% to 20% in 78 patients and from 21% to 40% in 22. Using multiple-step logistic regression analysis, the independent relative influences of clinical, exercise, and angiographic data on the presence of ^{201}Tl perfusion defects were assessed.

Significant predictors of a positive stress ^{201}Tl test result included percent maximal coronary stenosis ($P < .0005$), propranolol use ($P < .01$), interaction of propranolol use and percent maximal stenosis ($P < .005$), and stress-induced chest pain ($P = .05$). No other patient variable had a significant influence. Patients with maximal stenosis of 21% to 40% had ^{201}Tl perfusion defects (59%) more often than did patients with maximal stenosis of 20% or less (27%) ($P < .01$). Among patients with 21% to 40% stenosis, a positive ^{201}Tl test result was more common when 85% predicted maximal heart rate was achieved (75%) than when it was not (40%) ($P < .05$). Of the 16 nonapical perfusion defects in patients with 21% to 40% stenosis, 14 (88%) corresponded to the myocardial territory of a 21% to 40% coronary stenosis. Patients taking propranolol were more likely to have a positive ^{201}Tl test response (45%) than patients who did not (22%) ($P < .05$). Although patients with stress-induced chest pain more commonly had a positive ^{201}Tl test response than those without chest pain had, this did not reach statistical significance. However, ^{201}Tl perfusion defects were more common when typical angina pectoris was elicited (75%) than when atypical chest pain developed (25%) ($P < .05$).

The high incidence of ^{201}Tl perfusion defects associated with stenosis of 21% to 40%, and the close correlation of such defects with the myocardial territory supplied by these stenoses, suggest that such lesions may have true hemodynamic impact, particularly at high levels of stress. In addition, the high incidence of positive ^{201}Tl test responses in patients taking propranolol suggests that an attempt be made to wean patients from β-blocker treatment before ^{201}Tl exercise testing is undertaken.

▶ Note that even lesions with luminal diameter narrowing of less than 50% may be associated with ischemia and particularly at high degrees of effort. Although the authors recommend weaning patients off β-adrenergic blocking drugs before undertaking exercise stress testing, and this is indeed theoretically correct, a sudden withdrawal may precipitate rebound effects on the heart rate and blood pressure to precipitate acute ischemia.—Leon Resnekov, M.D.

"Ischemia at a Distance" During Intermittent Coronary Artery Occlusion: A Coronary Anatomic Explanation
James F. Brymer, Fareed Khaja, Mario Marzilli, and Sidney Goldstein, with

the technical assistance of John Alban (Henry Ford Hosp., Detroit)
J. Am. Coll. Cardiol. 6:41–45, July 1985   4–23

Several studies have suggested that ECG changes in an ST segment remote from changes in the primary infarct zone, or "ischemia at a distance," simply reflect electric "reciprocity." Twenty-eight patients with single-vessel coronary artery disease were monitored continuously during coronary angioplasty with a six-lead ECG to determine the mechanism of such changes during acute coronary occlusion. Changes in the ST segment were assessed as to reproducibility on successive balloon inflations.

Twenty-three patients had changes in the ST segment in the primary zone of occlusion. Thirteen (57%) of the 23 had additional changes in the ST segment in a remote zone: ten had unusually extensive occluded coronary arteries that extended into remote areas, two had occluded adjacent normal arteries observed on balloon inflation, and one had no evident anatomical explanation for the changes in remote areas. Ten (43%) patients who had changes in the ST segment in the primary zone had no abnormality in the remote zone. Seven of the ten had nonextensive primary zone arteries and three had abundant preexisting collateral vessels. Five patients had no changes in the ST segment in the primary or remote zone; four had abundant preexisting collateral vessels and one had severe left ventricular hypertrophy on the baseline ECG.

It is believed that changes in the ST segment in a remote zone are usually determined anatomically by the size, distribution, and collateral supply of the coronary artery involved and are not simply reciprocal.

▶ Ischemia at a distance, or remote ischemia as it is sometimes termed, is important. It results from the inadequacy of segmental coronary flow at a distance from the primary site of occlusion. An inadequate epicardial coronary artery supply may cause this to emerge, but more commonly it is a critical lack of collateral myocardial circulation that causes the ischemia to manifest. Another mechanism for ischemia to be present longer than might have been expected is the process now known as the stunned myocardium. With it, segmental hypocontractility of the myocardium persists even after flow is restored to a temporarily hypoperfused area.—Leon Resnekov, M.D.

Increased Thallium Lung Uptake After Exercise in Isolated Left Anterior Descending Coronary Artery Disease

Peter Liu, Marla Kiess, Robert D. Okada, H. William Strauss, Peter C. Block, Gerald M. Pohost, and Charles A. Boucher (Massachusetts Gen. Hosp., Boston)
Am. J. Cardiol. 55:1469–1473, June 1, 1985   4–24

Increased uptake of thallium by the lungs during exercise has been associated with exercise-induced elevation in left ventricular filling pressure, particularly in patients with multivessel coronary artery disease

(CAD). To determine the implications of this finding in one-vessel CAD, thallium scans were analyzed from 48 patients with one-vessel left anterior descending (LAD) CAD before and after percutaneous transluminal coronary angioplasty.

Thirteen patients (27%) had increased thallium activity and 35 had normal uptake. Patients with increased thallium uptake had more severe narrowing of the luminal diameter of the LAD (mean, 90% vs. 81%; $P < .003$), a lower peak heart rate during exercise (mean, 100 beats per minute vs. 122 beats per minute; $P < .01$), more segments per patient with abnormal uptake based on visual and quantitative criteria ($P < .02$), and slower clearance of thallium from myocardial segments of the LAD (mean 13.5 hours vs. 6.5 hours; $P < .007$).

Using stepwise logistic regression analysis, the peak exercise heart rate achieved, percent of LAD stenosis, and number of LAD segments with abnormal thallium content according to quantitative criteria were the most significant and independent determinants of the probability of increased thallium uptake by the lungs. After angioplasty, thallium uptake returned to normal in 12 of the 13 patients with previously elevated uptake.

Increased thallium uptake by the lungs after exercise occurs in one-vessel LAD disease and is correlated with greater luminal stenosis by angiography and severity of ischemia by thallium imaging. Therefore, increased thallium uptake by the lungs identifies a subset of patients with one-vessel CAD who have a greater amount of myocardium at risk.

Relation of Coronary Artery Disease and Left Ventricular Systolic Dysfunction to Left Ventricular End-Diastolic Pressure After Left Ventriculography
Christopher L. Wolfe, Michael D. Winniford, Kevin R. Wheelan, Saul Schaefer, Brian G. Firth, and L. David Hillis (Univ. of Texas at Dallas)
Am. J. Cardiol. 55:1622–1623, June 1, 1985   4–25

Several studies suggest that the magnitude of increase of left ventricular end-diastolic pressure (LVEDP) after the injection of iodinated contrast material may be related to the presence and severity of coronary artery disease (CAD) or systolic LV dysfunction. To assess this relationship in patients with and without CAD and no valvular or congenital heart disease, LVEDP was measured in 81 consecutive patients before and after left ventriculography. End-diastolic and end-systolic volumes and ejection fraction were calculated.

The mean baseline LVEDP was 14 mm Hg for 24 patients without and 17 mm Hg for 57 with CAD. Although LVEDP increased in all patients after left ventriculography, there was no difference in the mean $\triangle$LVEDP (peak minus baseline) between those without (9 mm Hg) and those with (8 mm Hg) CAD, regardless of the severity of the narrowing of the coronary artery. There was no relationship between $\triangle$LVEDP and LV ejection fraction, end-systolic volume index, cardiac index, or differential LV pressure.

The measurement of LVEDP after left ventriculography in patients without associated valvular or congenital heart disease has no value in identifying those with CAD or systolic LV dysfunction.

▶ Note that, contrary to popular belief, in this study measuring LVEDP after left ventriculography had little diagnostic value in the diagnosis of coronary artery disease or systolic hypofunctioning of the ventricle.—Leon Resnekov, M.D.

Simultaneous Assessment of Left Ventricular Systolic and Diastolic Dysfunction During Pacing-Induced Ischemia
Julian M. Aroesty, Raymond G. McKay, Gary V. Heller, Henry D. Royal, Ann V. Als, and William Grossman (Beth Israel Hosp., Boston, and Harvard Univ.)
Circulation 71:889–900, May 1985   4–26

Both systolic and diastolic dysfunction occur during pacing-induced myocardial ischemia, but the temporal sequence has not been established, partly because of technical difficulties in serial pressure-volume analyses at different pacing rates. Radionuclide ventriculography was used to evaluate 22 patients with coronary artery disease who were paced at increasing heart rates. Hemodynamic monitoring and ECG recording were carried out simultaneously. Sequential pressure-volume diagrams were constructed by using synchronized left ventricular pressure tracings and radionuclide volume curves. The 15 men and 7 women in the study had a mean age of 59 years. Nine had a myocardial infarction previously. Atrial pacing was carried out at an intermediate heart rate and at the maximum rate, either 85% of the age-predicted rate or the rate at which marked angina or atrioventricular block developed.

Eleven patients (group I) had nonischemic responses to pacing tachycardia; the other 11 (group II) had ischemic responses at the maximum pacing rate. None of the latter had angina or ischemic ST segment changes on intermediate pacing. Group I patients had a progressive decline in left ventricular end-diastolic pressure and volume and end-systolic volume, and no change in left ventricular ejection fraction. Pressure-volume diagrams suggested increased contractility and a slight increase in left ventricular distensibility. Group II patients had increased left ventricular end-diastolic pressure and volume after initial reduction, and a fall in ejection fraction. Decreased left ventricular distensibility was evident on intermediate-rate pacing before the onset of systolic dysfunction with maximum-rate pacing.

Both systolic and diastolic dysfunction are observed during ischemic responses to pacing tachycardia in patients with coronary artery disease. Diastolic impairment often precedes systolic depression in this setting.

▶ Although much emphasis has been placed on demonstrating systolic dysfunction of the left ventricle as an index of ischemia, considering diastolic function can also provide important insight into the pathophysiologic mechanisms associated with significant ischemia.—Leon Resnekov, M.D.

Usefulness of Transstenotic Coronary Pressure Gradient Measurements During Diagnostic Catheterization

Peter Ganz, Richard Abben, Peter L. Friedman, J. Daniel Garnic, William H. Barry, and David C. Levin (Brigham and Women's Hosp. and Harvard Med. School)
Am. J. Cardiol. 55:910–914, April 1, 1985   4–27

A method was devised of measuring phasic transstenotic coronary pressure gradients at routine catheterization. A 2 F polyvinyl chloride catheter with a radiopaque tip was used. Thirty-two transstenotic pressure gradients were measured in 25 patients seen between 1982 and 1984 who were candidates for primary percutaneous transluminal coronary angioplasty (PTCA) and 7 being considered for repeat PTCA. Patients with coronary collateral vessels and variant angina were excluded.

Fifteen patients had moderate angiographic stenoses of 25% to 75%. Seven of them had relatively large mean transstenotic gradients of 11–30 mm Hg at rest, increasing to 23–37 mm Hg when Renografin was injected, which increased coronary blood flow (Figs 4–3 and 4–4). All of these patients were well after technically successful PTCA. The eight patients with gradients of 0–6 mm Hg at rest and 0–21 mm Hg after injection of contrast material did not have PTCA. Two of the five with atypical angina

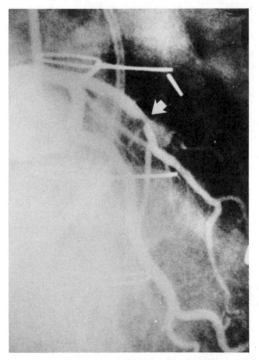

Fig 4–3.—Coronary arteriogram in anteroposterior view showing stenosis in left anterior descending coronary artery *(arrow)*. (Courtesy of Ganz, P., et al.: Am. J. Cardiol. 55:910–914, April 1, 1985.)

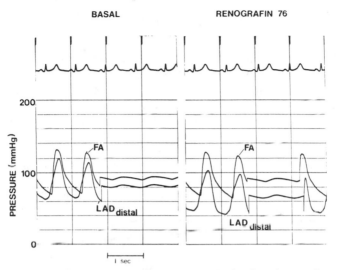

BASAL   RENOGRAFIN 76

Fig 4–4.—Mean transstenotic pressure gradient was 11 mm Hg basally and increased to 23 mm Hg after Renografin 76. FA, sidearm of femoral artery sheath; LAD$_{distal}$, left anterior descending coronary artery pressure beyond stenosis. (Courtesy of Ganz, P., et al.: Am. J. Cardiol. 55:910–914, April 1, 1985.)

were found to have esophageal disease. Another patient had a subtotally occluded marginal circumflex branch. Gradient measurements helped avoid invasive treatment in these patients. The 17 patients with angiographically severe stenoses had a mean resting gradient of 36 mm Hg and a mean gradient of 47 mm Hg after injection of contrast material. All patients did well after PTCA or, if it was necessary, coronary bypass grafting.

This is a safe and useful means of determining the physiologic significance of coronary stenoses. Transstenotic pressure gradient measurement at diagnostic catheterization may be especially useful when deciding on treatment in patients with angiographically moderate coronary stenoses.

▶ The determination of pressure gradients across stenotic coronary arteries is an extremely useful measurement for assessing the significance of arteriosclerotic narrowing of coronary arteries. In practice, however, treatment decisions, particularly those concerning PTCA and even aortocoronary bypass graft surgery, are unfortunately often made without any physiologic demonstration that a particular lesion has a hemodynamic effect.—Leon Resnekov, M.D.

Early Detection of Restenosis After Successful Percutaneous Transluminal Coronary Angioplasty by Exercise-Redistribution Thallium Scintigraphy
William Wijns, Patrick W. Serruys, Johan H. C. Reiber, Pim J. de Feyter, Marcel van den Brand, Maarten L. Simoons, and Paul G. Hugenholtz, with the statistical assistance of Jan G. P. Tüssen (Erasmus Univ. and Univ. Hosp. Dijkzigt, Rotterdam, The Netherlands)
Am. J. Cardiol. 55:357–361, Feb. 1, 1985   4–28

The value of exercise testing and thallium scintigraphy in predicting recurrence of angina pectoris and restenosis after primary successful percutaneous transluminal coronary angioplasty (PTCA) was evaluated prospectively. Symptom-limited exercise ECG and thallium scintigraphy were performed in 89 patients 4 weeks after they underwent successful PTCA. These patients were followed for 6.4 ± 2.5 months (mean, ± SD) or until recurrence of angina. They all underwent repeat coronary angiography at 6 months, or earlier if symptoms recurred. If the patients had no symptoms and if the stenosis was reduced to less than 50% of the luminal diameter, PTCA was considered successful. Restenosis was defined as an increase of the stenosis to more than 50% of the luminal diameter.

The ability of the thallium scintigram (presence of a reversible defect) to predict recurrence of angina was 66% vs. 38% for the exercise ECG (ST segment depression or angina at peak workload). Restenosis was predicted in 74% of patients by thallium scintigraphy, but in only 50% by exercise ECG.

Thallium scintigraphy was highly predictive, but the exercise ECG was not. These results suggest that, if restenosis was going to occur, it would have done so to some extent within 4 weeks after PTCA.

▶ Because, at present, there is a 30% incidence of restenosis after PTCA, a reliable noninvasive test could have great importance. In this study, note that thallium myocardial scintigraphy was more predictive than exercise ECG was. Unfortunately, not infrequently when restenosis occurs following PTCA, the process begins within the early weeks after treatment.—Leon Resnekov, M.D.

Assessment of Hemodynamic Significance of Isolated Stenoses of The Left Anterior Descending Coronary Artery Using Thallium-201 Myocardial Scintigraphy

Victor Kalff, Michael J. Kelly, Alan Soward, Richard W. Harper, Philip J. Currie, Yean L. Lim, and Aubrey Pitt (Alfred Hosp., Melbourne)
Am. J. Cardiol. 55:342–346, Feb. 1, 1985   4–29

The hypothesis was tested that results of stress thallium-201 myocardial perfusion scans (^{201}Tl) are related to the mean transstenotic pressure gradient of coronary stenoses independent of the percent of luminal diameter narrowing seen at angiography. The study patients included 20 men and 2 women, with a mean age of 47 years who had no previous myocardial infarction. Each underwent a symptom-limited, erect bicycle ^{201}Tl test when not taking antianginal therapy, shortly before percutaneous transluminal coronary angioplasty (PTCA) was performed in treatment of isolated left anterior descending coronary artery stenosis. The percent of narrowing, mean gradient at PTCA, and presence of a visually apparent ^{201}Tl defect were independently evaluated and results compared.

Four patients with 90% or more narrowing of the luminal diameter had positive ^{201}Tl responses with a mean gradient of 72 mm Hg. Among 18 patients with diameter narrowing of less than 90% the mean gradient was higher in the 11 whose ^{201}Tl response was positive (63 mm Hg) than in the 7 whose ^{201}Tl response was negative (33 mm Hg); however, the percent of narrowing did not differ significantly. Multiple regression analysis showed that the presence of a ^{201}Tl defect was a strong ($P = .003$), and percent narrowing a weak ($P = .048$), independent predictor of gradient. When the mean gradient was normalized for prestenotic pressure, both percent of narrowing ($P = .003$) and ^{201}Tl defects ($P = .006$) were significant independent predictors.

It would seem that ^{201}Tl adds valid information concerning the hemodynamic significance of a stenosis independent of percent of luminal diameter narrowing; this may be of value when the percent of narrowing is less than 90% and the clinical significance of a coronary stenosis is uncertain.

Prognostic Significance of Progression of Coronary Artery Disease

Alain Moise, Martial G. Bourassa, Pierre Théroux, Yves Taeymans, André Pasternac, Lucien Campeau, Marc A. Bois, Ihor Dyrda, and Paul Robert David (Montreal Heart Inst.)
Am. J. Cardiol. 55:941–946, April 1, 1985   4–30

Progression of coronary artery disease (CAD) is frequently seen on repeat cardiac catheterization, but its prognostic importance is uncertain. The influence of progressive disease on survival was studied in 313 patients with CAD who were catheterized twice, a mean of 39 months apart, and were followed for a mean of 41 months after the second study. The repeat study was most often done because of persistent stable angina, but 52 patients had unstable angina and 15 had recent acute infarction.

Progression of coronary disease was documented in 44% of patients, with at least 20% more stenosis in a segment initially narrowed by 50%

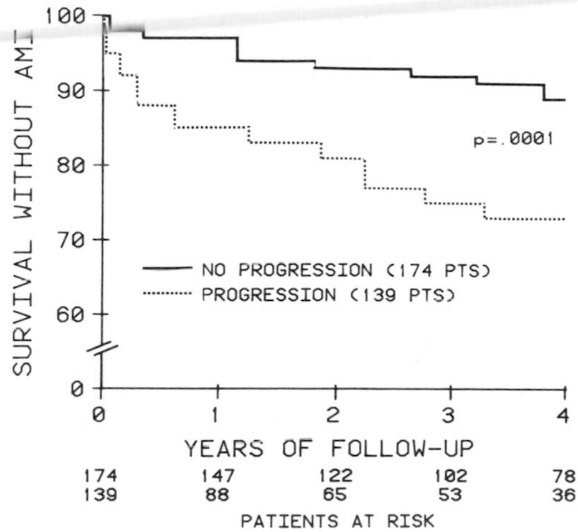

Fig 4–5.—Cumulative survival without acute myocardial infarction (AMI) in patients with and without progression. Comparison is performed by log-rank test. (Courtesy of Moise, A., et al.: Am. J. Cardiol. 55:941–946, April 1, 1985.)

or more or at least 30% more stenosis in an initially less narrowed segment. Coronary bypass grafting was performed in 116 patients after the second angiogram. The estimated 4-year survival was 89.5%. The 4-year survival without acute infarction was 82.5%. Progression was the most prominent predictor of survival without infarction on univariate analysis (Fig 4–5). Progression was also the best predictor of fatal or nonfatal infarction. Survival and survival without infarction did not differ significantly in the medical and surgical groups, even when perioperative events were excluded. The predictive value of progression for major events persisted.

Progression of coronary disease is an important prognostic factor for acute infarction; patients with progressive disease are at high risk of infarction. Measures designed to prevent infarction or slow atherogenesis, or both, might be targeted for these patients.

▶ Note that progression of coronary atherosclerosis was documented in almost half of the patients studied at a mean time of 39 months after the initial investigation. In addition, those in whom the lesions progressed were at much greater risk of myocardial infarction and other acute cardiac events occurring within a relatively short period of time.—Leon Resnekov, M.D.

Clinical and Angiographic Predictors of New Total Coronary Occlusion in Coronary Artery Disease: Analysis of 313 Nonoperated Patients
Alain Moise, Jacques Lespérance, Pierre Théroux, Yves Taeymans, Claude Goulet, and Martial G. Bourassa (Montreal Heart Inst.)
Am. J. Cardiol. 54:1176–1181, Dec. 1, 1984   4–31

Although the definition of progression in coronary artery disease (CAD) may vary, it usually includes the occurrence of a new occlusion as a qualifying criterion for progression. To identify clinical and angiographic predictors of new total coronary occlusion in CAD, data were analyzed concerning 313 consecutive patients who were treated medically and underwent catheterization twice, a mean of 39 months apart.

A new coronary artery occlusion was found in 98 (31%) patients on the repeat angiogram. Multivariate logistic regression analysis showed eight independent predictors of new occlusion. Four variables were identified at the time of the second angiogram: interval between the two studies ($P = .005$), decrease in ejection fraction ($P < .01$), appearance of bundle branch block ($P < .01$), and interim myocardial infarction ($P < .05$).

Four other predictors identified at the time of the first angiogram included two angiographic characteristics, one related to CAD severity (presence of 80% to 90% stenosis that jeopardized a nonakinetic left ventricular segment) ($P < .005$), and one related to extent of CAD (count of the lesions narrowed 75% or less in luminal diameter in a 15-segment coding system) ($P < .05$). The two other risk factors were smoking ($P < .05$) and male sex ($P < .05$). The 140 male smokers with at least one stenosis of 80% or more that jeopardized a contractile left ventricular segment or an extent score of 4 or more had higher incidence of occlusion than found in the 173 low-risk patients after intervals of less than 2 years (13/53 vs. 7/74, $P < .001$), 2–4 years (23/40 vs. 10/47, $P < .005$), and more than 4 years (27/47 vs. 18/54, $P < .05$). An interim myocardial infarction, new akinesia, and a 10% or greater decrease in ejection fraction were also more frequent in the high-risk group, suggesting that the predicted occlusions actually contributed to the worsening of left ventricular function. The appearance of a new coronary artery occlusion can be predicted by a combination of two angiographic and two clinical characteristics at the time of the first evaluation.

Evolving Myocardial Infarction

▶ ↓ The seven abstracts that follow document early and late results after thrombolytic therapy for evolving myocardial infarction, about which much concern and uncertainty remain. Based on the results of many large randomized trials, there seems little doubt that thrombolytic therapy succeeds in lysing coronary artery thrombi in many patients. The time for administering therapy may be critical. If administered intravenously within 90 minutes of onset of symptoms, streptokinase succeeds in a very high proportion of patients, but there is no absolute time of administration beyond 90 minutes that negates any chance of success. The shorter the time from onset of symptoms to receiving treatment, the better the results, not only of lysing thrombi but also, and equally important, of ensuring improvement in the acutely depressed ventricular function. Recombinant tissue plasminogen activator yields results even more impressive than those of streptokinase in lysing thrombi, and there are several newer compounds that may succeed equally or be even more efficient.

Whether percutaneous transluminal coronary angioplasty (PTCA) should be attempted (and if so, when) after thrombolytic therapy is as yet uncertain. Many patients who sustain evolving myocardial infarction have thrombi superimposed on severe atherosclerotic coronary artery narrowing. Lytic therapy, of course, cannot reduce the degree of atherosclerosis, and the questions being asked about PTCA after lytic therapy are by no means unimportant. This is particularly so because a need for proceeding rapidly after thrombolysis to PTCA might require cardiac catheterization laboratories to be available for such methods at any time during the day or night, something that logistically is difficult to achieve in practice and is also very costly. Studies are required to determine the need for and timing of PTCA in association with thrombolytic therapy. Results should be considered both in the short-term and long-term, particularly the effects of therapy and its timing on ventricular function.—Leon Resnekov, M.D.

Intracoronary Thrombolytic Therapy in Acute Myocardial Infarction: A Prospective, Randomized, Controlled Trial
Albert E. Raizner, Francisco A. Tortoledo, Mario S. Verani, and Richard E. van Reet, with James B. Young, Frank D. Rickman, W. Richard Cashion, David A. Samuels, Craig M. Pratt, Mohammed Attar, Howard S. Rubin, John M. Lewis, Milton S. Klein, and Robert Roberts (Baylor College of Medicine)
Am. J. Cardiol. 55:301–308, Feb. 1, 1985   4–32

A prospective, randomized trial was conducted to assess the efficacy of intracoronary thrombolytic therapy with streptokinase in AMI in 64 patients who were randomized within 6 hours of onset of symptoms to one of three groups. A control group of 16 patients received conventional treatment. Nineteen patients underwent coronary arteriography and received corticosteroids as well as the intracoronary and intravenous administration of nitroglycerin. Twenty-nine patients received management identical to that of the nitroglycerin group, with the addition of the intracoronary administration of streptokinase.

Recanalization occurred in 21 of 29 patients (72%) given streptokinase. The global and regional ejection fraction (EF) was determined by radionuclide ventriculography before any intervention and 7–10 days later. No significant improvement in global EF was achieved in controls or in those given nitroglycerin. The global EF did not increase significantly in those given streptokinase. However, in patients recanalized with the latter drug, the EF improved from 42% to 49%. Responses in all groups varied widely. Improvement in global EF of more than 5% was noted in 44% of patients recanalized with streptokinase. When subgrouped on the basis of initial global EF of 45% or less, or more than 45%, only patients recanalized with streptokinase and an initial EF of 45% or less had an improved global EF. The regional EF of all involved infarct regions was improved only in the streptokinase group and in the streptokinase-recanalized subgroup. When only the most involved infarct regions were analyzed, the control, nitroglycerin-treated, and streptokinase-treated groups improved, with patients recanalized with streptokinase having the greatest degree of improvement.

This study demonstrates a beneficial effect of thrombolytic therapy on global and regional function in patients in whom recanalization with streptokinase is successful, with predominant benefit in those with initially depressed left ventricular function.

Intravenous Versus Intracoronary Streptokinase in Acute Myocardial Infarction

Russell P. Valentine, Douglas E. Pitts, Jo Ann Brooks-Brunn, James G. Williams, Eugene Van Hove, and Paul E. Schmidt (Methodist Hosp. of Indiana, Inc., Indianapolis)

Am. J. Cardiol. 55:309–312, Feb. 1, 1985   4–33

Studies were made in 164 consecutive patients with AMI in a prospective trial of coronary thrombolysis with streptokinase. The first 98 patients were treated with the intracoronary (ic) administration of streptokinase after coronary angiography, and the next 66 patients received a high-dose rapid infusion of streptokinase [900,000 international units (IU)] intravenously (iv) before angiography. The average total drug dose in ic patients was 213,000 ± 82,000 IU. First-pass radionuclide ejection fraction (EF) was determined within 24 hours of admission and 10–14 days afterward to evaluate left ventricular function.

In the iv group, 42 of 66 infarct-related arteries were patent on the initial angiogram and 6 opened with subsequent ic streptokinase. In the ic group, 13 of 98 infarct-related arteries were patent on the initial angiogram and 50 of 85 opened with the ic streptokinase. The iv and ic groups did not differ in time from onset of chest pain to presentation, type of infarct, or underlying severity of coronary artery disease. In the iv group, streptokinase therapy was begun 67 minutes earlier than in the ic group. In 62 patients in whom reperfusion was successful, the mean EF increased from 39% early to 48% late. The mean EF increased from 36% to 40% in 30 patients in whom reperfusion was unsuccessful. The increase in EF was significantly greater in patients in the reperfused group. The mean EF increased by 11% in 18 iv streptokinase-reperfused patients, whereas in 44 patients who had reperfusion by ic streptokinase the mean EF increased by 9% (difference not significant). Complications of the lysis procedure were similar in the two groups. Streptokinase whether given by the ic or iv route is of comparable efficacy and safety in establishing reperfusion of the infarct-related artery in patients with AMI.

Effects of Intracoronary Streptokinase and Intracoronary Nitroglycerin Infusion on Coronary Angiographic Patterns and Mortality in Patients With Acute Myocardial Infarction
K. Peter Rentrop, Frederick Feit, Heinrich Blanke, Peter Stecy, Richard Schneider, Mariano Rey, Steven Horowitz, Martin Goldman, Karl Karsch, Henry Meilman, Marc Cohen, Stephen Siegel, Joseph Sanger, James Slater, Richard Gorlin, Arthur Fox, Richard Fagerstrom, and W. Ford Calhoun (Mt. Sinai School of Medicine and New York Univ.)
N. Engl. J. Med. 311:1457–1463, Dec. 6, 1984   4–34

In all, 124 patients seen from 1981 to 1982 with a clinical diagnosis of AMI were assigned to intracoronary streptokinase or nitroglycerin administration, both treatments, or conventional management without initial angiography. The dose of streptokinase was 2,000 units per minute, and that of nitroglycerin, 0.01 mg/minute. Coronary angiography was performed after the intravenous administration of heparin. The study patients subsequently received nitroglycerin intravenously in standard doses for 72 hours, followed by isosorbide dinitrate orally. All patients were fully anticoagulated with heparin acutely and then given warfarin for 3 months.

All but two patients had ECG or enzymatic evidence of AMI. Total coronary occlusion was found on initial angiography in 67% of the 91 patients examined. Acute recanalization occurred in 74% of 43 streptokinase-treated patients, but in only 6% of 18 nitroglycerin-treated patients. Comparable patency rates (77%) were found in all groups after 10–14 days. Mortality at 6 months was 21% in streptokinase-treated patients and 10% in patients not given streptokinase, not a significant difference. Mortality at 6 months was significantly related to both previous infarction and anterior wall infarction. No deaths were clearly related to intervention, but one was a complication of angiography. Serious bleeding was similarly frequent in all groups.

Potential benefit from early recanalization of total coronary obstruction was possible in only about half of the present series. Because thrombolytic therapy carries a risk of hemorrhage and has not been confirmed to improve either left ventricular function or survival, continued evaluation by prospective randomized trials is required before the method is generally adopted for clinical use.

Late Effects of Intracoronary Streptokinase on Regional Wall Motion, Ventricular Aneurysm, and Left Ventricular Thrombus in Myocardial Infarction: Results From the Western Washington Randomized Trial
John R. Stratton, Sarah M. Speck, James H. Caldwell, Michael L. Stadius, Charles Maynard, Kathryn B. Davis, James L. Ritchie, and J. Ward Kennedy (Seattle VA Med. Ctr. and Univ. of Washington)
J. Am. Coll. Cardiol. 5:1023–1028, May 1985   4–35

Although intracoronary streptokinase reestablishes coronary artery patency in 60% to 80% of patients with AMI, its role in preserving left ventricular function is controversial. In addition, its effect on left ventricular aneurysm or thrombus formation has not been established.

To determine whether intracoronary streptokinase improves late regional wall motion or reduces left ventricular aneurysm or thrombus formation in patients with AMI, two-dimensional echocardiography was performed at 8 ± 3 weeks after infarction in 83 patients randomized to receive streptokinase (n = 45) or standard therapy (n = 38) in the Western Washington Intracoronary Streptokinase Trial. Regional wall motion was evaluated in nine left ventricular segments in at least two views on a scale of 1 to 4 (normal, hypokinetic, akinetic, and dyskinetic). Left ventricular thrombus formation was interpreted as positive, equivocal, or negative. All patients received anticoagulant therapy in the hospital and 52 continued to receive it after discharge.

Among the patients treated with streptokinase, the average time to treatment was 4.7 ± 2.5 hours after onset of symptoms; 67% had successful reperfusion. There was no significant difference between streptokinase-treated and control patients in mean global (1.5 ± 0.4 in both groups) and regional wall motion. The prevalence of left ventricular aneurysm was 16% in both groups. There were four definite left ventricular thrombi and one equivocal thrombus, all in the streptokinase-treated group (difference not significant). There was no benefit of streptokinase therapy in any of the echocardiographic variables in subgroups of patients with anterior infarction, inferior infarction, no prior infarction, or reperfusion with streptokinase.

Intracoronary streptokinase, when given relatively late in the course of AMI, does not result in improved global or regional wall motion or a reduction in left ventricular aneurysm or thrombus formation in 8-week survivors. These findings contrast with those of prior studies that report sustained improvement at 1 month and at 6 months. However, the echocardiographic findings are concordant with the results of late global and regional radionuclide ejection fraction studies in the entire cohort of patients in the Western Washington Intracoronary Streptokinase Trial.

Factors That Determine Recovery of Left Ventricular Function After Thrombolysis in Patients With Acute Myocardial Infarction
Florence H. Sheehan, Detlef G. Mathey, Joachim Schofer, Harold T. Dodge, and Edward L. Bolson, with the technical assistance of Suzanne Mitten and Jane Wygant (Univ. of Washington and Univ. Hosp. Eppendorf, Hamburg)
Circulation 71:1121–1128, June 1985   4–36

An attempt was made to determine the factors influencing recovery of regional left ventricular function after reperfusion in patients given streptokinase by the intracoronary route in treatment of AMI. All patients were seen within 3 hours of onset of chest pain. Streptokinase was infused at a rate of 4,000 units per minute to reperfusion, and then at a rate of 2,000 units per minute for at least 45 minutes longer. Angiography was repeated an average of 45 days later, and 13 patients were again evaluated 8–24 months after thrombolytic therapy. Hypokinesis in the region of infarction was measured by the centerline method.

Patients with circumflex artery thrombosis had less regional hypokinesis early after infarction than the others had, and they had no functional recovery after reperfusion. In the other patients, hypokinesis improved more after thrombolysis in those with a minimal stenosis diameter exceeding 0.4 mm than in those with severe residual stenosis. Hypokinesis also improved more in patients treated within 2 hours of onset of symptoms. Patients with the most depressed regional function initially had the greatest improvement.

Thrombolysis can salvage left ventricular function in patients with AMI, but reperfusion alone may not be adequate. It must be achieved early in the course of infarction, and definitive revascularization may be necessary to produce maximum functional recovery.

Coronary Thrombolysis With Recombinant Human Tissue-Type Plasminogen Activator: A Prospective, Randomized, Placebo-Controlled Trial
Désiré Collen, Eric J. Topol, Alan J. Tiefenbrunn, Herman K. Gold, Myron L. Weisfeldt, Burton E. Sobel, Robert C. Leinbach, Jeffrey A. Brinker, Philip A. Ludbrook, Isunehiro Yasuda, Bernadine H. Bulkley, Alice K. Robison, Adolph M. Hutter, Jr., William R. Bell, James J. Spadaro, Jr., Ban An Khaw, and Elliott B. Grossbard (Genetech, Inc., South San Francisco; Univ. of Leuven, Belgium; Johns Hopkins and Baltimore City Hosps.; Washington Univ.-Barnes Hosp. Med. Ctr.; and Massachusetts Gen. Hosp.)
Circulation 70:1012–1017, December 1984   4–37

Human tissue-type plasminogen activator (t-PA), which can induce thrombolysis without systemic fibrinogenolysis, is now available in recombinant form (rt-PA) for widespread use if desired. A collaborative study of rt-PA thrombolysis was undertaken in 45 consecutive patients seen within 6 hours of onset of symptoms of myocardial infarction. An intravenous dose of 0.5 mg/kg is now given over 1 hour and an intracoronary dose of 0.375 mg/kg over 30 minutes. Recent patients have received another 0.25 mg/kg intravenously in another hour.

One of 14 patients given placebo had complete recanalization and 1 had partial recanalization. Three fourths of patients given 0.5 mg of rt-PA per kg intravenously had complete recanalization within 90 minutes. Five patients had early reocclusion. All four patients with partial recanalization did well with intracoronary streptokinase treatment. There was no mortality during the study, and no patient required transfusion. Reperfusion arrhythmias were benign and readily treated. No patient had a fall in fibrinogen concentration to less than 100 mg/dl.

Both intravenous and intracoronary infusion of rt-PA can reliably produce coronary thrombolysis without compromising systemic hemostasis, generally within 90 minutes. Early reocclusion has occurred in about one fifth of the patients, but only after discontinuance of the infusion. Intravenous rt-PA administration holds considerable promise for coronary thrombolysis in patients seen soon after onset of myocardial infarction.

Regional Wall Motion Improvement After Coronary Thrombolysis With Recombinant Tissue Plasminogen Activator: Importance of Coronary Angioplasty
Eric J. Topol, James L. Weiss, Jeffrey A. Brinker, Kenneth P. Brin, Sidney O. Gottlieb, Lewis C. Becker, Bernadine H. Bulkley, Nisha Chandra, John T. Flaherty, Gary Gerstenblith, Sheldon H. Gottlieb, Alan D. Guerci, Pamela Ouyang, Michaelene P. Llewellyn, Myron L. Weisfeldt, and Edward P. Shapiro (Johns Hopkins Hosp. and Francis Scott Key Med. Ctr., Baltimore)
J. Am. Coll. Cardiol. 6:426–433, August 1985   4–38

The efficacy of coronary thrombolysis with recombinant tissue plasminogen activator (rt-PA) in restoring myocardial function was examined in 20 consecutive patients seen within 6 hours of onset of chest pain caused by myocardial infarction. Patients received rt-PA intravenously in a dose of 0.25–0.75 mg/kg in 30–120 minutes or a saline placebo. Three patients without recanalization during placebo infusion received rt-PA by intracoronary infusion in a dose of 0.375 mg/kg in 15–30 minutes.

Reperfusion with rt-PA succeeded in 65% of patients. Only one of three patients treated by the intracoronary route had reperfusion. Two of nine patients with reperfusion who returned for coronary angioplasty had reocclusion at that time, without symptoms; angioplasty failed in these patients. A patient with total left anterior descending artery occlusion died in cardiogenic shock. Another patient had an intracoronary thrombus at the time of surgical revascularization. The most functional improvement was seen at 10 days in patients who had both successful thrombolysis and coronary angioplasty. However, early reperfusion could not be related to the functional recovery of infarct segments.

Angioplasty has an important role in enhancing regional myocardial function after acute coronary occlusion and coronary thrombolysis. Thrombolysis with rt-PA provides for safe, definitive revascularization by coronary angioplasty.

Myocardial Infarction: Acute and Later Phases

Acute Myocardial Infarction: Period Prevalence, Case Fatality, and Comparison of Black and White Cases in Urban and Rural Areas of South Carolina

Julian E. Keil, Donald E. Saunders, Jr., Daniel T. Lackland, Martin C. Weinrich, Murray B. Hudson, John A. Gastright, Naseeb B. Baroody, E. C. O'-Bryan, Jr., and Ronald W. Zmyslinski (Medical Univ. of South Carolina; Richland Mem. Hosp., Columbia, S.C.; Univ. of South Carolina; and South Carolina Dept. of Health and Environmental Control, Columbia)

Am. Heart J. 109:776–784, April 1985   4–39

Community surveillance may explain the relative roles of prevention (in terms of AMI incidence data) and improved medical care practice (in terms of case fatality rate) in the recent significant decline in cardiovascular disease mortality. It may also offer information on geographic patterns of manifestations of cardiovascular disease and the effect of environmental factors. To examine the feasibility of establishing community surveillance of cardiovascular disease in two geographically distinct areas of South Carolina, patient charts were reviewed for baseline data of AMI occurrence in blacks and whites, in-hospital case fatality, out-of-hospital mortality attributed to AMI, location of infarction, and racial and gender differences from the rural Pee Dee area and urban Columbia. Selected data were also secured from death certificates. The diagnosis of AMI (definite, probable, unvalidated, or negative) was based on certain criteria, including ECG findings, retrosternal pain, lactate dehydrogenase concentration, and creatine phosphokinase activity.

Community surveillance revealed 1,085 prevalent AMIs during 1978 in both areas. Based on the criteria described, 658 hospitalized patients had definite or probable AMI. Death certificates identified 427 who died before admission to the hospital and whose disease was classified as unvalidated. This indicated a need to verify death certificate diagnosis in out-of-hospital deaths, which occurred in approximately two thirds of all black patients and about one third of whites. White males had higher AMI rates among rural Pee Dee residents than in urban Columbia, whereas blacks of both sexes had higher rates in Columbia. White females had similar AMI rates in both areas. For definite and all criteria AMI in both Columbia and the Pee Dee area, white males had the highest period prevalence rates, at least double the black male rates except for all criteria AMI in Columbia, where white male and black male rates were similar. Out-of hospital AMI rates were higher in blacks than in whites in both areas, and were four times higher than in the Minneapolis-St. Paul area. Urban-living patients experienced more anterior infarctions than did those living in rural areas, which may partly explain the higher in-hospital case fatality in urban Columbia.

This study demonstrates the feasibility of assessing patient records in private and community hospitals in urban and rural areas of South Carolina. The data indicate those areas that need to be approached to improve survival after cardiovascular events, e.g., better access to emergency care (transportation to hospitals), particularly in the black population.

▶ It is known that hypertension is more common in blacks living in the United States. This is an interesting study comparing the prevalence and mortality of AMI among blacks and whites and in rural and urban areas of South Carolina. Curiously, there were more anterior infarctions in urban patients. A worrisome finding was the higher out-of-hospital rates of AMI in blacks. Further demographic studies of this type may provide more insight into racial differences of cardiac disease and provide help in planning effective medical coverage in areas at present deficient.—Leon Resnekov, M.D.

Use of the Initial Electrocardiogram To Predict In-Hospital Complications of Acute Myocardial Infarction
John E. Brush, Jr., Donald A. Brand, Denise Acampora, Bruce Chalmer, and Frans J. Wackers (Yale Univ. and Univ. of Vermont)
N. Engl. J. Med. 312:1137–1141, May 2, 1985   4–40

The initial ECG was evaluated as a predictor of complications in 469 patients with suspected AMI to determine whether ECG interpretation can be used to identify those having a low likelihood of complications who could be safely hospitalized in an intermediate care unit. An ECG recording was classified as positive if it showed one or more of the following: evidence

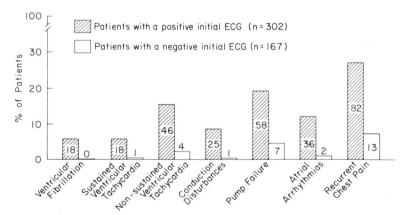

Fig 4–6.—Percentages of patients with individual complications of acute myocardial infarction, according to the initial ECG. Numbers of patients are shown within or above the bars. The differences in complication rates between the two ECG groups are all statistically significant ($P < .01$). (Courtesy of Brush, J.E., Jr., et al.: N. Engl. J. Med. 312:1137–1141, May 2, 1985. Reprinted by permission of The New England Journal of Medicine.)

of infarction, ischemia, or strain; left ventricular hypertrophy; left bundle branch block; or paced rhythm.

Forty-two (14%) of 302 patients with positive ECGs had at least one life-threatening complication (ventricular fibrillation, sustained ventricular tachycardia, or heart block), as compared with only 1 (0.6%) of 167 patients with a negative ECG. Figure 4–6 represents the rates of individual complications of AMI. Life-threatening complications were 23 times more likely if the initial ECG was positive ($P < .001$). Other complications were three to ten times more likely ($P < .01$), and the need for interventions was four to ten times more likely ($P < .05$). Death was 17 times more likely ($P < .001$) in patients with a positive ECG.

Patients with a negative initial ECG have a low likelihood of complications and could be treated in an intermediate care unit rather than a coronary care unit. This would reduce admissions to the coronary care unit by 36%, thus reducing hospital costs without compromising patient care.

Q Wave, S-T Segment, and T Wave Myocardial Infarction: Useful Clinical Distinction
Michael J. Zema (Brookhaven Meml. Hosp. Med. Ctr., Patchogue, N.Y.)
Am. J. Med. 78:391–398, March 1985   4–41

Abundant experimental and clinical evidence now suggests that the presence or absence of Q waves on surface ECG does not permit distinction between pathologic transmural and subendocardial myocardial infarction. It has been recommended that the use of certain ECG descriptors of myocardial infarction be avoided. To establish clinical subsets, studies were made in 114 consecutive patients with first myocardial infarction. The table presents the incidence of various ECG infarction types and the in-hospital patient mortality associated with them.

The lack of development of Q waves accompanying AMI delineated

---

INCIDENCE OF ELECTROCARDIOGRAPHIC
MYOCARDIAL INFARCTION TYPES AND ASSOCIATED
IN-HOSPITAL MORTALITY

Types	Incidence (percent)	Mortality (percent)
Normal electrocardiographic	3/114 (3)	0/3 (0)
S-T segment	3/114 (3)	1/3 (33)
T wave	22/114 (19)	0/22 (0)*
Non-Q wave	28/114 (25)	1/28 (4)†
Q wave (total)	86/114 (75)	13/86 (15)
Q wave (inferior)	50/114 (44)	6/50 (12)
Q wave (anterior)	36/114 (32)	7/36 (19)

*$P = .03$.
†$P = .07$.
(Courtesy of Zema, M.J.: Am. J. Med. 78:391–398, March 1985.)

those patients with low in-hospital mortality. The left ventricular ejection fraction was less after Q wave than after non-Q wave infarction ($P <$ .0001). Left ventricular end-diastolic pressure was greater after Q wave than after non-Q wave infarction ($P < .02$). Fixed thallium perfusion scintigraphic defects were more common in survivors of Q wave (98%) than in survivors of non-Q wave (64%) infarction ($P < .002$). Objectively demonstrable myocardial ischemia was more common after non-Q wave (68%) than after Q wave (32%) infarction ($P < .01$). The incidence of late cardiac events (sudden death plus reinfarction) did not differ after Q wave or non-Q wave infarction. Patients with Q wave, ST segment, and T wave myocardial infarction differed physiologically, clinically, and prognostically.

It is of little consequence to the clinician managing patients whether or not these useful ECG descriptors also accurately define groups that differ anatomically with regard to the thickness of the injured myocardial wall. Based on this study, the author cannot support those who would recommend abandoning such useful terms as "Q wave," "ST segment," and "T wave" myocardial infarction.

Prognostic Significance of Precordial ST-Segment Depression During Inferior Acute Myocardial Infarction

Mark A. Hlatky, Robert M. Califf, Kerry L. Lee, David B. Pryor, Galen S. Wagner, and Robert A. Rosati (Duke Univ.)
Am. J. Cardiol. 55:325–329, Feb. 1, 1985   4–42

To assess the mechanism and prognostic importance of precordial ST segment depression during inferior AMI, studies were made in 162 patients hospitalized between 1969 and 1982. Those with ST segment depression in leads V_1, V_2, and V_3 had significantly larger infarctions as assessed by a QRS scoring system. Hospital mortality was 4% (3 of 75) among patients without ST depression and 13% (11 of 87) in those with ST segment depression. The relationship between the amount of ST segment depression and hospital mortality was significant ($P < .001$ by logistic regression) and remained significant ($P < .003$) after adjusting for other potentially prognostic factors. Among patients discharged from the hospital, the 5-year survival was 92% in those without precordial ST segment depression and 80% in those with precordial ST depression ($P = .058$ by the Cox model).

The precordial ST segment depression observed on the admission ECG during inferior AMI indicates a larger infarction, predicts a higher hospital mortality, and suggests a poorer long-term prognosis after discharge. Precordial ST changes during inferior AMI may provide a valuable noninvasive method of classifying patients into high-risk or low-risk groups.

▶ The preceding three abstracts all consider the use of the ECG to provide information about prognosis, type of ischemia, and complication rates. Because the ECG is readily available at the moment of entry into the hospital, such studies are important and helpful. Note that in those with a negative initial ECG the risk of subsequent complications is extremely low. If this is indeed the case, the patients can be cared for in an intermediate care area rather than the more expensive coronary care unit. The cost of providing quality care under these circumstances is greatly reduced.—Leon Resnekov, M.D.

Comparison of Enzymatic and Anatomic Estimates of Myocardial Infarct Size in Man

D. B. Hackel, K. A. Reimer, R. E. Ideker, E. M. Mikat, T. D. Hartwell, C. B. Parker, E. B. Braunwald, M. Buja, H. K. Gold, A. S. Jaffe, J. E. Muller, D. S. Raabe, R. E. Rude, B. E. Sobel, P. H. Stone, R. Roberts, and the MILIS Study Group (Duke Univ.)
Circulation 70:824–835, November 1984   4–43

Enzymatic estimates of myocardial infarct size were compared with anatomical measurements in 49 patients enrolled in the Multicenter Investigation of Limitation of Infarct Size (MILIS) study program within 18 hours of onset of acute infarction at five centers. Infarct size was estimated from serial plasma MB creatine kinase (MB-CK) measurements. Thirty-seven hearts were anatomically evaluable, and adequate samples for MB-CK estimation were available in 25 of these.

The overall correlation coefficient between enzymatic estimates of infarct size and anatomical measurements in the 25 study cases was 0.87. The coefficient for total CK was 0.86. Correlation coefficients for peak MB-CK and peak total CK estimates were 0.76 and 0.79, respectively. Interobserver variability in estimating anatomical infarct size was 19%, but the correlation between estimates was 0.96. The possible role of reperfusion of certain infarcts in the findings is unclear.

Close correlation was found between enzymatic and anatomical estimates of myocardial infarct size in this study, but neither is a perfect measure of true infarct size. Enzymatic estimates appear to be acceptable when groups of patients are compared in clinical trials of interventions for limiting infarct size. The use of infarct size rather than mortality as an end point considerably reduces the number of patients needed to document efficacy.

Measurement of Myocardial Infarct Size by Technetium Pyrophosphate Single-Photon Tomography

James R. Corbett, Samuel E. Lewis, Christopher L. Wolfe, Donald E. Jansen, Margaret Lewis, James S. Rellas, Robert W. Parkey, Robert E. Rude, L. Maximilian Buja, and James T. Willerson (Univ. of Texas at Dallas)
Am. J. Cardiol. 54:1231–1236, Dec. 1, 1984   4–44

Infarct size and the extent of previous infarction are the chief prognostic determinants after AMI. Single-photon emission computed tomography (SPECT) with ^{99m}Tc-pyrophosphate was used to evaluate data on 38 men

CLINICAL CHARACTERISTICS AND INFARCT MASSES FOR INDIVIDUAL INFARCT GROUPS

Location of MI	Previous MI	Peak Serum CK (IU)	Infarct Mass (g)	Cardiac Events*	
				First MI	All Pts
Anterior TM (n = 14)	2	1,525 ± 942	38.6 ± 19.6	6	7
Inferior TM (n = 16)	2	1,525 ± 987	35.6 ± 15.1	6	7
Nontransmural (n = 16)	10	392 ± 264+	17.5 ± 11.1+	1	6

*Mean follow-up period was 12.0 ± 4.7 months.
†$P < .05$ compared with other groups.
CK, creatine kinase; MI, myocardial infarction; TM, transmural.
(Courtesy of Corbett, J.R., et al: Am. J. Cardiol. 54:1231–1236, Dec. 1, 1984.)

and 8 women with documented AMI whose mean age was 52 years. Fourteen patients had a past history of infarction. Sixteen control patients with chest pain but no evidence of infarction also were studied. The SPECT studies were performed an average of 3 days after admission within 2–4 hours after injection of 25 mCi of ^{99m}Tc-pyrophosphate. The distribution of nuclide uptake was determined using an overlay of pyrophosphate on the ungated cardiac blood pool. Areas of increased pyrophosphate uptake within infarcts were thresholded at 65% of peak activity. The blood pool was thresholded at 50% and subtracted.

Both death and congestive heart failure were more frequent in patients without previous infarction who had acute infarcts weighing more than 40 gm. Correlation between measured infarct mass and the peak serum creatine kinase value was 0.83, $P < .001$. Comparable correlation was obtained for anterior, inferior, and nontransmural infarcts (table).

It would appear that SPECT with ^{99m}Tc-pyrophosphate has clinical prognostic value in sizing AMIs. More than 200 studies have been done without adverse consequences, but patients in severe congestive failure or shock are not candidates for this examination. Acquisition times should be considerably less with newer SPECT systems.

▶ Single-photon emission computed tomography (SPECT) is capable of providing quantified information not only in regard to infarct size, the subject of this abstract, but also when used in conjunction with thallium myocardial scintigraphy for heart muscle perfusion studies. Whether the clinician requires information about infarct size rather than areas of the myocardium at ischemic risk can be questioned. Therapy should be provided to regions at risk of further myocardial ischemic damage, because the area of the infarct is, of course, beyond therapeutic help.—Leon Resnekov, M.D.

Assessment of Potentially Salvageable Myocardium During Acute Myocardial Infarction: Use of Postextrasystolic Potentiation
John McB. Hodgson, William W. O'Neill, Nathan Laufer, Patrick D. V. Bourdillon, Joseph A. Walton, Jr., and Bertram Pitt (Univ. of Michigan)
Am. J. Cardiol. 54:1237–1244, Dec. 1, 1984   4–45

Thrombolytic therapy for AMI has gained widespread acceptance despite poor documentation of myocardial salvage. To determine the role of postextrasystolic (PES) potentiation in assessing the potential for myocardial salvage before attempting thrombolytic therapy, 23 patients with evolving AMI undergoing catheterization for thrombolytic therapy had interventional contrast ventriculography with programmed atrial stimulation. Using an area method based on a right anterior oblique segmental projection, three segments of the ventricle were defined and ejection area and the normalized segmental contraction index (NSC) were calculated. Segmental PES potentiation was present if an increase in NSC index for a given segment of at least 1 normal SD occurred between the normal cycle beat and the PES beat.

Postextrasystolic potentiation was present in 56% of infarct-related segments within an average of 5.1 hours and was seen for as long as 9 hours after onset of AMI. The presence or magnitude of segmental potentiation was not related to time from onset of pain to ventriculography, initial ejection fraction, presence of collaterals, left ventricular end-diastolic pressure, or PES delay. Successful reperfusion with the intracoronary administration of streptokinase was achieved in 18 patients within an average of 6.2 hours after onset of AMI. Repeat contrast ventriculography was performed an average of 11 days after AMI in these patients. Only a positive segmental PES response ($P < .0001$) and the presence of collaterals to the infarct-related segment ($P < .02$) were significantly correlated with improved chronic segmental ventricular function. The predictive value of PES analysis was highest in affected segments without visible collateral supply ($r = .80$, $P < .0001$). No significant complications resulted from acute ventriculography or atrial stimulation.

The presence of acute segmental PES potentiation is predictive of improved chronic segmental ventricular function if reperfusion is successful, particularly in segments without collaterals. Analysis of segmental PES potentiation, therefore, allows prospective determination of those patients with evolving AMI who are most likely to benefit from acute thrombolytic therapy.

Precordial ST Segment Depression During Acute Inferior Myocardial Infarction: Early Thallium-201 Scintigraphic Evidence of Adjacent Posterolateral or Inferoseptal Involvement

Allan S. Lew, A. Teddy Weiss, Prediman K. Shah, Jamshid Maddahi, Thomas Peter, William Ganz, H. J. C. Swan, and Daniel S. Berman (Cedar-Sinai Med. Ctr. and Univ. of California at Los Angeles)
J. Am. Coll. Cardiol. 5:203–209, February 1985   4–46

Recent studies demonstrated that precordial ST segment depression during AMI is associated with more extensive necrosis and reduced left ventricular function. However, whether these findings reflect the extent of coronary artery disease or disease of the left anterior descending artery is uncertain. To assess the clinical significance of precordial ST segment depression during inferior AMI, a 12-lead ECG tracing was correlated with closely timed thallium-201 scintigraphic findings and coronary angiographic findings in 44 patients hospitalized with their first inferior AMI.

Thirty-six patients had precordial ST segment depression (group 1) and 8 did not (group 2). All 44 patients had an inferior wall perfusion defect. Additional perfusion defects of the adjacent posterolateral wall (n = 20), the ventricular septum (n = 9), or both (n = 6), were present in 35 patients (97%) in group 1 as compared with only 1 patient (13%) in group 2 (P < .001). The frequency of multivessel coronary artery disease and disease of the left anterior descending artery did not differ significantly between the two groups or between patients with and without a thallium-201 perfusion defect involving the ventricular septum.

Precordial ST segment depression during an inferior AMI may be indicative of more extensive ischemia or infarction of adjacent posterolateral or inferoseptal myocardial segments. This involvement is independent of coexistent multivessel or left anterior descending coronary artery disease. It reflects the extent and pattern of distribution of the artery of infarction for the following reasons: (1) involvement is always adjacent to and continuous with a perfusion defect of the inferior wall, and (2) the patterns of perfusion defects are consistent with the anatomy of the right and circumflex coronary arteries, the posterolateral wall being supplied by either artery and the inferoseptum supplied by the posterior descending artery, which is a branch of the right coronary artery in 90% of individuals.

▶ Adjacent, neighboring, and more distant ischemia are all important when considering the total ischemic damage after myocardial infarction. The interpretation of precordial ST segment depression in the presence of inferior AMI results from more extensive ischemia. In turn, this comes about because of the anatomical distribution of the coronary arterial supply, therefore suggesting more extensive involvement than otherwise.—Leon Resnekov, M.D.

Ventricular Septal Rupture Complicating Acute Myocardial Infarction: Identification of Simple and Complex Types in 53 Autopsied Hearts
Brooks S. Edwards, William D. Edwards, and Jesse E. Edwards (United Hosps., St. Paul, Univ. of Minnesota, and Mayo Clinic and Found.)
Am. J. Cardiol. 54:1201–1205, Dec. 1, 1984   4–47

Ventricular septal rupture is a recognized serious complication of AMI. To determine whether there are clinical features that may favor the occurrence of either of the two types of septal rupture, simple or complex, a pathologic analysis was made of 53 autopsied hearts with rupture of the ventricular septum complicating AMI. The simple type of rupture was defined as a direct through-and-through opening connecting the two ventricles. Complex ruptures were associated with serpiginous dissection tracts, hemorrhagic tracts, and myocardial disruption. Specimens were classified as to the location of the underlying AMI and the level of the septum (apex to base) at which the rupture occurred.

Inferior AMI was found in 29 hearts and anterior AMI in 24. Complex ruptures occurred in 20 of the inferior AMIs (69%) and in 5 of the anterior AMIs (21%) (P < .001). Ruptures that involved the inferobasal portion of the septum were more likely to be complex (94%) than were ruptures in all other locations (27%) (P < .001). Among the 28 hearts with simple rupture, inferior AMI was observed in 9 (32%) and anterior AMI in 19 (68%). Rupture of a second structure, in addition to the ventricular septum, occurred in 11 hearts, including 9 with involvement of the left ventricular free wall and 2 of the papillary muscle. Significant three-vessel obstructive coronary arterial atherosclerosis was present in 48 hearts. The interval from onset of the AMI to rupture of the septum, estimated in 22 patients, averaged 4 days (median, 2.5 days). Complete heart block occurred in six patients during hospitalization. Five had inferior AMI and four of these had complex septal rupture.

Predictors for a simple type of ventricular rupture are anterior AMI or inferoapical AMI, whereas for complex ruptures, the predictor is inferior AMI, particularly in the inferobasal portion. Furthermore, the clinical combination of inferior AMI, complete heart block, and rupture of the ventricular septum may provide a preoperative diagnosis of complex septal rupture.

▶ This is a useful analysis of one of the acute complications of myocardial infarction, i.e., ventricular septal rupture. Other anatomical disruptions that may occur after AMI include damage to papillary muscles with precipitation of hemodynamically severe mitral regurgitation usually associated with considerable hemodynamic compromise. Aneurysms also may occur rapidly, especially after extensive anterior myocardial infarction resulting from proximal occlusion of the left anterior descending artery. All of these lesions are amenable to surgery; this may involve repair of the acute myocardial damage, removal of the aneurysm, mitral valve replacement or repair, and associated aortocoronary bypass grafting as needed. Such extensive surgery in the presence of AMI is associated with a significant mortality, however, and patients need to be chosen with care for such approaches.—Leon Resnekov, M.D.

Right Ventricular Myocardial Infarction in Patients With Chronic Lung Disease: Possible Role of Right Ventricular Hypertrophy

Harry A. Kopelman, Mervyn B. Forman, B. Hadley Wilson, Frank D. Kolodgie, Raphael F. Smith, Gottlieb C. Friesinger, and Renu Virmani (Vanderbilt Univ.)
J. Am. Coll. Cardiol. 5:1302–1307, June 1985   4–48

The occurrence of right ventricular myocardial infarction in patients with chronic lung disease and right ventricular hypertrophy remains controversial. Findings in 28 patients with chronic lung disease, inferior myocardial infarction, and significant coronary artery disease without (group Ia) or with (group Ib) right ventricular hypertrophy were compared with those in 20 patients with chronic lung disease with right ventricular hypertrophy but without evidence of inferior myocardial infarction or significant coronary artery disease (group II). The data were analyzed retrospectively to determine the relationship between right myocardial infarction and right ventricular hypertrophy in these patients. Chronic lung disease was diagnosed on the basis of clinical criteria and findings in chest radiograhs and pulmonary function tests.

Right ventricular wall thickness was 3.3 mm ± 0.5 in group Ia, 6.0 mm ± 1.1 in group Ib, and 8.8 mm ± 2.4 in group II (group Ia vs. Ib, $P < .001$; group Ia vs. II, $P < .001$; group Ib vs. II, $P < .001$). Right ventricular infarction was significantly higher in incidence among patients with inferior myocardial infarction and right ventricular hypertrophy (group Ib) than among patients with infarction but without right ventricular hypertrophy (Ia) (11 vs. 3, $P < .008$). There was no significant difference in the extent of anatomical coronary disease at autopsy in groups Ia and Ib. The incidence of right ventricular infarction did not differ significantly between groups Ia and II. Isolated right ventricular infarction occurred in four patients (20%) in group II. The cause of death was directly related to right ventricular myocardial infarction in 6 of 18 patients (33%), 4 of whom were from group Ib and 2 from group II. None of the right ventricular infarctions in group Ia appeared to be directly related to mortality.

Patients with right ventricular hypertrophy caused by chronic lung disease are at risk for the development of right ventricular myocardial infarction, particularly in the setting of inferior myocardial infarction. In addition, patients with chronic lung disease and right ventricular hypertrophy, but with insignificant coronary artery disease, may sustain isolated right ventricular infarction. Both increased myocardial oxygen demand and a decreased supply may play a role in this relationship.

▶ There continues to be a great deal of interest in right ventricular myocardial infarction. Most patients have infarction of the left ventricle that involves neighboring regions of the right ventricle, the lesion often spreading through the posterior portion of the ventricular septum. Isolated right ventricular infarction is much less common. This abstract provides information about right ventricular infarction in patients with previous right ventricular hypertrophy a result of chronic lung disease. Isolated right ventricular infarction is a potential risk in such patients and should be borne in mind when assessing acute infarction in individuals known to have chronic obstructive lung disease and right ventricular hypertrophy.—Leon Resnekov, M.D.

Embolic Potential of Left Ventricular Thrombus After Myocardial Infarction: A Two-Dimensional Echocardiographic Study of 119 Patients
Cees A. Visser, Gerard Kan, Richard S. Meltzer, Arend J. Dunning, and Jos Roelandt, with the technical assistance of Marga Van Corler and Harry de Koning (Univ. of Amsterdam; Erasmus Univ., Rotterdam; and Interuniversitary Cardiology Inst., Utrecht)
J. Am. Coll. Cardiol. 5:1276–1280, June 1985   4–49

Left ventricular thrombus is a common complication after AMI. The clinical course of 119 patients with left ventricular thrombus that complicated myocardial infarction was reviewed to determine the role of two-dimensional echocardiography in delineating the embolic potential. A thrombus was considered to be protruding if its luminal edge had a curvature that was opposite in sign to that of the adjacent left ventricular wall, or was considered freely mobile if the thrombus edge moved independently (and on occasion, erratically) of the adjacent wall.

The site of the infarct was anterior in 108 patients and inferior in 11. Embolism occurred more frequently in patients with an acute infarct (12 of 46, 26%) than in those with a chronic infarct (14 of 73, 19%); however, the difference was not significant. Systemic embolism occurred in 26 patients: stroke in 18, lower limb embolism in 7, and mesenteric embolism in 1. A protruding type of thrombus was seen in 23 of 26 patients with embolism (88%) and in 17 of 93 of those without (18%). Free mobility of the thrombus was found in 15 of 26 patients with embolism (58%), compared with 3 of 93 of those without (3%). The finding of a protruding thrombus had greater sensitivity in predicting systemic embolization than did free mobility (88% vs. 58%), but was less specific (82% vs. 97%). The positive and negative predictive accuracy of a protruding configuration was 57% and 96%, respectively, and of a free mobility, 85% and 89%, respectively.

Of 46 patients treated with oral anticoagulants, 12 had systemic embolism, including 2 who died. Full-dose oral anticoagulant therapy had been given before embolism occurred in seven patients; in five it was started after an embolic event. Repeat echocardiograms showed a decrease in size or disappearance of the thrombus in six patients. There was no change in thrombus configuration in four patients, including two who had recurrence of emboli despite anticoagulation.

The embolic potential of a left ventricular thrombus that complicates myocardial infarction can be identified by two-dimensional echocardiography on the basis of a protruding configuration, particularly in association with free mobility of the free edge of the thrombus. These features may be of value in outlining the benefits and disadvantages of oral anticoagulant therapy.

▶ Because the presence of a left ventricular thrombus, particularly after anterior myocardial infarction, is an indication for anticoagulant therapy for at least the first 3 months following the acute episode, tests of precision are needed in the diagnosis of thrombus. Apart from two-dimensional echocardiography, noninvasive testing includes radionuclear angiography and isotopic labeling of platelets to demonstrate adherence by nuclear imaging to the left ventricular thrombus.—Leon Resnekov, M.D.

Prediction of Mortality During the First Year After Acute Myocardial Infarction From Clinical Variables and Stress Test at Hospital Discharge
Paolo Fioretti, R. W. Brower, Maarten L. Simoons, Robert J. Bos, Taco Baardman, Anita Beelen, and Paul G. Hugenholtz (Erasmus Univ., Univ. Hosp. Dijkzigt, Interuniversity Cardiology Inst., Rotterdam)
Am. J. Cardiol. 55:1313–1318, May 1, 1985   4–50

Although many studies have examined the prognostic value of predischarge stress testing after AMI, only a few studies have included patients who could not perform the bicycle ergometry test, or have tried to analyze the prognostic value of the stress test independent of other clinical data. A prospective study was designed to determine the predictive value during the first year of a predischarge symptom-limited stress test in 405 consecutive survivors of AMI. On an average of 13 days after AMI, 300 patients performed bicycle ergometry; 105 others were judged ineligible for the test: 43 because of cardiac limitations (angina or heart failure) and 62 because of noncardiac limitations.

Mortality was 57% (24 of 43) in the cardiac-limited group. In contrast, mortality in the noncardiac-limited group and in those eligible for the test was only 8% (5 of 62) and 7% (20 of 300), respectively. Using univariate analysis, the best stress test predictor of mortality was the extent of blood pressure increase: 42 ± 24 mm Hg in 280 survivors compared with 21 ± 14 mm Hg in 20 nonsurvivors ($P < .001$). Among the 212 patients who had a blood pressure increase of at least 30 mm Hg, mortality was 3% (6 patients), whereas it was 16% (14 patients) among 88 with an increase in blood pressure of less than 30 mm Hg. Angina, ST changes, and arrhythmias were not significantly associated with mortality. An inadequate blood pressure increase was an independent predictor of mortality, based on exercise stress data alone; a history of healed AMI and the use of digitalis on discharge were independent predictors based on clinical data only. For predicting cardiac events in patients eligible for stress testing, combining both clinical and exercise test results improved the predictive accuracy for late mortality (sensitivity, 85%; specificity, 76%) compared with using each variable alone. When nonfatal reinfarction was added to mortality as the endpoint, stress test results lost their independent predictive value relative to clinical variables. However, stress test results appeared to have independent predictive value when other endpoints were added, e.g., late coronary artery bypass surgery, coronary angioplasty, and persistent congestive heart failure.

At discharge, patients who are not eligible for stress testing because of cardiac limitations have a high risk of dying during the subsequent year. Patients who are eligible for stress testing can be further stratified into low-risk and intermediate-risk groups by a combination of clinical variables and extent of blood pressure increase during exercise. This combination improves the accuracy of prognosis. Such attempts at stratification allow better utilization of increasingly costly health resources in that patients at very low risk need not require further investigation.

Prognostic Significance of Left Ventricular Ejection Fraction After Acute Myocardial Infarction: A Bedside Radionuclide Study
Michael J. Kelly, Peter L. Thompson, and Michael F. Quinlan (Queen Elizabeth II Med. Center, Nedlands, Australia)
Br. Heart J. 53:16–24, January 1985   4–51

Angiographic studies have evaluated the prognostic significance of left ventricular ejection fraction in patients with AMI. Because the invasive nature of such measurements limits their application, a prospective study was undertaken to assess the prognostic significance of left ventricular ejection in myocardial infarction as measured by the bedside first-pass portable probe radioisotope method described by Steele et al. The initial ejection fraction was measured in 171 patients with confirmed AMI within a mean 23.5 hours of onset of major symptoms. The results were related to the subsequent incidence of ventricular fibrillation in the hospital, and to hospital and postdischarge mortality in a mean follow-up period of 15 months (range, 9–21 months).

The mean ejection fraction was 0.36 (range, 0.12–0.62). Eight episodes of primary ventricular fibrillation, all 12 hospital deaths caused by pump failure, and 12 of 13 postdischarge deaths occurred among the 81 patients with an initial postinfarction left ventricular ejection fraction of less than 0.35. Ejection fraction was related to the number of previous myocardial infarctions, peak creatine phosphokinase activity, and ECG indicators of the site and severity of myocardial infarction. However these variables had no significant independent prognostic significance when ejection fraction results were known, suggesting that their prognostic significance could largely be explained by their association with depressed left ventricular ejection fractions.

Left ventricular ejection fraction measured within the initial 24 hours after AMI predicts prognosis throughout the subsequent year. The use of the first-pass portable radioisotope method allows bedside measurements to be obtained more promptly, more conveniently, and less expensively than with radionuclide ventriculography.

Value of Radionuclide Angiography for Predicting Specific Cardiac Events After Acute Myocardial Infarction

Kenneth G. Morris, Sebastian T. Palmeri, Robert M. Califf, Ray A. McKinnis, Michael B. Higginbotham, R. Edward Coleman, and Frederick R. Cobb (Duke Univ. and Durham VA Med. Ctr.)
Am. J. Cardiol. 55:318–324, Feb. 1, 1985   4–52

The value of rest and exercise radionuclide angiography in predicting specific events including death, recurrent AMI, coronary care unit readmission for unstable chest pain, and medically refractory angina after AMI was studied in 106 consecutive survivors of AMI. The study protocol consisted of radionuclide angiography at rest and during upright bicycle exercise 3 weeks after AMI.

Analysis of the radionuclide angiographic variables using the Cox proportional hazards regression model yielded significant associations of the time to death with ejection fraction at rest and during exercise. Both variables added significant prognostic information to the clinical assessment. The change in ejection fraction from rest to exercise predicted the time to coronary artery bypass grafting for medically refractory angina before and after adjustment for the clinical descriptors, but did not predict death or other nonfatal events. Significant correlations were found between radionuclide angiographic variables and a variety of clinical descriptors previously reported to have prognostic significance. Both rest and exercise ejection fracture were correlated indirectly with mortality. Clinical and radionuclide angiographic variables that measured left ventricular function were predictive of subsequent mortality, whereas those reflecting residual potentially ischemic myocardium were predictive of subsequent nonfatal ischemic events. Rest and exercise radionuclide angiography after AMI provides significant prognostic information about specific events during the follow-up period independent of that provided by clinical assessment.

Regional Left Ventricular Wall Motion Assessment: Comparison of Two-Dimensional Echocardiography and Radionuclide Angiography With Contrast Angiography in Healed Myocardial Infarction
Anthony P. Freeman, Robert W. Giles, Warren F. Walsh, Richard Fisher, I. Provan, C. Murray, and David E. L. Wilcken (Prince of Wales and Prince Henry Hosps., Sydney)
Am. J. Cardiol. 56:8–12, July 1, 1985   4–53

Accurate evaluation of regional left ventricular (LV) function is important in the management of patients with coronary artery disease. The diagnostic ability of radionuclide angiography and two-dimensional echocardiography in assessing regional LV wall motion was compared with that of contrast angiography in 52 patients with healed myocardial infarction. When 5 patients with inadequate two-dimensional echocardiography studies were excluded, the LV images of 47 patients obtained by all three techniques were divided into seven segments for analysis: anterobasal, anterolateral, apical, inferior, posterobasal, septal, and posterolateral.

Radionuclide angiography and two-dimensional echocardiography results were in close agreement with findings on contrast angiography in assessing normal and abnormal wall motion in the anterobasal (91%, 91%, respectively), anterolateral (87%, 79%), and apical (94%, 81%) segments. Two dimensional echocardiography and radionuclide angiography were more sensitive in detecting abnormalities in the anterolateral (83%, 77%, respectively) and apical (95%, 84%) segments, and were least sensitive in detecting abnormalities of the inferior segment (48%, 48%). The specificity for all segments ranged from 94% in the anterolateral wall to 71% in the septal segment for echocardiography, and from 93% in the anterobasal segment to 73% in the apical segment for radionuclide angiography. Major discrepancies with contrast angiography occurred more often in the posterobasal, posterolateral, inferior, and septal LV segments.

Both noninvasive techniques, two-dimensional echocardiography and radionuclide angiography, are reliable in detecting the more common anteroapical wall motion abnormalities. However, they are relatively less sensitive in evaluating inferior, posterior, and septal LV segments.

▶ The preceding four abstracts all deal with various investigations that provide information about prognosis during the first year following AMI. On average, mortality rates are double within the first 6 months after discharge from the hospital at about 10%, and are 5% at 1 year; subsequently, the average annual rate is about 3%. The cause of the higher mortality during the initial post-hospital 6-month period is uncertain, but it seems to relate to a higher incidence of ventricular rhythm disturbances emerging during this time. There is evidence accruing that about 20% of patients during this early recovery phase may be experiencing episodes of silent ischemia. These permit dangerous ventricular dysrhythmias to emerge acutely and threaten life. Other mechanisms have to do with the extent of total and segmental ventricular ischemia. In turn these depend on the nature and extent of arteriosclerotic lesions of the various coronary arteries and their branches, and the presence or absence of adequate collateral circulation.

Fortunately, many of the investigations providing guidance about prognosis can be undertaken noninvasively, relying on exercise ECG and radionuclear techniques. It is more difficult, however, to obtain evidence about phasic silent ischemia, although exercise thallium scintigraphy may be helpful as may long term ECG ambulatory monitoring; these studies may have to be repeated several times before evidence of phasic ischemia is obtained.—Leon Resnekov, M.D.

Effect of Digitalis Treatment on Survival After Acute Myocardial Infarction
J. Thomas Bigger, Jr., Joseph L. Fleiss, Linda M. Rolnitzky, Jacques P. Merab, and Kevin J. Ferrick (Columbia Univ. and Columbia Presbyterian Med. Ctr.)
Am. J. Cardiol. 55:623–630, March 1, 1985   4–54

Data from 504 patients enrolled in a postinfarction natural history study were assessed to determine whether treatment with digitalis is associated with decreased survival after AMI. At time of discharge, 229 patients (45%) were taking digitalis.

After 3 years of follow-up observation, the cumulative survival rate for patients discharged taking digitalis was 66%, compared with 87% for those not treated. Univariate analysis showed that statistically significant differences existed between the two groups for age, previous AMI, left ventricular failure in the coronary care unit, atrial fibrillation in the coronary care unit, peak creatine kinase levels, enlarged heart and pulmonary vascular congestion observed on the discharge chest x-ray film, ventricular arrhythmias, and treatment with diuretic, antiarrhythmic, and β-blocking drugs. Survival analysis using Cox's regression model indicated that the association between digitalis and decreased survival was of borderline significance after adjustment for atrial fibrillation and left ventricular failure. The serum digoxin concentration was measured in 83% of patients who took digitalis; survival was inversely and significantly related to the serum digoxin level, i.e., the higher the serum digoxin level, the lower the long-term survival. After adjusting for atrial fibrillation and left ventricular failure, the serum digoxin level was not significantly related to survival.

Taken together with the results of three other large, nonrandomized studies of digitalis treatment after AMI, this study suggests that digitalis treatment may have adverse effects on survival during the follow-up period. Until this question is definitively answered by controlled, randomized clinical studies, clinicians should assess whether treatment is really needed for left ventricular dysfunction after AMI in each individual patient, and, if it is, which treatment has the best risk-benefit ratio.

▶ Over the years there has been a great deal of interest and much investigation into the use of digitalis preparations during and after AMI. What has emerged, and is confirmed by this study, is that far from being beneficial, such therapy may even be detrimental. The facts seem to be that as a positive inotropic intervention, digitalis is relatively weak; its main effect is to slow the heart rate. Digitalization also permits ventricular rhythm disturbances to emerge, particularly in the presence of segmental myocardial ischemia and any disturbance of intracellular and extracellular electrolytes. Caution is therefore needed in deciding whether to digitalize a patient during the acute phase of myocardial infarction and subsequently.—Leon Resnekov, M.D.

Long Term Survival of Patients Mobilised Early After Acute Myocardial Infarction
R. R. West and A. H. Henderson (Welsh Nat. School of Medicine, Cardiff, Wales)
Br. Heart J. 53:243–247, March 1985   4–55

A previous Welsh multicenter trial of early (fifth day) compared with late (tenth day) mobilization of 742 patients after uncomplicated myocardial infarction found that there were no significant differences in survival during the first year; however, partial follow-up observation subsequently showed significantly reduced survival during the second and third years among patients mobilized early. A full 10-year follow-up study was made of all patients admitted to the trial.

Ten years after admission to the study, 51% of those mobilized early and 55% of those mobilized late survived. This overall difference in survival was not statistically significant. Sixteen of the patients were lost to follow-up study before 8 years. Comparison of survival rates of patients, mobilized early and late showed that several subgroups had different mortality rates. Patients with higher mortality about 1 year after infarction in the early mobilization group included those admitted to hospital "F," patients with a previous history of hypertension, and those with arrhythmia or bradycardia on admission. Causes of death after 10 years of follow-up observation included heart disease (71%), other circulatory diseases (hypertension, cerebrovascular disease, arteriosclerosis) (18%), and others (mostly cancer). The evidence from this study is not sufficient to contraindicate mobilization as early as the fifth day after uncomplicated myocardial infarction.

▶ As each year goes by, articles appear recommending earlier and earlier discharge from the hospital after AMI. No doubt there will soon appear an article recommending ambulatory care! The fact is, however, that it all depends on the severity of the infarction, extent of damage to the myocardium, regions of ischemia at a distance, and electrophysiologic parameters. In essence, therefore, decisions about early mobilization have to be individualized according to the patient's presentation. When the patient is truly complication free, early discharge may be perfectly in order. Indeed, when one considers the fact that so many patients with acute infarction have no symptoms and are ambulatory throughout the event, the diagnosis having to be established retrospectively, there is little to wonder about the safety of early discharge in the complication-free patient. On the other hand, it should be recollected that mortality during the first hour of AMI remains distressingly high. These individuals, of course, rarely enter the medical care system.—Leon Resnekov, M.D.

Early Exercise Training in Patients Older Than Age 65 Years Compared With That in Younger Patients After Acute Myocardial Infarction or Coronary Artery Bypass Grafting
Mark A. Williams, Carl M. Maresh, Dennis J. Esterbrooks, James J. Harbrecht, and Michael H. Sketch (Creighton Univ., Omaha; and St. Luke's Hosp., and Midwest Res. Inst. Kansas City, Mo.)
Am. J. Cardiol. 55:263–266, Feb. 1, 1985   4–56

To evaluate potential benefits that elderly cardiac patients might gain from early exercise programs, 361 such patients were studied: Group I included 60 patients aged 44 years or less; group II, 114 patients aged 45–54 years; group III, 111 patients aged 55–64 years; and group IV, 76 elderly patients aged at least 65 years. All of the patients participated in a 12-week exercise program within 6 weeks of AMI or coronary artery bypass grafting. All patients participated in symptom-limited exercise tests before and after completion of the exercise program.

Between tests, elderly patients had significant differences in body weight, percent of body fat, heart rate at rest (77–68 beats per minute), maximal heart rate, maximal physical work capacity (METs), submaximal average double product, and submaximal average rating of perceived exertion. Magnitudes of change were similar among groups, although the elderly patients had a significantly lower absolute physical work capacity at testing after training than the other three groups had ($P < .05$). In 25 elderly patients who received β-blocking drugs, METs increased from 5.1 to 7.8 ($P < .05$). In the remaining 51 elderly patients not receiving β-blocking drugs, METs increased from 5.4 to 8.2 ($P < .05$).

Elderly male cardiac patients benefit from participation in early exercise programs through enhanced functional capacity and improved psychological responses to exertion. As a result of decreased submaximal myocardial oxygen demand, they may be less symptomatic during their daily routines, which should enhance the quality of their lives. Elderly patients appear to be at no greater risk from participation in exercise programs than younger patients are and should not be excluded from early rehabilitation exercise programs simply on the basis of age.

▶ Certainly, there seems no reason to deny the benefit of early exercise programs to patients of more advanced years recovering from AMI. Benefit comes about irrespective of age.—Leon Resnekov, M.D.

Type A Behavior and Survival After Acute Myocardial Infarction
Robert B. Case, Stanley S. Heller, Nan B. Case, Arthur J. Moss, and the Multicenter Post-Infarction Research Group (St. Luke's-Roosevelt Hosp. Ctr., Columbia Univ., and Cornell Univ. Med. College, New York; North Shore Univ. Hosp., Manhasset, N.Y.; and Univ. of Rochester, N.Y.)
N. Engl. J. Med. 312:737–741, March 21, 1985   4–57

To ascertain the influence of personality factors on the course of coronary artery disease, type A behavior was assessed in 516 patients within 2 weeks after AMI using the Jenkins Activity Survey questionnaire. None of the survivors of AMI had other major illnesses, and all were younger than age 70 years.

During a follow-up period of 1–3 years, no relationship was discovered between the type A score and total mortality, cardiac mortality, time to death for nonsurvivors, left ventricular ejection fraction, or duration of stay in the coronary care unit. These negative findings were not changed by restricting the analyses to men younger than age 61 or by comparing extreme score categories. When the contributions of behavioral, demographic, and cardiac physiologic factors to postinfarction mortality were evaluated by multivariate survivorship analyses, the physiologic factors were the only ones that contributed a significant and independent mortality risk; the type A score did not enter the survivorship model.

Thus, no association was found between type A behavior and the long-term outcome of AMI. Certain behavior characteristics (e.g., hostility and unexpressed anger) may have an adverse influence on established coronary disease. An investigation of this possible association may be warranted. Such specific characteristics need not be part of the discretely defined type A personality.

▶ There has always been considerable interest in emotional and personality factors regarding the precipitation of acute cardiac events in those prone to coronary artery disease. There is difficulty, however, in assessing the significance of such factors and in accurately measuring stress and personality change. Such studies are important, however, because emotional stress has already been shown to precipitate acute myocardial ischemia with or without symptoms that can adversely affect the patient's outcome.—Leon Resnekov, M.D.

Ventricular Rhythm Disturbances

Prolonged Electrical Systole and QT > QS$_2$ Secondary to Coronary Artery Disease

Harisios Boudoulas, Charles A. Bush, Stephen F. Schall, Carl V. Leier, and Richard P. Lewis (Ohio State Univ.)

Am. J. Cardiol. 55:915–919, April 1, 1985   4–58

It has been proposed that dyssynchrony of the ventricular myocardial action potential may lead to QT prolongation and QT > QS$_2$, which are associated with high mortality in patients with coronary artery disease. Areas of viable myocardium within a left ventricular aneurysmal scar could result in slow or dyssynchronous depolarization-repolarization. Recordings of QT-QS$_2$ were made within 48 hours of cardiac catheterization in 41 patients with coronary disease and left ventricular aneurysm, 46 with a history of acute infarction but no left ventricular aneurysm, and 52 with coronary disease only. Patients receiving class I antiarrhythmia drugs were excluded.

The incidences of QT > QS$_2$ were 71% in the patients with aneurysm and 20% to 22% in the control groups. Long QT, corrected for heart rate, was also significantly greater in the aneurysm group. Among other patients with previous infarction, QT > QS$_2$ was more frequent in those receiving digitalis. Rates of long QT and QT > QS$_2$ did not differ significantly between patients with previous acute infarction and those with coronary disease but no past infarction.

The finding of QT > QS$_2$ or long QT in a patient with left ventricular aneurysm probably reflects dyssynchronous depolarization or repolarization within the aneurysm or in the border zone. The question of an increased incidence of ventricular arrhythmias and death in patients with left ventricular aneurysm and QT > QS$_2$ remains to be clarified. Previous studies in patients recovering from acute infarction have shown that the presence of QT > QS$_2$ is a risk factor in sudden death, independent of left ventricular function or the number of obstructed coronary vessels.

► Electrophysiologic parameters in patients with coronary artery disease are of extreme importance. Changes of the ventricular action potential that may clinically be associated with prolongation of a QT time and prolongation of electrical ventricular systole may have an ominous prognosis. Dangerous ventricular rhythm disturbances including torsade-de-pointes may emerge. Further investigations are needed to elucidate the complex relationship between anatomical damage, extent of coronary artery disease and AMI, and electrical parameters.—Leon Resnekov, M.D.

Significance of Exercise-Induced Ventricular Arrhythmia in Stable Coronary Artery Disease: A Coronary Artery Surgery Study Project

Magdi Sami, Bernard Chaitman, Lloyd Fisher, David Holmes, David Fray, and Edwin Alderman (Stanford Univ., Montreal Heart Inst., Mayo Clinic and Found., and Univ. of Washington)

Am. J. Cardiol. 54:1182–1188, Dec. 1, 1984   4–59

Whether exercise-induced ventricular arrhythmias are merely markers of more advanced coronary artery disease (CAD) or whether they carry an independent prognostic risk of cardiac death is unknown. To determine the prognostic significance of exercise-induced ventricular arrhythmias in patients with stable CAD, 1,486 patients who were enrolled in the multicenter patient registry of the Coronary Artery Surgery Study between September 1975 and May 1979 were examined retrospectively. The patients had CAD established by angiography, underwent a standard Bruce exercise test at entry, and were followed up for a mean of 4.3 years. Patients with minimal CAD (group I) and patients with significant CAD (group II) were divided into subgroups IA (with exercise-induced ventricular arrhythmia, 16 patients), IB (without such arrhythmia, 229 patients), IIA (with such arrhythmia, 130 patients), and IIB (without such arrhythmia, 1,111 patients). Significant CAD was defined as a reduction in diameter of at least 70% in any major coronary artery, or narrowing of at least 50% in the left main artery.

Groups IA and IB had similar clinical and angiographic characteristics; however, group IA had a significantly lower mean ejection fraction (EF) than found in group IB (50% vs. 64%), respectively. Group IIA had a higher prevalence of previous myocardial infarction, a lower mean EF, and a higher proportion of patients with at least two coronary arteries that were significantly more narrow than in group IIB.

The 5-year event-free survival (76% and 88% in groups IA and IB, respectively, and 71% and 76% in groups IIA and IIB, respectively) was not significantly influenced by the presence of exercise-induced ventricular arrhythmias. The 5-year incidence of cardiac death was also not affected by the presence of exercise-induced ventricular arrhythmias. Stepwise Cox regression analysis of selected clinical and angiographic factors showed that the only significant independent risk factors for all cardiac events were the number of coronary arteries that were narrowed and the left ventricular EF. These findings suggest that exercise-induced ventricular arrhythmias, although associated with more advanced CAD, do not carry a prognostic risk independent of other risk factors.

▶ This study confirms previous investigations documenting that exercise-precipitated ventricular rhythm disturbances are not an independent prognostic risk. Prognosis is determined particularly by left ventricular function and by the nature and extent of CAD.—Leon Resnekov, M.D.

Ventricular Arrhythmia Induced by Programmed Ventricular Stimulation After Acute Myocardial Infarction

Pietro Santarelli, Fulvio Bellocci, Francesco Loperfido, Mario Mazzari, Rocco Mongiardo, Annibale S. Montenero, Ugo Manzoli, and Pablo Denes (Catholic Univ., Rome; and Rush-Presbyterian St. Luke's Med. Ctr., Chicago)
Am. J. Cardiol. 55:391–394, Feb. 1, 1985   4–60

The prevalence, characteristics, and clinical significance of ventricular electric instability with programmed ventricular stimulation were studied in 49 men and 1 woman (mean age, 53 years) who were hemodynamically stable within 17–40 days after AMI. Double extrastimuli at 2-mA and 10-mA intensity were used, so were two right ventricular sites. Ventricular electric instability was defined as induction of ten or more consecutive intraventricular reentrant beats.

Of 50 patients, 23 (46%) had ventricular electric instability; ten of these patients had sustained induced ventricular tachycardia (VT). No significant differences were observed between patients with and without ventricular electric instability with respect to age, site of AMI, coronary prognostic index, maximal level of creatine kinase, number of narrowed coronary arteries, and presence of severe wall motion abnormalities. During a mean follow-up period of 11.2 months, no patient died suddenly. During repeated Holter recordings, patients with ventricular electric instability had a higher incidence of nonsustained VT than did patients without ventricular electric instability.

In patients who are hemodynamically stable after AMI, programmed ventricular stimulation can be performed safely. In these patients there is a high prevalence of inducible sustained and nonsustained VT that does not correlate with the clinical or angiographic data. After discharge, those with ventricular electric instability have a higher incidence of nonsustained VT during Holter monitoring than found in those without ventricular electric instability. The predictive value of programmed ventricular stimulation in sudden death was not addressed by this study because of the low incidence of fatal events and the high prevalence of therapy.

Sudden Coronary Death: Comparison of Patients With to Those Without Coronary Thrombus at Necropsy

Carole A. Warnes and William C. Roberts (Natl. Heart, Lung, and Blood Inst., Bethesda, Md.)
Am. J. Cardiol. 54:1206–1211, Dec. 1, 1984   4–61

Most necropsy studies of victims of sudden coronary death (SCD) report a relatively low frequency of coronary thrombus. Among 70 victims of SCD, certain clinical and morphological findings in 13 victims with coronary thrombus were compared with the findings in 57 victims without coronary thrombus to determine the frequency and significance of coronary thrombus in SCD. In addition, the composition of the thrombi and their contribution to luminal narrowing were described.

Patients with a coronary thrombus were significantly younger than those without it (mean age, 43 vs. 51 years; $P < .02$), had a higher mean percent of segments of the four major epicardial coronary arteries minimally narrowed (0% to 25%) in cross-sectional area (XSA) by atherosclerotic plaque (27% vs. 19%; $P < .001$), and had a lower mean percent of XSA narrowing by plaque at the site of maximal coronary stenosis (89% vs. 95%; $P < .01$). Twelve patients with a thrombus (92%) had near-total occlusion of one or more coronary arteries by plaque alone, or plaque plus thrombus, as did 34 of the patients without thrombus (60%). The two groups did not differ in sex, previous angina pectoris or clinical AMI, healed myocardial infarction at necropsy, mean heart weight, number of major coronary arteries narrowed by 76% to 100% in XSA by atherosclerotic plaque, or the mean percent of segments of the coronary arteries narrowed by 76% to 100% in XSA by atherosclerotic plaque. The thrombus was located in the left anterior descending (LAD) artery in six, in the left circumflex in five, the left main artery in one, and the right coronary artery in 1. As for the location of the thrombus within the artery, it was located in the proximal half of the LAD or left circumflex artery in 11, in the left main artery in 1, and in the distal half of the right coronary artery in 1. In five patients, the thrombus occurred at the site of maximal narrowing by atherosclerotic plaque, and in another five in the area that contained the most severe degree of narrowing by plaque. It occurred in another coronary artery in three patients. The coronary thrombus consisted predominantly of fibrin in six patients and platelets in seven, suggesting the possibility of usefulness of antiplatelet agents in preventing thrombus formation. All seven patients with predominantly platelet thrombi were younger than the patients with fibrin (mean age, 34 vs. 53 years). None had previous angina pectoris or AMI, whereas all six of the other group did.

Coronary thrombi are infrequent in victims of SCD. When observed, their significance is uncertain, because victims of SCD without coronary thrombi have similar amounts of severe coronary narrowing.

Acute Hemodynamic and Antiischemic Effects of Intravenous Amiodarone
William J. Remme, Diederik C. A. Van Hoogenhuyze, X. Hanno Krauss, Albert Hofman, Dick A. C. M. Kruyssen, and Cock J. Storm (Zuiderziekenhius, Rotterdam, The Netherlands)
Am. J. Cardiol. 55:639–644, March 1, 1985   4–62

Acute hemodynamic and anti-ischemic properties of amiodarone, a widely used antiarrhythmic agent, were studied in 15 men and 1 woman with reduction of a left coronary artery of more than 70%. The mean age was 53 years. Two successive atrial pacing stress tests (APST I and II) were performed, with an interval of 40 minutes between tests. Amiodarone, 5 mg/kg infused during a 5-minute period, was administered 30 minutes after APST I.

Hemodynamic changes during amiodarone administration consisted of a 20% decrease in left ventricular (LV) systolic pressure, a 13% decrease in systemic vascular resistance, and an 18% decrease in stroke work. Coronary vascular resistance was reduced by 19% and coronary sinus flow increased by 23%. Despite a secondary 14% increase in heart rate, contractility decreased by 21%, and was accompanied by a 45% increase in LV end-diastolic pressure that persisted until APST II. Although most hemodynamic changes were observed only during infusion, contractility and LV systolic pressure remained diminished at the beginning of APST II and during pacing, resulting in a reduction in myocardial oxygen compared with findings in APST I. Amiodarone treatment significantly reduced pacing-induced myocardial ischemia. Lactate metabolism remained normal during APST II at maximal pacing rates, whereas ST segment depression, LV end-diastolic pressure after pacing, and angina were significantly reduced during APST II. Amiodarone was generally well tolerated.

Intravenously administered amiodarone reduces vascular resistance and contractility and inhibits pacing-induced myocardial ischemia in human beings, presumably by reducing myocardial oxygen demand.

▶ Amiodarone has now been released by the Federal Drug Administration for general use, but not without dire warnings about possible serious side effects emerging. It is an extremely useful drug for managing ventricular rhythm disturbances that are otherwise difficult to prevent, and for slowing conduction across the atrioventricular node. Unfortunately, many side effects, some of which are very serious indeed, may emerge; these include important lung changes, hepatic and renal effects, as well as changes in thyroid function. In addition, amiodarone has hemodynamic effects. It is a peripheral vasodilator and, as demonstrated in this article, it significantly reduces myocardial oxygen demand. Thus, amiodarone antidysrhythmic therapy may be indicated and may be successful even in the presence of LV dysfunction.—Leon Resnekov, M.D.

5 Cardiac Surgery

Coronary Revascularization

Twelve-Year Experience With Internal Mammary Artery for Coronary Artery Bypass

Hendrick B. Barner, John W. Standeven, and Jeffrey Reese (St. Louis Univ.)
J. Thorac. Cardiovasc. Surg. 90:668–675, November 1985   5–1

At least one internal mammary artery (IMA) was used for coronary revascularization in 1,000 patients between 1972 and 1984, and 103 of these had bilateral IMA grafting. There were 1,395 associated vein grafts and 1,158 IMA anastomoses, for an average of 2.5 grafts per patient. Sequential IMA grafts were used in 58 patients. The IMA was used as a free graft in 20 patients. Mean follow-up period was 6½ years.

Operative mortality was 1.4%; 11 of 14 deaths occurred in the first 240 patients treated. Actuarial survivals were 93% at 5 years, 84% at 10 years, and 77% at 12 years, including all deaths. The 10-year survival for

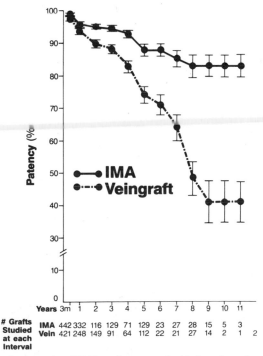

# Grafts Studied at each Interval	3m	1	2	3	4	5	6	7	8	9	10	11
IMA	442	332	116	129	71	129	23	27	28	15	5	3
Vein	421	248	149	91	64	112	22	21	27	14	2	1	2

Fig 5–1.—Actuarial patency for all IMA grafts compared with the vein grafts, with the number of grafts entering interval indicated. (Courtesy of Barner, H.B., et al.: J. Thorac. Cardiovasc. Surg. 90:668–675, November 1985.)

patients who had IMA bypass to the left anterior descending artery only was 88%. Chest pain recurred at a mean rate of 6% per year. Perioperative infarction occurred in 4% of the patients, and late infarction occurred at a mean rate of 1.5% per year. Thirty-five reoperations were performed for recurrent symptoms, including six percutaneous transluminal angioplasties. The overall potency rates for IMA grafts and vein grafts at 1 year were 96% and 93%, respectively. The rates at 10 years were 83% and 41%, but only a small number of grafts were available for study.

The IMA is now widely considered to have advantages over the saphenous vein for myocardial revascularization (Fig 5–1). There is little tendency for atherosclerosis to develop in the IMA after 10 years, in contrast to results in vein grafts. Use of the right IMA should become routine. Further, wider use of the IMA is possible through sequential IMA grafting.

▶ This study clearly demonstrates the feasability and safety of using the IMA for revascularization of single or multiple coronary arteries. Its application is widened by the use of free IMA grafts and sequential anastomoses. The improved graft patency and resulting improved longevity and freedom from recurrence of angina that this and other studies demonstrated requires reevaluation of the long-term results of surgical therapy. Results of the CASS study require reassessment because IMA grafts were used relatively infrequently during the period studied. The improved long-term results will further improve the comparison of surgical vs. medical therapy.—Hillel Laks, M.D.

Left Thoracotomy for Reoperative Coronary Artery Bypass Procedures
Ross M. Ungerleider, Noel L. Mills, and Andrew S. Wechsler (Duke Univ. and Ochsner Clinic, New Orleans)
Ann. Thorac. Surg. 40:11–15, July 1985   5–2

Nine patients underwent saphenous vein bypass grafting to the circumflex coronary artery system by means of left thoracotomy. This approach avoids adhesions that make a repeat sternotomy time consuming and possibly dangerous when previously patent saphenous vein or internal mammary grafts are present. In these procedures the descending thoracic aorta generally is cannulated for arterial inflow, and the main pulmonary artery is cannulated for venous return. Positioning of the pericardial incision is illustrated in Figure 5–2. The proximal end of the graft usually is readily placed on the left subclavian artery. Coronary anastomosis is done on the cold, fibrillating heart. Aortic cross clamping and cardioplegic arrest have not been necessary. Venting is possible through the left atrial appendage if filling pressures increase. All nine patients recovered uneventfully, and none had postoperative bleeding, respiratory problems, or infectious complications.

This approach is especially useful for patients who require grafting to the circumflex coronary artery system, especially if the patient is relatively unstable and would benefit from rapid institution of cardiopulmonary bypass. Increased use of the internal mammary artery to revascularize the

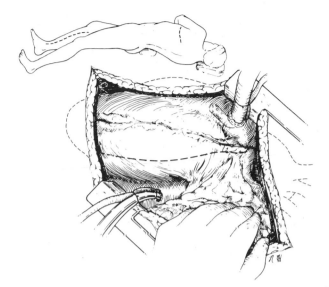

Fig 5–2.—Positioning of patient and pericardial incision used to approach the circumflex coronary artery by using left thoracotomy technique. (Courtesy of Ungerleider, R.M., et al.: Ann. Thorac. Surg. 40:11–15, July 1985.)

left anterior descending (LAD) artery system may create more situations in which patients with patent LAD artery grafts require revascularization of the circumflex system. Patients have had consistently good results after cardiopulmonary bypass times of 40–97 minutes. This approach may also be useful in patients with prosthetic valves because the back of the heart can be grafted without torsion or lifting the heart. Multiple grafts can be made to the circumflex coronary artery system.

▶ This technique of approaching the circumflex coronary artery system via a left thoracotomy appears to be a valuable addition to the surgeon's armamentarium. In specific situations the median sternotomy may provide a less desirable approach to the circumflex coronary artery system in patients with previously placed patent grafts to the left anterior descending and right coronary systems, particularly when the internal mammary artery is used. Examples include patients with previous mediastinal irradiation and mediastinitis, and those undergoing simultaneous pulmonary procedures through the left chest.—Hillel Laks, M.D.

Detrimental Effect of Perioperative Myocardial Infarction on Late Survival After Coronary Artery Bypass: Report From the Coronary Artery Surgery Study: CASS

Hartzell V. Schaff, Bernard J. Gersh, Lloyd D. Fisher, Robert L. Frye, Michael B. Mock, Thomas J. Ryan, Richard B. Ells, Bernard R. Chaitman, Edwin L. Alderman, George C. Kaiser, David P. Faxon, Martial G. Bourassa, and participants in the Coronary Artery Surgery Study (Coordinating Ctr. for Collaborative Studies in Coronary Artery Surgery, Univ. of Washington)
J. Thorac. Cardiovasc. Surg. 88:972–981, December 1984   5–3

The effects of perioperative infarction on the outcome of coronary artery bypass grafting were assessed by using data from the Coronary Artery Surgery Study (CASS) concerning 9,777 patients who were operated on between 1974 and 1979. A ventricular aneurysm was resected or plicated in 489 of these patients, and 53 had mitral valve replacement as well as

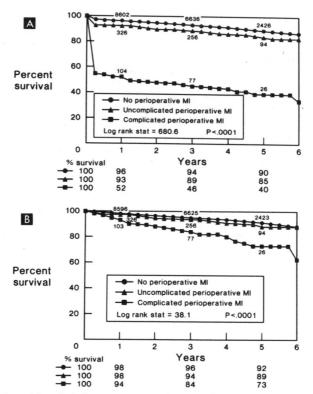

Fig 5–3.—Actuarial survival after coronary artery bypass grafting. Patients who had a perioperative myocardial infarction are stratified according to presence or absence of complications. **A,** important effect of perioperative myocardial infarction on early mortality is evident; only 52% of patients were alive 1 year after operation in group with complicated perioperative myocardial infarction. **B,** survivorship includes only patients who were dismissed from hospital. Late survival for patients with uncomplicated perioperative infarction was virtually the same as that for patients who had no perioperative infarction but was significantly reduced for patients with complicated perioperative infarction. MI, myocardial infarction. (Courtesy of Schaff, H.V., et al.: J. Thorac. Cardiovasc. Surg. 88:972–981, December 1984.)

myocardial revascularization. Perioperative infarction was diagnosed in 561 patients, or 5.7% of the series. The incidence declined during the study to 4.1% in 1979.

Overall hospital mortality was 2.8%; for patients with perioperative infarction mortality was 19%. When infarction was diagnosed during operation mortality was 25%. Perioperative infarction was associated with female gender, class IV (Canadian Cardiovascular Society) or unstable angina, and severe stenosis of the left main coronary artery. Affected patients more often had three-vessel disease and cardiomegaly before operation.

Complications were noted in 35% of patients with perioperative infarction; ventricular tachyarrhythmias and cardiogenic shock were most frequent. Additional procedures were associated with higher operative mortality but not with more frequent perioperative infarction. Late survival was significantly compromised by perioperative infarction because of infarction-related complications (Fig 5–3). Perioperative infarction was found on multivariate analysis to be an important independent predictor of late survival after coronary artery bypass surgery; only left ventricular function, age, and number of associated medical disorders were more significant factors.

Perioperative myocardial infarction has been a significant factor in late mortality after coronary artery bypass surgery in the CASS. However, hospital survivors with uncomplicated periopertive infarction have an excellent long-term outlook.

▶ There have been previous reports of smaller series suggesting that perioperative myocardial infarction does not influence long-term survival or symptomatic status. This excellent report of a large number of patients (almost 10,000) from multiple centers shows clearly that patients with a perioperative myocardial infarction overall have a higher early mortality (19%) and a reduced long term survival (85% at 5 years). It also shows that patients with a perioperative myocardial infarction may be divided into two groups: The one third who have a complication from the myocardial infarction, including ventricular tachyarrhythmias, bradyarrhythmias, supraventricular tachyarrhythmias, cardiogenic shock and congestive cardiac failure have a high rate of early mortality (45%) and high rate of late survival (73% for hospital survivors at 5 years), whereas the two thirds who have an uncomplicated perioperative myocardial infarction have a low rate of early mortality (5%) and high rate of late survival (80% for hospital survivors at 5 years) that is similar to patients who do not sustain a myocardial infarction. Because complications of myocardial infarction are more common in patients with preoperatively impaired left ventricular function, this report explains the results of previous smaller studies showing little effect of perioperative myocardial infarction on survival.—Hillel Laks, M.D.

Twelve-Year Experience With Bilateral Internal Mammary Artery Grafts

David L. Galbut, Ernest A. Traad, Malcolm J. Dorman, Paul L. DeWitt, Parry B. Larsen, Deborah Weinstein, Joan M. Ally, and Thomas O. Gentsch (Miami Heart Inst., Miami Beach)
Ann. Thorac. Surg. 40:264–270, September 1985   5–4

The efficacy of bilateral internal mammary artery (IMA) grafting was reviewed in 227 patients (201 men) operated on with supplemental autologous vein grafting between 1972 and 1984. The mean age was 55 years. Triple-vessel disease was present in 73% of the patients, and 12% had left main coronary stenosis. There were 725 coronary grafts placed, averaging 3.2 per patient. All patients received bilateral IMA grafts.

Operative mortality was 4%, falling to 1% in the last 4 years of the study period. Five patients required reoperation for bleeding. Perioperative infarction occurred in 7.5% of the patients. Late mortality was 8%. Twelve patients (5%) had late nonfatal myocardial infarction. Of 68 patients followed for a mean of 10½ years, 69% were asymptomatic and only two were in New York Heart Association functional class III or class IV. Patency rates in 30 patients studied a mean of 4½ years after operation, usually for recurrent chest pain, were 92% for left IMA grafts and 87% for right IMA grafts.

These findings confirm the superior long-term patency of IMA grafts. Use of the IMA can be extended with sequential grafts and by placing the right IMA through the transverse sinus for circumflex artery revascularization. Bilateral IMA grafting is associated with a low operative risk and

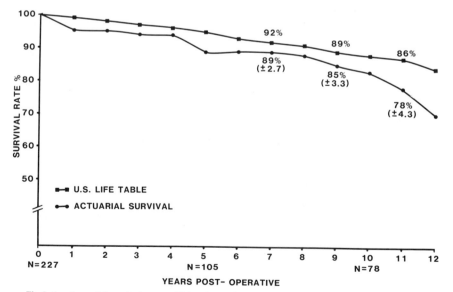

Fig 5–4.—Actuarial survival among 204 patients after coronary revascularization with bilateral IMA and occasional saphenous vein grafts compared with age-matched population from U.S. life table. (Courtesy of Galbut, D.L., et al.: Ann. Thorac. Surg. 40:264–270, September 1985.)

can provide excellent long-term functional improvement and survival (Fig 5–4).

▶ This important experience with a 12-year follow-up period describes the expanded use of bilateral internal mammary artery (IMA) grafts. Both detached mammary arteries and sequential grafts were used successfully. Again, late patency was superior to that of vein grafts, and the complications of bilateral IMA takedown were not significantly increased.—Hillel Laks, M.D.

Surgical Survival in the Coronary Artery Surgery Study (CASS) Registry
William O. Myers, Kathryn Davis, Eric D. Foster, Charles Maynard, and George C. Kaiser (Marshfield Clinic, Wis.; Univ. of Washington; Albany Med. College; and St. Louis Univ.)
Ann. Thorac. Surg. 40:245–260, September 1985   5–5

Nonrandomized surgical survival data were obtained from the Coronary Artery Surgery Study (CASS) registry. A total of 8,991 patients in the registry part of the CASS had primary isolated coronary bypass grafting, and 8,971 were followed for longer than 30 days. The 5-year survival for this group was 90%, and operative mortality was 2.4%. Patients with left main coronary disease had a 5-year survival of 85%, compared with 91% for those with other lesions. The respective operative mortality rates were 3.8% and 2.1%. Results were comparable in patients with left main coronary disease and those with triple-vessel disease. Patients with single- and double-vessel disease had respective 5-year survival rates of 93% and 92% and operative mortality rates of less than 2%.

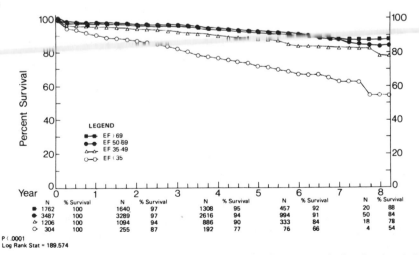

Fig 5–5.—Left ventricular dysfunction rated by ejection fraction (EF) shows markedly reduced survival in patients with EF of less than 35%, moderately impaired survival in group with EF from 35% to 49%, and nearly identical survival in categories considered to be normal or greater than 50%. (Courtesy of Myers, W.O., et al.: Ann. Thorac. Surg. 40:245–260, September 1985.)

Patients with normal or nearly normal left ventricular function had a 5-year survival of 92% and an operative mortality of 2%. The respective figures for patients with moderate impairment were 80% and 4.2% and for those with poor left ventricular function, 65% and 6.2% (Fig 5–5). The differences in survival were significant. Significant factors in long-term survival, excluding hospital mortality, included left ventricular wall motion score, congestive heart failure score, age, number of operable vessels, smoking, left ventricular end-diastolic pressure, and percent of left main coronary stenosis.

Nonrandomized surgical survival data from the CASS indicate that good left ventricular function is the preoperative factor most predictive of improved long-term survival.

▶ As shown in this study, left ventricular function is so important to long-term survival that greater efforts should be directed toward detecting and adequately treating coronary artery disease before left ventricular impairment has occurred.—Hillel Laks, M.D.

Determinants of 10-Year Survival After Primary Myocardial Revascularization
Delos M. Cosgrove, Floyd D. Loop, Bruce W. Lytle, Carl C. Gill, Leonard A. R. Golding, Christopher Gibson, Robert W. Stewart, Paul C. Taylor, and Marlene Goormastic (Cleveland Clinic Found.)
Ann. Surg. 202:480–490, October 1985   5–6

Information on the first 1,000 patients undergoing primary elective myocardial revascularization at the Cleveland Clinic each year from 1971 through 1978 was analyzed in an attempt to identify determinants of long-term survival. Operative mortality was 1%, and 0.2% of patients were lost to follow-up study. The mean follow-up period was nearly 9 years.

The 5-year and 10-year survival rates were 93% and 79%, respectively. Five-year rates ranged from 96% for patients with single-vessel disease to 91% for those with left main coronary disease; the 10-year survival was also related to extent of coronary disease. Survival at both 5 years and 10 years declined with the degree of left ventricular impairment. Patients with severe impairment had a 5-year survival of 81% and a 10-year rate of 54%. Internal mammary artery grafts were associated with better survival than was the use of vein grafts only (Fig 5–6). Incomplete revascularization compromised survival. Advancing age was the most significant factor in late survival. Risk factors for all age groups included left main coronary disease, three-vessel disease, abnormal ECG findings, hypertension, and smoking. Overall survival was equivalent to that of the age-matched and sex-matched United States population at 5 years, but slightly lower at 10 years.

Advancing age was by far the most important risk factor in survival after primary myocardial revascularization in this series. The superiority of the internal mammary artery is increasingly apparent. Complete revas-

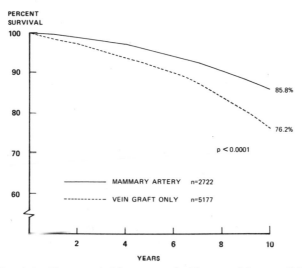

Fig 5–6.—Cumulative 10-year survival for artery grafts. (Courtesy of Cosgrove, D.M., et al.: Ann. Surg. 202:480–490, October 1985.)

cularization is also important. Moderate or severe left ventricular impairment continues to be a highly important determinant of long-term survival.

▶ The findings in this report were similar to those found in the Coronary Artery Surgery Study. Most striking was the demonstration that there was a higher long-term survival in patients who had internal mammary artery grafts than in patients with saphenous vein grafts.—Hillel Laks, M.D.

The Coronary Artery Surgery Study (CASS): A Critical Appraisal
Gerald S. Weinstein and Bruce Levin (Lenox Hill Hosp. and Columbia Univ.)
J. Thorac. Cardiovasc. Surg. 90:541–548, October 1985   5–7

The Coronary Artery Surgery Study (CASS) has had a great impact on current thinking regarding surgery for coronary artery disease, but there is considerable misunderstanding of its applicability to clinical practice. The randomized, controlled prospective study of 780 patients involves only a small subset of those with chronic, stable angina and mild symptoms. Patient groups that were not included in the study are listed in the table. Only 13% of patients initially included in the registry fulfilled the criteria for randomization, and only 5% of the patients screened originally actually participated in the study.

Fewer than 70% of these patients were followed for 5 years. Of the 390 who were assigned to have surgery, 91.5% were operated on; of the 390 who were assigned to receive medical therapy, only 74.4% actually had the assigned treatment. The crossover rate from the medically assigned group to surgery was 25.6%, and in the important group with triple-vessel disease, the crossover rate was 38%. Despite this, these patients were

---

PATIENTS TO WHOM CASS DOES NOT APPLY*

Clinical criteria

  Unstable angina, defined as:

   1. More severe, prolonged, or frequent angina ("crescendo" pattern) superimposed on preexisting pattern of relatively stable, exertion-related angina[4]

   2. Angina at rest as well as with minimal exertion[4]

   3. New-onset angina brought on by minimal exertion[4]

  Angina more severe than Class II

  Congestive heart failure (NYHA Class III or IV).

  Age > 65 yr

  Asymptomatic, but with positive exercise stress test[9]

  Known coronary artery disease and arrhythmia or congestive heart failure, but no angina[9]

  No coronary angiogram performed[9]

Angiographic criteria

  Left main coronary artery narrowing >70% luminal diameter

  Ejection fraction <0.35

  Ventricular aneurysm likely to require resection

  Valvular disease likely to require valve replacement

*NYHA, New York Heart Association.
(Courtesy of Weinstein, G.S., and Levin, B.: J. Thorac. Cardiovasc. Surg. 90:541–548, October 1985.)

---

included in the "medical" group for statistical analysis. The 5-year mortality was 5.5% in the surgical group and 8% in the medical group. Medically treated patients with an ejection fraction of less than 0.5 had poorer survival rates than did those with higher ejection fractions, but no statistically significant difference was apparent in the surgically treated group.

The CASS and its conclusions are relevant to only a small proportion of patients with coronary artery disease. Noncompliance with the assigned treatment casts some doubt on the validity of the results. The statistical power of the study is so low that a real difference is likely to have been overlooked. The conclusion that patients who resemble those in the CASS can safely defer surgery is not warranted. The study did not address the possibility that a delay in surgery may compromise long-term survival. The long-term results of the study may, however, still be of interest.

▶ This well thought out and analytical appraisal of the CASS is particularly critical of the conclusions drawn from the randomized portion of the study. It is important reading for those confronted with the unwarranted conclusions drawn by physicians and the lay public from an otherwise valuable assessment of coronary artery surgery as it was practiced between 1974 and 1979. It is important to note also the improvements in coronary revascularization that have occurred during the last 5 years, particularly the increased use of the internal mammary artery with its improved early and late graft patency.—Hillel Laks, M.D.

Intermediate-Term Results of Coronary Artery Bypass Grafting for Acute Myocardial Infarction

James K. Kirklin, E. H. Blackstone, George L. Zorn, Jr., Albert D. Pacifico, John W. Kirklin, Robert B. Karp, and William J. Rogers (Univ. of Alabama at Birmingham)
Circulation 72 (Suppl. 2):175–178, September 1985   5–8

A prospective study of emergency surgical treatment for AMI in conjunction with other reperfusion measures was begun in 1982. Intermediate-term results now are available for the first 35 patients who were operated on within 48 hours of infarction. The 29 men and 6 women had a mean age of 55 years. In the 30 patients who presented with an infarct syndrome, mean duration of pain at the time of surgery was 12 hours. Thirteen patients received intravenous injections or, in most cases, intracoronary injections of streptokinase. Seven of the 13 had clot lysis. In two patients an attempt at emergency angioplasty was unsuccessful, and five others had elective angioplasty that was complicated by acute vessel occlusion.

Hospital mortality was 3%. All four patients who were in cardiogenic shock before operation survived, but with morbidity. The actuarial survival 2 years after operation was 93%. No patient required repeat revascularization, but one underwent cardiac transplantation because of persistent left ventricular failure. Angina was uncommon after revascularization, and no patient has had a subsequent infarction. Most patients were in New York Heart Association class I at follow-up examination.

The early and intermediate-term results of emergency myocardial revascularization warrant its continued use in higher risk patients with AMI. A small number of patients with cardiogenic shock were successfully operated on. Most patients were free of angina and in good physical status at follow-up study.

▶ This report of 35 patients undergoing coronary revascularization within 48 hours of infarction includes those with failed angioplasty (7) and failed streptokinase therapy (13). The low early mortality rate of 3% and the excellent late survival of 93% at 2 years confirms previous reports that coronary revascularization can be undertaken with relatively low risk and excellent results soon after myocardial infarction. Coronary revascularization should be considered as one of the safe and effective options in selected patients sustaining a myocardial infarction. In some cases, particularly in patients with triple-vessel disease, it may be preferable to the intravenous infusion of streptokinase or to angioplasty as the primary intervention.—Hillel Laks, M.D.

Sequential Internal Mammary Artery Grafts: Expanded Utilization of an Ideal Conduit

M. Laxman Kamath, Linda S. Matysik, Donald H. Schmidt, and Linda L. Smith (Mount Sinai Med. Ctr., Milwaukee)
J. Thorac. Cardiovasc. Surg. 89:163–169, February 1985   5–9

Sequential internal mammary artery (IMA) grafting represents an attempt to overcome the limited availability of these arteries for multiple coronary bypass grafting. Between 1980 and 1983, 87 patients had sequential anastomoses in which one or both IMAs were used at myocardial revascularization. In 49 patients, one IMA was used as a sequential anastomosis; in 31 others, one IMA was used in this way and the other as a single end-to-side anastomosis. Seven patients had both IMAs used sequentially to revascularize four myocardial areas. The clinical outcome was similar in these groups. The 77 men and 10 women had a mean age of 59 years. No IMA less than 1 mm in diameter at the site of anastomosis was used. There were 94 sequential anastomoses.

There was no hospital mortality. The patency rates on coronary angiography in the first postoperative year were 90% for 83 vein grafts and 93% for 84 IMA grafts, not a significant difference. One of two abnormal pyrophosphate scans was in relation to an IMA graft. Seven of 64 patients had equivocal exercise stress test results but none had definitely positive findings. All but 4 of 83 patients had complete symptomatic relief. Three others improved considerably. One patient failed to improve after operation.

Sequential anastomosis of the IMA is technically feasible and is a practical approach to myocardial revascularization. Sequential IMA grafting adequately meets the nutritional demands of the myocardium.

▶ This report studies the results of sequential IMA grafts. It is important to recognize that sequential grafts were used only in selected patients. Thus, of 774 patients operated on during the study period, 376 received one or two IMA grafts and only 87 had sequential IMA grafts. The size of the IMA was a major determinant in the decision to use sequential anastomoses, and these were performed only when the IMA diameter exceeded 2 mm. In this report, vein graft and IMA patency were not significantly different, but the numbers were too small to conclude that the early sequential IMA anastomosis patency is lower than the single IMA anastomosis patency is. This study also demonstrates that in selected patients, the IMA was adequate to provide the increased myocardium supplied by the sequential anastomosis.—Hillel Laks, M.D.

Analysis of Morbidity and Mortality in Patients 70 Years of Age and Over Undergoing Isolated Coronary Artery Bypass Surgery
Daniel M. Rose, Joseph Gelbfish, Israel J. Jacobowitz, Marshall Kramer, Zvi Zisbrod, Anthony Acinapura, Paula Cappabianca, and Joseph N. Cunningham, Jr. (Maimonides Med. Ctr., Brooklyn, and St. Vincent's Med. Ctr., New York)
Am. Heart J. 110:341–346, August 1985   5–10

Many elderly patients now are referred for coronary artery bypass surgery, but recent studies generally have found increased morbidity and mortality in this age group. Since 1981, 144 men and 57 women, mean age 74 years, have been operated on. Those who had valve replacement or repair were excluded. More elderly than younger patients had a history of congestive heart failure and diabetes, and more had surgery for unstable symptoms. Also, more older patients had triple-vessel disease and left main coronary artery disease, and more had a depressed left ventricular ejection fraction.

Slightly fewer grafts were used in older than in younger patients. Older patients had more postoperative myocardial infarcts, more strokes, and more episodes of renal failure that required dialysis. Mortality was 6% in the older group and 2% in the younger group. Patients with perioperative infarction had respective mortality rates of 44% and 27%. Mortality was similar in the two groups for patients who required intra-aortic balloon support before or after operation.

Patients aged 70 years and older can be operated on relatively safely for coronary artery disease, although they do have increased preoperative risk factors; also, increased postoperative morbidity and mortality can be expected. Serious postoperative complications are more likely in this population. The inability to provide complete revascularization may contribute to increased postoperative morbidity and mortality.

▶ The combination of an aging population and enhanced expectations of activity and life-style has resulted in an increase in the number of patients over 70 years of age undergoing coronary revascularization. This study shows that this population is at increased risk only partly because they have more severe disease, as evidenced by the lower ejection fraction, higher prevalence of triple-vessel disease, left main coronary disease, and unstable angina. Excluding these risk factors, age per se was associated with a higher mortality rate. This increased risk is generally related to noncardiac causes; only 3 of the 12 deaths were cardiac related. In the elderly, there is an increased incidence of cerebral vascular accidents, sepsis, and respiratory failure. It is clear that age per se is a significant consideration in undertaking bypass surgery in the elderly, particularly in women (early mortality of 8.8% vs. 4.8% for men).—Hillel Laks, M.D.

Aspirin or Dipyridamole Individually Prevents Lipid Accumulation in Primate Vein Bypass Grafts
Lawrence E. Boerboom, Gordon N. Olinger, Lawrence I. Bonchek, Ilhan I. Gunay, and Ahmed H. Kissebah (Med. College of Wisconsin, Milwaukee)
Am. J. Cardiol. 55:556–559, Feb. 15, 1985   5–11

Aspirin and dipyridamole often are used together as antithrombotic agents, but it is not clear whether their combined use is necessary for antilipid effects. Combined and single-drug therapy was compared in studies of stump-tailed macaque monkeys who had cephalic vein grafts that were interposed in the femoral arteries and that were fed a normolipemic diet. Aspirin was given in a dose of 80 mg daily; the dose of dipyridamole was 50 mg daily. The same doses were used during combination treatment.

None of the grafts had overt evidence of stenosis, kinking, or gross atherosclerotic lesions when they were removed 3 months after insertion.

Concentrations of cholesterol and apolipoprotein-B in grafts were similar to concentrations in ungrafted veins; in each of the treated groups concentrations were significantly lower than in grafts from untreated animals. In grafts from control monkeys concentrations of cholesterol were 250% higher, and concentrations of apolipoprotein-B were 925% higher, than in ungrafted veins. There were no significant differences in concentrations among the treated groups.

Treatment with aspirin or dipyridamole reduces the uptake of cholesterol and apolipoprotein-B by vein bypass grafts in monkeys. The effect is comparable to that obtained by using both drugs together. Aspirin and dipyridamole may be expected to reduce clinically manifest atherosclerotic degeneration of grafts with delayed occlusion. Either of these drugs may be used alone over the long term to mitigate graft atherosclerosis.

▶ This paper shows that aspirin and dipyridamole are individually effective in reducing the deposition of lipids in the walls of vein grafts placed in the arterial system. Clinical studies have already shown that aspirin and Persantine are effective in reducing graft occlusions during the first year when occlusions are generally thrombotic. This study holds out promise that late occlusion caused by atherosclerosis may be prevented by antiplatelet therapy. Meanwhile, the long-term use of aspirin combined with Persantine seems warranted for patients after coronary revascularization.—Hillel Laks, M.D.

Coronary Artery Bypass Following Percutaneous Transluminal Coronary Angioplasty
Duncan A. Killen, William R. Hamaker, and William A. Reed (St. Luke's Hosp., Kansas City, Mo.)
Ann. Thorac. Surg. 40:133–138, August 1985   5–12

Patients in whom percutaneous transluminal coronary angioplasty (PTCA) is unsuccessful usually require coronary artery bypass grafting, sometimes on an emergency basis. Review was made of data on 286 patients who had at least one PTCA procedure and underwent coronary artery bypass grafting during a 4-year period. The 214 men and 72 women had a mean age of 60 years. Forty-two patients had previous coronary artery bypass surgery. Twenty-nine patients underwent emergency PTCA for evolving infarction. Sixty-one patients had more than one PTCA procedure before bypass surgery.

Ninety-three patients were taken directly from the catheterization laboratory to the operating room for immediate coronary artery bypass grafting. The most frequent indications for such a procedure were prolonged chest pain that was consistent with AMI and worsening of coronary obstruction seen at angiography after PTCA. In 32 patients cardiogenic shock or pulmonary edema developed. All but 2 of the 115 emergency bypass operations were done within 24 hours of PTCA. Perioperative infarction occurred in 46 patients treated on an emergency basis (43.5%) and in 7 treated electively (4.1%). The 30-day mortality was 11% in the emergency group and 3% in the elective group. Five late infarctions occurred during an average follow-up period of 1½ years. Two patients required repeat coronary artery bypass grafting, and one had repeat PTCA. Of the survivors, 73% were free of angina 3 years postoperatively. Late mortality in early survivors was 1.4% per year.

The results of emergency coronary artery bypass grafting after failed PTCA are poor in patients with previous coronary bypass, multivessel disease, and other complex forms of coronary artery disease. Prompt bypass grafting may be preferable to persistent attempts to salvage a PTCA procedure when it is not going well.

▶ This study describes the results of coronary revascularization undertaken both electively and emergently after coronary balloon angioplasty. It is clear that the results of the emergency procedures are significantly worse than those of elective surgery. In addition, the mortality and perioperative infarction rates were increased in high-risk patients, i.e., those with multivessel disease, cardiogenic shock, and previous coronary bypass surgery. This report underlines the need for a randomized study to evaluate the place of balloon angioplasty, particularly in these high-risk groups.—Hillel Laks, M.D.

Determinants of Operative Mortality and Long-Term Survival in Patients With Unstable Angina: The CASS Experience
John R. McCormick, Edgar C. Schick, Jr., Carolyn H. McCabe, Richard A. Kronmal, and Thomas J. Ryan (Univ. Hosp., Boston, and Univ. of Washington)
J. Thorac. Cardiovasc. Surg. 89:683–688, May 1985   5–13

Determinants of long-term survival were sought in a series of 3,311 patients who underwent coronary revascularization for unstable angina in the Coronary Artery Surgery Study (CASS) between 1974 and 1979. All patients had new or recurrent episodes of angina at rest that lasted longer than 30 minutes and did not respond promptly to standard treatment. The mean age was 56 years, and 80% of the group were men. Also, 52% had previous myocardial infarction. New-onset angina was present in 39%. Further, 50% of the patients had three-vessel disease and 14% had left main coronary artery disease.

Operative mortality was 4%. Significant factors in operative mortality included advanced age, severe left ventricular (LV) dysfunction, and stenosis of at least 50% in the left main coronary artery in a left dominant circulation. The type of clinical presentation was not a significant factor in operative mortality. Thus, patients with rest angina or acute coronary insufficiency (pain lasting for more than 30 minutes with ECG changes) had a similar mortality to those with new-onset or changing-pattern angina. Survival at 7 years was 70%. Indices of LV dysfunction were the most important predictors of long-term outcome. The number of diseased vessels and associated illness also were significant factors, and cardiomegaly was a useful prognostic factor. Patients with one-vessel and two-vessel disease had comparable cumulative survival rates, but those with three-vessel disease had a substantially worse outlook.

Operative mortality after coronary artery bypass surgery in patients with unstable angina is low and is chiefly influenced by LV function, age, and stenosis of the left main coronary artery in a left dominant circulation. Long-term survival is lower in patients with clinical or angiographic evidence of poor LV function. It remains to be determined whether bypass prolongs life in comparable groups of patients who are managed medically. The optimal timing of bypass surgery in patients with unstable angina also requires further study.

▶ This is a definitive review of the surgical results of treatment of unstable angina pectoris. Although the early mortality was slightly increased (4%) compared with that after elective coronary revascularization, the determinants of survival are similar to those in other patients in the CASS study, namely, age, ventricular function, and the presence of left main coronary artery disease. Long-term survival studies over 7 years showed an average yearly mortality of 4.7% with similar determinants, namely, ventricular function, associated illness, and context of coronary disease. The impact of expanded use of the internal mammary artery on early and late mortality remains to be established.—Hillel Laks, M.D.

Valve Repair

Results of Valve Reconstruction for Mitral Regurgitation Secondary to Mitral Valve Prolapse

Patricia A. Penkoske, F. Henry Ellis, Jr., Sidney Alexander, and Elton Watkins, Jr. (Lakey Clinic Med. Ctr., Burlington, Mass.; New England Deaconess Hosp. and Harvard Univ., Boston)
Am. J. Cardiol. 55:735–738, Mar. 1, 1985   5–14

Mitral valve prolapse (MVP), the leading cause of isolated mitral regurgitation, is often the result of myxomatous degeneration of the mitral valve. Reconstruction of the valve rather than replacement is often more feasible technically, but it is not often used in the United States. A review was made of a 14-year experience with mitral valve reconstruction for mitral regurgitation in patients who had MVP with and without ruptured chordae tendinae. A total of 479 patients with mitral valve disease underwent surgery, 82 (17%) of whom had mitral regurgitation secondary to MVP. Thirty-one patients (6%) had valve reconstruction by a technique of leaflet plication and posteromedial annuloplasty. Twenty-seven of these patients were in New York Heart Association (NYHA) class III. Eleven patients had associated cardiac disease that required correction at the time of valvuloplasty: two required aortic valve replacement and nine had coronary artery bypass grafting procedures.

One (3%) hospital death and six late deaths (19%) occurred among the 31 patients. Only three deaths were related to cardiac factors. The mean adjusted 5-year survival rate was 89%. Major complications included persistent or recurrent mitral regurgitation in five patients (16%) and cerebral embolus in one. The degree of anular dilatation was not appreciated at the time of surgery in three of four patients with persistent mitral regurgitation. All 24 surviving patients are in NYHA class I or class II. The overall survival rate free of cardiac-related complications was 73% after an average follow-up period of almost 4 years.

Mitral valve reconstruction has demonstrable advantages over valve replacement in the surgical management of patients with mitral regurgitation that is secondary to MVP. Persistent or recurrent mitral regurgitation can be reduced by correction of anular dilatation at the time of operation.

▶ This is a relatively small experience with valve repair for MVP. In fact, 19 of the 31 patients had chordal rupture. The technique used consisted of plication of the involved segment and posteromedial annuloplasty with a figure of eight suture. Although 5 of 30 survivors had significant residual or recurrent mitral regurgitation, the remainder had good hemodynamic results. Whether the results would have been improved with use of the Carpentier ring remains controversial, but the outcome does demonstrate that the Carpentier ring is not essential for all types of valve repair.—Hillel Laks, M.D.

Carpentier's Flexible Ring Versus De Vega's Annuloplasty: A Prospective Randomized Study
R. Rivera, E. Duran, and M. Ajuria (Univ. of Madrid)
J. Thorac. Cardiovasc. Surg. 89:196–203, February 1985   5–15

Carpentier's flexible ring and De Vega's semicircular annuloplasty are the two most popular techniques of tricuspid annuloplasty. To evaluate their effectiveness in controlling mitral regurgitation, 159 patients who had mitral valve disease with moderate to severe tricuspid regurgitation were prospectively randomized to undergo one of the two procedures. Seventy-six had Carpentier's tricuspid annuloplasty with the flexible open ring and 83 had De Vega's semicircular annuloplasty. Comparison of the results was based on clinical and angiographic (right ventriculography or aortography, or both) measurement of tricuspid regurgitation and its relation to the condition of the left side of the heart and to the pulmonary vascular resistance capable of inducing significant pressure overload in the right ventricle.

There were no significant differences in mean age, proportion of male patients, type of mitral lesion, incidence of aortic valvulopathy, and other preoperative and postoperative characteristics between the two groups. Although organic tricuspid damage was more common in the Carpentier group, the incidence of tricuspid commissurotomy was similar (eight in the Carpentier group and six in the De Vega group). After an average follow-up period of 64 months, clinical signs of tricuspid regurgitation and right-sided heart failure were significantly more common among patients with De Vega's annuloplasty who did not have residual lesions of the left side of the heart and in those with residual lesions who had re-operation or late death. Hemodynamic and angiographic studies in 76 patients showed that the incidence of moderate to severe tricuspid regurgitation after operation was high with both annuloplasty techniques in patients with either high total pulmonary resistance or organic tricuspid damage; however, when patients with these characteristics were excluded, the incidence was significantly lower in the Carpentier group (1 of 18, or 5%) than in the De Vega group (9 of 19, or 47%). The incidence of reoperation and late death was similar in both groups.

The Carpentier's flexible ring annuloplasty is a more efficacious means of controlling tricuspid regurgitation, especially if there is no organic tricuspid damage and pulmonary resistance decreases after operation.

▶ There has been much controversy about the need for the Carpentier ring as opposed to the DeVega technique of tricuspid annuloplasty. This randomized study concludes that the Carpentier ring tricuspid annuloplasty is superior to the DeVega method and ascribes this improvement to preservation of the normal tricuspid valve shape with the ring. In our own experience, we have found that the DeVega annuloplasty can be performed rapidly and is very satisfactory for patients without organic disease of the tricuspid valve or severe pulmonary hypertension.—Hillel Laks, M.D.

Long-Term Results of Open Mitral Valve Reconstruction for Mitral Stenosis
Lawrence H. Cohn, Elizabeth N. Allred, Leslie A. Cohn, Verdi J. Disesa, Richard J. Shemin, and John J. Collins, Jr. (Harvard Univ. and Brigham and Women's Hosp., Boston)
Am. J. Cardiol. 55:731–734, March 1, 1985   5–16

With the development of improved cardiopulmonary perfusion techniques, open mitral valve reconstruction has almost totally replaced closed mitral commissurotomy in the management of mitral stenosis (MS). A review was made of the long-term results in 120 consecutive patients aged 22–75 years who underwent open mitral valvuloplasty for rheumatic MS during a 12-year period. Nine patients were in functional class II, 106 were in class III, and 5 were in class IV. Before operation, 107 patients underwent cardiac catheterization; 13 had only noninvasive studies. Atrial fibrillation was present in 66 patients. At catheterization the mean mitral valve area was 1.09 sq cm, and the mean pulmonary wedge to left ventricular diastolic gradient was 14 mm Hg.

Indications for operation were congestive heart failure in 92 patients and thromboembolic events in 28. Cardiopulmonary bypass was used in all patients for open reconstruction under direct vision. Superior commissurotomy was done in 115 patients and inferior commissurotomy in 114; the papillary muscles were incised and the chordae were lengthened in 39, and calcium was removed from valve leaflets in 23. Suture or ring annuloplasty was not required. The mean follow-up period was 53 months (range, 6–143 months).

OPEN MITRAL VALVE OPERATIONS FOR
MITRAL STENOSIS

Report	No. of Pts	Operative Mortality (%)	Mean Follow-Up (mo)	T (%/ patient-year)	Reoperation Rate (%/patient-year)
Laschinger et al	150	0	46	0.7	0
Vega et al	155	1.2%	36	0.6	0.5
Housman et al	100	1	46	0.5	4.6
Aaron and Lower	106	0.9	36*	0.6	0.9
Cohn et al	120	0	53	1.8	1.7

T, thromboembolism.
*Assumed from partial data presented.
(Courtesy of Cohn, L.H., et al.: Am. J. Cardiol. 55:731–734, March 1, 1985.)

There were no operative deaths, but five late deaths occurred, all from noncardiac causes. The actuarial probability of survival at 10 years was 95 ± 2%. Thromboemboli occurred in nine patients. The actuarial probability of freedom from thromboembolism at 10 years was 91 ± 3%, and the linearized rate was 1.8% emboli for each patient-year of follow-up study. Conversion to sinus rhythm occurred in 25 of 50 patients in atrial fibrillation before operation; 12 of 42 patients in preoperative sinus rhythm experienced atrial fibrillation. Reoperation that necessitated valve replacement was performed in nine patients, for an absolute incidence of 7.5% and an annual incidence of 1.7% per patient-year. At 10 years the probability of freedom from reoperation was 84 ± 5%.

The table shows that in open mitral valvuloplasty for MS there has been low operative mortality, and long-term results have been excellent, based on freedom from thromboemboli and need for reoperation. These findings suggest that earlier surgery should be considered in patients with MS to prevent the development of chronic atrial fibrillation. The onset of atrial fibrillation or clinical thromboembolism, even in a functional class II patient, may be an indication for open mitral valvuloplasty. With the incidence of reoperation being less than 10% during a mean follow-up period of more than 4 years, it is believed that reoperation should be performed before severe functional impairment develops.

► This report confirms the excellent results that can be obtained with open mitral valve reconstruction for isolated MS and therefore supports the trend away from closed mitral commissurotomy.—Hillel Laks, M.D.

Intraoperative Contrast Two-Dimensional Echocardiography: Evaluation of the Presence and Severity of Aortic and Mitral Regurgitation During Cardiac Operations

Manuel G. Eguaras, Javier Pasalodos, Venancio Gonzalez, Anastasio Montero, Miguel A. Garcia, Ignacio Moriones, Jorge Granados, Federico Valles, and Manuel Concha (Univ. of Cordoba)

J. Thorac. Cardiovasc. Surg. 89:573–579, April 1985   5–17

It has been difficult to assess the degree of mitral or aortic regurgitation in the nonbeating or fibrillating heart. Contrast two-dimensional echocardiography was used in the intraoperative study of valve regurgitation in 35 patients undergoing cardiac operations with conventional cardiopulmonary bypass. All 35 patients, whose mean age was 47 years, had been catheterized previously. Echocardiography was performed after sternotomy and opening of the pericardium. A real-time mechanical digital scanner was used. A 5-ml volume of 5% dextrose in water served as the contrast material.

No patient had complications from the procedure. Eleven required two contrast injections for visualization of microbubbles. Contrast material was visualized as microbubbles flowing retrograde through the incompetent valve. The findings agreed with the angiographic results in 34 instances. One patient with mild aortic regurgitation observed on angiography had moderate regurgitation seen on echocardiography. No false positive or false negative results were obtained. Contrast echocardiography can be a useful means of evaluating the presence and severity of valve regurgitation during operation, making it possible to avoid preoperative cardiac catheterization in some patients.

▶ This study demonstrates the accuracy of intraoperative contrast echocardiography to assess mitral and aortic valvular regurgitation. With increased use of valve repair operations, particularly for the mitral valve, a method of assessing the repair intraoperatively assumes great importance.—Hillel Laks, M.D.

Experiences With the Carpentier Techniques of Mitral Valve Reconstruction in 103 Patients (1980–1985)

Frank C. Spencer, Stephen B. Colvin, Alfred T. Culliford, and O. Wayne Isom (New York Univ.)

J. Thorac. Cardiovasc. Surg. 90:341–350, September 1985   5–18

A total of 103 patients aged 2–77 years underwent some type of Carpentier reconstruction for mitral insufficiency. Nearly all patients with mitral insufficiency are now operated on, regardless of age or etiology, and associated procedures (e.g., triple bypass surgery) have been done increasingly often. A ring annuloplasty was used in all patients except for three small children. Elongated chordae were shortened by implantation into a papillary muscle in 18 patients, and 5 others had chordae transposed from the mural to the aortic leaflet. Shortened, fused chordae were divided in 13 patients with rheumatic heart disease. Most patients required procedures other than prosthetic ring annuloplasty. Large amounts of calcium were removed from the mitral anulus in a few cases. The Carpentier self-retaining mitral retractor was especially helpful in operative exposure of the mitral valve.

Myocardial ischemia was required for 1–2 hours in most patients. Two hospital deaths occurred, both apparently unrelated to the technique of repair. Residual mitral insufficiency occurred in only one patient. Most of the patients were asymptomatic at follow-up examination, with little or no restriction of activity. Nearly all are in New York Heart Association classes I and II. There were no late recurrences of insufficiency. One patient was reoperated on for deshiscence of the prosthetic ring. Another was reoperated on because of acute valvulitis caused by recurrent rheumatic fever; and a heroin addict had recurrent endocarditis. Thromboembolism was of only minor importance, and only one patient sustained permanent neurologic deficit.

These gratifying results are nearly identical with those reported by Carpentier. Extensive calcification of the anulus may or may not contraindicate this procedure. Aortic leaflet involvement was seen as a persistent challenge.

▶ This excellent experience with mitral valve repair confirms the applicability of Carpentier's technique to nonrheumatic disease of the mitral valve. The discussion of this paper by Dr. Carpentier and others is worth reading. Dr. Carpentier points out the effectiveness of chordal transposition from the posterior to the anterior leaflet as a method of treating anterior leaflet prolapse.—Hillel Laks, M.D.

Valve Replacement

In Vivo Hemodynamic Comparison of Porcine and Pericardial Valves
Delos M. Cosgrove, Bruce W. Lytle, Carl C. Gill, Leonard A. R. Golding, Robert W. Stewart, Floyd D. Loop, and George W. Williams (Cleveland Clinic Found.)
J. Thorac. Cardiovasc. Surg. 89:358–368, March 1985   5–19

The Carpentier-Edwards bovine pericardial valve and the Carpentier-Edwards SupraAnnular porcine valve were developed to improve the hemodynamic function of tissue valves. To evaluate the relative performance of the standard Carpentier-Edwards procine valve, the Carpentier-Edwards SupraAnnular porcine valve, and the Carpentier-Edwards bovine pericardial valve in the aortic position, 100 patients who had aortic valve replacement were studied during operation. Peak-to-peak systolic gradients, mean systolic gradients, effective valve orifice areas, and performance indices were calculated. Nine patients underwent simultaneous mitral valve replacement with the use of a porcine bioprosthesis.

The mean gradient across the valve decreased as valve size increased for standard and pericardial valves. The mean area of the valve orifice increased for all valves as size increased. Valve function curves showed that the transvalvular gradient for both pericardial and SupraAnnular valves increased as flow increased and valve size decreased. The mean area of the orifice of both pericardial and SupraAnnular valves increased as flow and valve size increased. At the same flow rate, the 23-mm pericardial valves had larger orifice areas, higher performance indices, and lower gradients than the 23-mm SupraAnnular valve had.

The Carpentier-Edwards SupraAnnular valve is hemodynamically superior to the standard Carpentier-Edwards porcine bioprosthesis. However, the Carpentier-Edwards bovine pericardial valve is less obstructive in the aortic position than either of the porcine valves. The excellent hemodynamic performance results from a design that does not include the aortic anulus in the mounting mechanism and from the absence of the muscle bar that is present to varying degrees in porcine valves.

▶ This study confirms previous reports that have demonstrated the hemodynamic superiority of the bovine pericardial valve over the porcine aortic xenograft. The Carpentier-Edwards bovine pericardial valve incorporates an improved attachment of the pericardial leaflet to the strut. Whether this will improve its longevity in comparison with the Ionescu-Shiley pericardial valve remains to be seen. The bovine pericardial valve may be the valve of choice for the elderly patient with a small anulus.—Hillel Laks, M.D.

Transseptal Control of the Difficult Aortic Anulus
John D. Rumisek, William R. Berry, Michael J. Barry, and John S. Clarke (Letterman Army Med. Ctr., San Francisco)
Ann. Thorac. Surg. 39:385–386, April 1985   5–20

Control of the aortic root in extensive erosive endocarditis, with or without mycotic ventricular septal defect, often requires secure prosthetic fixation to the interventricular septum. Suture placement deep within the left ventricular outflow tract is impeded by the overlying right ventricular outflow tract and the composite graft; subsequent suture laxity or pull-through can lead to uncontrollable bleeding, recurrent aneurysm, or an intracardiac fistula. A simple and rapid means of firmly securing a prosthetic composite graft to the diseased septum in the difficult aortic root was developed.

TECHNIQUE.—With cardiopulmonary bypass and cold cardioplegia, a low sigmoid aortotomy is extended inferiorly toward the noncoronary cusp, the aortic valve is removed, and nonviable tissue is débrided. Bolstered mattress sutures of 2–0 Tevdek or Ti-Cron are passed through intact areas of the posterior aortic anulus or anterior mitral anulus from the ventricular aspect to the prosthetic sewing ring. A short vertical or transverse incision is then made in the pulmonary infundibulum just below the valve, and horizontal mattress sutures are passed through the anterior prosthetic sewing ring and then through the interventricular septum from left to right (Fig 5–7). Sutures are placed above the level of the papillary

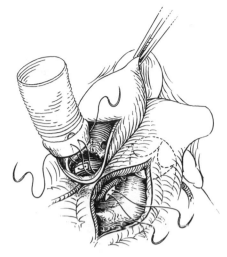

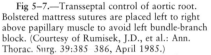

Fig 5–7.—Transseptal control of aortic root. Bolstered mattress sutures are placed left to right above papillary muscle to avoid left bundle-branch block. (Courtesy of Rumisek, J.D., et al.: Ann. Thorac. Surg. 39:385 386, April 1985.)

muscle of the conus if possible. The transseptal sutures are tied last, within the right ventricular outflow tract over felt bolsters, or incorporated as part of a mycotic ventricular septal defect patch repair. The infundibular incision is closed with running Prolene sutures.

Aortic root repair with a composite graft, ventricular septal defect patch, and coronary translocation was recently carried out successfully in a patient with aortic prosthetic valve endocarditis and septal involvement, by the right ventricular outflow tract approach. Early use of this method is recommended to reconstruct the destroyed aortic root in patients with erosive infective endocarditis.

▶ This is an excellent technique that may prove invaluable for the patient with a friable aortic anulus caused by endocarditis or other conditions.—Hillel Laks, M.D.

Comparison of Bioprosthetic and Mechanical Valve Replacement for Active Endocarditis
Michael S. Sweeney, George J. Reul, Jr., Denton A. Cooley, David A. Ott, J. Michael Duncan, O. H. Frazier, and James J. Livesay (Texas Heart Inst., Houston)
J. Thorac. Cardiovasc. Surg. 90:676–680, November 1985   5–21

Relatively low rates of recurrent endocarditis in nonaddicted patients have raised questions regarding the assumption that foreign material should not be placed into an actively infected site. Data were reviewed on 185 patients who underwent valve replacement for active valvular endocarditis between 1979 and 1984. Eighty-eight received a bioprosthetic Ionescu-Shiley pericardial valve, and the other 97 received a mechanical St. Jude Medical valve prosthesis. The groups were similar in age and sex distribution. Two thirds of the patients had life-threatening active bacterial or fungal endocarditis of a native valve; the other third had involvement of a prosthetic valve. A bioprosthesis was placed 12 patients with prosthetic valve endocarditis.

Early mortality was similar in the two groups. Seventy-nine percent of patients with bioprostheses and 88% of those with mechanical prostheses were in New York Heart Association functional class I or class II postoperatively. Fifteen patients with bioprostheses were reoperated on, ten for recurrent endocarditis and five because of sterile perivalvular leakage. Only five patients with a mechanical prosthesis had reoperation, four for recurrent endocarditis and one for sterile leakage. Two nonfatal thromboembolic events occurred in both groups. Three late deaths in the bioprosthesis group occurred during hospitalization for reoperation.

Mechanical prosthetic valves were more resistant to reinfection and the need for reoperation was less likely in this series. Bioprostheses are more likely to fail in an actively infected bed. Mechanical prostheses seem to be preferable for use in patients with active endocarditis.

▶ This is the first report that we are aware of concluding that the mechanical valve is preferable to the tissue valve for patients with active endocarditis. The data are persuasive that the mechanical valve is better able to withstand the sequelae of residual infection. Further studies of this important question are needed.—Hillel Laks, M.D.

Experience With Outlet Strut Fracture of the Björk-Shiley Convexoconcave Mitral Valve Prosthesis

Che-keung Mok, Jan Wai-Tsun Lee, Siu-Ming Kong, and Kenneth Kin-Kong Hui (Univ. of Hong Kong)
Am. Heart J. 110:814–818, October 1985   5–22

Outlet strut fracture (OSF) with dislodgement and embolization of the tilting disk is a recognized complication in patients with a Björk-Shiley convexoconcave valve prosthesis (BSCP). Seven such patients have been reported in the English language literature, six of whom had a mitral prostheses and one an aortic prosthesis. Five further instances of OSF in a mitral BSCP were encountered, all within a 15-month period. All five patients had acute left heart failure and pulmonary edema. Both the outlet strut and the tilting disk were missing from the mitral prostheses. Three patients had emergency operations, and two survived. The risk of OSF in a series of 237 patients with a BSCP was 1.7%, or 0.076/100 patient-months of experience.

Design features in the outlet strut elevation angle of the BSCP complicate its welding to the orifice ring, and a small area of phase segregation in the weld zone could reduce the ductility and endurance of the outlet strut. Neither poor valve handling nor undesirable implantation techniques were implicated in the authors' five patients. The monostrut valve designed by Björk, in which all parts of the valve are integral with the flange and no welds are present, may overcome any drawbacks of the BSCP while retaining its good qualities.

Outlet strut fracture should be considered in patients with acute palpitations, worsening dyspnea, evidence of peripheral circulatory failure, and marked pulmonary edema. Immediate replacement of the broken prosthesis is necessary. Unless the outlet strut or tilting disk is present in the left side of the heart, it is probably best not to attempt to retrieve it until the patient's condition stabilizes.

▶ For several years the Björk-Shiley valve has been the most commonly used mechanical valve. The convexoconcave modification was released in 1979. In 1983 there was a voluntary recall of mitral valves sizes 29 mm, 31 mm, and 33 mm that had been processed between February 1981 and March 1982. In this report the incidence of strut fracture in valves processed after March 1982 was 3.5%, or 0.2/100 patient-months. This study would suggest a much higher incidence of strut fracture than previously reported. Whether the incidence will increase with time remains to be seen. If it rises progressively, elective replacement of these valves may become necessary.—Hillel Laks, M.D.

Mitral Valve Replacement Combined With Myocardial Revascularization: Early and Late Results for 300 Patients, 1970 to 1983
Bruce W. Lytle, Delos M. Cosgrove, Carl C. Gill, Robert W. Stewart, Leonard A. R. Golding, Marlene Goormastic, Paul C. Taylor, and Floyd D. Loop (Cleveland Clinic Found.)
Circulation 71:1179–1190, June 1985   5–23

Information was reviewed on the first 300 consecutive patients undergoing primary mitral valve replacement combined with coronary bypass grafting between 1970 and 1983 at the Cleveland Clinic. Intermittent ischemic arrest was used until 1976 and St. Thomas solution cardioplegia was used thereafter. Bioprostheses were used in 54% of the patients and mechanical prostheses in 46%. Myxoid degeneration and rheumatic disease were the most frequent indications for valve replacement.

Hospital mortality was 7%. Significant risk factors included cardiomegaly, paced rhythm or atrial fibrillation, left main coronary obstruction, and an elevated serum bilirubin concentration. Follow-up study of 278 patients for a mean of 4 years showed event-free survival rates at 2 years, 5 years, and 10 years of 65%, 46%, and 21%, respectively. Long-term survival was compromised by in-hospital ventricular arrhythmia, left ventricular dysfunction, and a rheumatic or ischemic basis for mitral valve disease. Patients with bioprostheses who did not receive warfarin had a better event-free survival rate than did those given warfarin and those with mechanical prostheses whether or not warfarin was given. No patient had worse symptoms after operation, and all but two were in New York Heart Association functional class I or class II at follow-up study.

Warfarin anticoagulation may not be indicated for patients with mitral bioprostheses even if atrial fibrillation is present, but studies of more patients are needed. Bioprostheses in this position appear positively to affect survival and event-free survival for at least 6 years.

▶ This is an excellent study of early and late results for the combined operation. Other groups have reported a mortality as high as 18% for the combined operation in those patients with acute ischemia undergoing emergency operation. In this study, only 47 of the 300 patients had mitral regurgitation of ischemic origin and it is not specified as to how many had emergency procedures. The 10-year survival of 31% and event-free survival of 21% demonstrates the poor prognosis of the combined lesion after surgery. Greater attention should be directed toward improving this dismal outlook both by improving the timing of surgery and by reducing the causes of late death, e.g., arrhythmias.—Hillel Laks, M.D.

The Starr-Edwards Valve
Albert Starr (Oregon Health Sciences Univ.)
J. Am. Coll. Cardiol. 6:899–903, October 1985   5–24

Current models of the Silastic ball valve, models 6120 mitral and 1200/1260 aortic, have been in use for nearly two decades. Data were obtained prospectively on 318 mitral model 6120 prostheses and on 603 aortic model 1260 prostheses placed from 1965 to 1984. Totals of patient-years of follow-up for mitral and aortic valves are 783 and 1,318, respectively, from 1965 to 1972, and 586 and 1,512 from 1973 to 1984.

Actuarial rates of thromboembolism compared favorably with those recently reported for other currently used prostheses. There have been seven valve thromboses, five in the mitral position. One mitral and one aortic thrombosis were fatal. The rates were 0.4% and 0.1% per patient-year, respectively. Rates of all valve failures were 1.9% per patient-year for mitral prostheses in the earlier period and 1.2% per patient-year in the later period. Respective rates for aortic prostheses were 1.5% and 1.1%.

Dramatically improved results are obtained today with the Silastic ball valve compared with those obtained in the late 1960s with the same valve models. The results obtained after 1973 compare favorably with those reported for other contemporary prostheses introduced in the early 1970s. The difference is especially marked for valve thromboembolism. Newer mitral tissue valves may prove to be more durable, but the Silastic ball valve is presently preferred for patients whose life expectancy exceeds 10 years.

▶ This unique report reviews the results of the Silastic ball valve, which has been in use for a longer period of time than any other valve. It clearly indicates that for patients with a projected survival of more than 10 years, the Silastic ball valve has advantages over the tissue valves used during the last 10–15 years. Newer generations of disk valves must still use this actual experience as a basis for comparison rather than projected survival. Unexpected valve failure may still occur in new valves, as demonstrated by the convexoconcave Björk-Shiley valve modification.—Hillel Laks, M.D.

The Monostrut Björk-Shiley Heart Valve
Viking O. Björk and Dan Lindblom (Karolinska Hosp., Stockholm)
J. Am. Coll. Cardiol. 6:1142–1148, November 1985   5–25

Since 1982, the Björk-Shiley valve prosthesis has been machined from a single piece of Haynes 25, a cobalt base alloy, in the form of a monostrut valve without welds to eliminate the risk of fracture of the welded two-armed outflow strut of the initial valve. Since 1982, 864 monostrut valves have been implanted, and 268 patients have been followed for 2–3 years. The flat disk has been changed to a convexoconcave disk to reduce the occurrence of thromboembolic complications. The average age at operation was 60 years.

Hospital mortality was 4%. Actuarial 2-year survivals, including operative mortality, were 93% for isolated aortic valve replacement and 91% for isolated mitral replacement. Bleeding complications occurred at a rate of 1.3% per patient-year. Thromboembolic complications occurred at rates of 0.6% per patient-year after aortic replacement and 2.6% per patient-year after mitral replacement in patients given anticoagulants. No valve thrombosis occurred. The proportion of patients in New York Heart Association functional classes III and IV decreased from 62% to 4% at 1 year after operation. Significant hemolysis did not occur.

The monostrut Björk-Shiley tilting-disk valve is more durable than the previous prosthesis was and is associated with a lower rate of thromboembolic complications. Hemodynamic performance is optimal at the 70-degree opening angle, and functional improvement was excellent after 2–3 years in this series.

▶ This latest modification of the Björk-Shiley valve appears to have solved the problem of valve durability and strut fracture while maintaining the advantages of the convexoconcave disk, which has excellent hemodynamics and is associated with only a low incidence of thromboembolism. Theoretically, this valve may have an advantage over the St. Jude valve in avoiding a the use of hinged pivot, which may be subject to eventual dysfunction because of continued wear at one point. For both valves, however, combined clinical experience is required to prove irrefutably their long-term durability.—Hillel Laks, M.D.

Valve Failure With the Ionescu-Shiley Bovine Pericardial Bioprosthesis: Analysis of 2,680 Patients
George J. Reul, Jr., Denton A. Cooley, J. Michael Duncan, O. H. Frazier, Grady L. Hallman, James J. Livesay, David A. Ott, and William E. Walker (Texas Heart Inst., Houston)
J. Vasc. Surg. 2:192–204, January 1985   5–26

The Ionescu-Shiley bovine pericardial bioprosthetic valve (BPV) was used in 2,680 patients between 1978 and 1983. They were followed for a mean of 22 months. The aortic valve was replaced in 1,427 patients, the mitral valve in 982, both in 258, and the tricuspid valve in 13. Associated procedures were performed in nearly half of the patients undergoing aortic valve replacement and in nearly one third of those undergoing mitral valve replacement. Almost 5,000 patient-years of follow-up study are available.

Actuarial 5-year survivals, including early mortality, were 77% in the aortic replacement group and 70% in the mitral group. For double-valve replacements, the actuarial 3-year survival was 70%. Thromboembolism was diagnosed or presumed in 88 patients, for a linearized rate of 1.87% emboli per patient-year, and occurred most often in the mitral and double-valve groups. Long-term anticoagulant therapy was not a significant factor. Valve failure necessitating reoperation occurred in 85 patients, most often in the aortic group. Distressing causes for valve failure were valve calcification (0.68% per patient-year) and leaflet disruption (0.23% per patient year). Endocarditis requiring reoperation was most frequent in the double-valve group. The most frequent cause of valve failure was calcification. Actuarial freedom from valve failure at 5 years was 86% in the aortic position, 91% in the mitral position, and 97% when both valves were replaced.

The Ionescu-Shiley BPV appears to be performing satisfactorily with regard to thromboembolism, perivalvular leakage, endocarditis, and hemodynamics. It should not be used in patients younger than age 30 years, or perhaps in those younger than age 50, because of accelerated calcification. The number of valves with leaflet disruption has increased and seems to be time related. At present, the BPV is limited to placement in elderly patients who have possible anticoagulation problems and patients with a small anulus.

▶ This valuable report of a large series of patients demonstrates the reduced longevity of this valve, particularly because of valve calcification and leaflet dehiscence; these events occur even in the age group older than 30 years and increase with the duration of follow-up observation. Leaflet dehiscence, thought to result from stress or abrasion at the base of the leaflet, may be prevented by modification of the valve design and structure. However, this valve does have excellent hemodynamics and should be considered particularly for older patients with a small anulus.—Hillel Laks, M.D.

Six Years of Experience With the St. Jude Medical Valvular Prosthesis
Kit V. Arom, Demetre M. Nicoloff, Thomas E. Kersten, William F. Northrup, III, and William G. Lindsay (Minneapolis Heart Inst. and United Hosps., St. Paul)
Circulation (Suppl. 2)72:II-153–II-158, September 1985   5–27

The results of valve replacement with the St. Jude prosthesis were reviewed in 680 patients operated on between 1977 and 1983. The group included 14 children. Two thirds of patients were in New York Heart Association (NYHA) functional class IV at the time of operation. Congestive heart failure accounted for 85% of the patients and occurred chiefly because of mechanical valve problems.

The operative mortality was 7% overall; it was 15.5% in patients who had mitral valve replacement combined with coronary bypass revascularization, but only 2% when aortic replacement was combined with bypass grafting. The mean follow-up period was 2 years. Late mortality was highest in mitral valve replacement patients having additional procedures and in patients having double valve replacement. No mechanical prosthetic failures occurred. All three valve thromboses were in double valve procedures. The incidence of thromboembolism was 0.7 per 100 patient-years in the aortic valve replacement group and 2.2 per 100 patient-years in the mitral valve replacement group. Three patients had bacterial endocarditis, and one of them died of sepsis. All five paravalvular leaks were in the mitral valve replacement group. Bleeding complications occurred in 42 patients, 30 of them in the aortic replacement group. The overall survival at 6 years was 86%. All but 4% of patients were in NYHA functional class I or class II at follow-up study.

The St. Jude valve appears to be the mechanical prosthesis of choice for use in disabled cardiac patients. All survivors in the present series improved functionally, and there have been no mechanical prosthetic failures.

▶ This report presents early and late results with the St. Jude valve. The mean follow-up period was 24 months, but it was as long as 60 months in some instances. These results are promising and the thromboembolism rate is very similar to that of the monostrut Björk-Shiley valve. The St. Jude valve is unique among tilting disk valves in having a hinged pivot. Because this concentrates the wear in one area, unlike in other disk valves, continued long-term follow-up study is essential to ensure that late pivot breakdown does not occur. Hemodynamically, this is an excellent valve, and because of its low profile it is well suited to the difficult anulus and to use in children.—Hillel Laks, M.D.

Surgery for Congenital Heart Disease

Repair of Anomalous Origin of the Left Coronary Artery in the Infant and Small Child

Frank M. Midgley, Donald C. Watson, Jr., Lewis P. Scott, III, Karen S. Kuehl, Lowell W. Perry, Frank M. Galioto, Jr., Roger N. Ruckman, and Stephen R. Shapiro (Children's Hosp. and Natl. Med. Ctr. and George Washington Univ.)
J. Am. Coll. Cardiol. 4:1231–1234, December 1985   5–28

An anomalous left coronary artery arising from the pulmonary artery is a rare defect that is associated with high mortality in infants; such conditions that are refractory to medical care require aggressive surgical treatment. Ten children were operated on between 1978 and 1983, five undergoing a new procedure described by Takeuchi et al. that is designed to direct aortic flow via an intrapulmonary baffle to the anomalous left coronary orifice. Surgery is performed with cardiopulmonary bypass, moderate systemic hypothermia, and cold potassium cardioplegia. A peninsula-like flap measuring 15 × 30 mm, created by incising the pulmonary artery, is sutured to an aortopulmonary window 6 mm in diameter to produce a tunnel directing blood flow to the coronary orifice. The defect in the pulmonary artery wall is repaired with a pericardial patch.

The median age of the five children was 12 months; three were younger than age 1 year, and two were younger than age 4 months. One early and one late death occurred. Two of the three survivors were well after 7–44 months, and one was lost to follow-up study. Postoperative catheterization in one child showed an intact repair.

This pulmonary artery neocoronary procedure is useful in infants and small children with anomalous origin of the left coronary artery from the pulmonary artery. The neocoronary vessel is made of viable pulmonary artery wall and can act as a high-pressure conduit without undergoing degenerative change. It is potentially capable of enlargement. No prosthetic materials are necessary. The left coronary artery is not manipulated, and its growth potential is preserved. The method is especially useful when reimplantation and subclavian artery procedures are not feasible.

▶ The authors obtained excellent early results using the technique described by Takeuchi et al. In the one child restudied, excellent repair was observed 10 months later. Long-term follow-up observation with cardiac catheterization is necessary to establish this procedure as the operation of choice for the anomalous left coronary artery arising from the pulmonary artery. This experience is certainly encouraging.—Hillel Laks, M.D.

Repair of Aortic Coarctation in Infants: Experience With an Intraluminal Shunt
D. Glenn Pennington, Hugh M. Dennis, Marc T. Swartz, Soraya Nouri, Suchiung Chen, Farrid Azzam, and John F. Schweiss (St. Louis Univ. and Cardinal Glennon Children's Hosp., St. Louis)
Ann. Thorac. Surg. 40:35–40, July 1985   5–29

Operative morbidity and mortality have declined in infants with coarctation. An intraluminal shunt has been used in those with poor collateral blood flow to provide added protection. Sixty-three infants aged 1 year or younger underwent repair of thoracic aortic coarctation between 1962 and 1984. Forty-seven were aged 3 months or younger at the time of operation. Nearly three fourths of the infants had associated cardiovascular anomalies other than patent ductus arteriosus, and these were often complex. Almost half of the infants had a ventricular septal defect. Emergency treatment for congestive failure was necessary in 34 children. Prostaglandin E_1 infusions were given to nine recent patients; also, subclavian aortoplasty

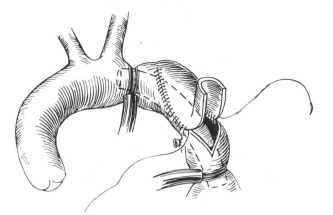

Fig 5–8.—Silastic intraluminal shunt in place with proximal end in transverse aorta. Occluding snares must be secured tightly enough to prevent bleeding without occluding shunt. (Courtesy of Pennington, D.G., et al.: Ann. Thorac. Surg. 40:35–40, July 1985.)

was used in the most recently treated patients. A Silastic intraluminal shunt (Fig 5–8) has been used in 15 patients since 1980.

Early mortality was 16%. None of 25 children operated on between 1981 and 1984 died postoperatively. Subclavian flap aortoplasty was associated with a lower mortality than resection and end-to-end anastomosis were. None of 15 infants who had subclavian aortoplasty with an intraluminal shunt died. One child operated on without a shunt is paraplegic. Four who had end-to-end anastomosis had an arm-leg pressure gradient of 20 mm Hg or higher at follow-up. No gradients were found in those who had the subclavian flap aortoplasty.

Even infants with complex associated defects can now safely undergo repair of coarctation of the aorta. Results have improved with the use of prostaglandin infusion, subclavian flap aortoplasty, and intraluminal shunting during operation. More precise anastomosis results in a lower incidence of recurrent coaractation.

▶ The technique of using an intraluminal shunt might prove useful in conjunction with the use of evoked potential monitoring of spinal cord function. Experimental evidence would suggest that if the evoked potential becomes abnormal, there is time to provide adequate spinal cord blood flow before irreversible changes occur. The intraluminal shunt might prove useful as a means of providing such flow.—Hillel Laks, M.D.

Long-Term Results of the "Palliative" Mustard Operation
Janardan P. Dhasmana, Jaroslav Stark, Marc de Leval, Fergus J. Macartney, Philip G. Rees, and James F. N. Taylor (The Hosp. for Sick Children, London)
J. Am. Coll. Cardiol. 6:1138–1141, November 1985   5–30

Forty-one children with pulmonary vascular disease and transposition or double-outlet right ventricle had the Mustard operation between 1973 and 1980. The mean age at operation was 9 years. One child underwent a palliative Senning procedure. Thirty-nine children had complete transposition of the great arteries, seven with an intact ventricular septum, and two had double-outlet right ventricle with a subpulmonary ventricular septal defect. Twenty-one had 34 previous operations. All of the children patients were severely cyanotic and had limited exercise tolerance, and all had evidence of moderate to severe pulmonary vascular disease. A pericardial baffle was used in 35 patients and a Dacron cloth baffle in 5.

There were three hospital deaths. Actuarial survival during a mean follow-up period of 77 months was 92%. Half of the survivors evaluated were in functional class I after operation. Only one child remained disabled. Systemic arterial oxygen saturation improved substantially after operation. Some increase in systemic vascular resistance was seen in the 21 recatheterized patients. The mean effective pulmonary blood flow increase to a highly significant degree.

Early hospital mortality after a palliative Mustard or Senning procedure is acceptable, and most long-term survivors have done well functionally. Early operation is best, before pulmonary vascular obstructive disease develops, but the palliative approach is a useful option if the patient's condition is not diagnosed or surgically treated before obstructive changes occur.

▶ This extensive follow-up study of patients undergoing a palliative Mustard procedure demonstrates the excellent long-term results that can be obtained with a relatively low operative risk. Interestingly, it was found that pulmonary vascular resistance did not fall after the procedure, although systemic resistance did.—Hillel Laks, M.D.

Congenital Aortic Stenosis With Hypoplasia of the Left Sinus of Valsalva: Anatomical Reconstruction of the Aortic Root
John L. Harlan, Edward B. Clark, and Donald B. Doty (Univ. of Iowa)
J. Thorac. Cardiovasc. Surg. 89:288–294, February 1985   5–31

Operative results were reviewed in 13 patients with congenital aortic stenosis who had asymmetry of the aortic root caused by a hypoplastic left sinus of Valsalva, associated with a supravalvular ridge above the left coronary ostium and dysplasia of the aortic valve. Folding and buckling of the left aortic cusp resulted. The aortic valve was bicuspid in all but two patients. The mean age was 8½ years. The average left ventricle-aorta systolic pressure gradient was 81 mm Hg. An oblique aortotomy was made in a spiral manner to the right and posteriorly into the left sinus of Valsalva, and in seven patients a second incision was made to the right of the posterior commissure into the noncoronary sinus. Slightly fused valve commissures were opened in 12 patients. The aortic root was reconstructed with a spiral Dacron patch and posterior commissure repositioning.

The mean follow-up period was 21 months. Twelve patients were asymptomatic on exertion after operation; one had occasional dyspnea. The average pressure gradients were 36 mm Hg at the end of operation and 28 mm Hg at follow-up catheterization 2 years after operation. Aortic root angiography showed a more symmetric appearance of the supravalvular area and left sinus of Valsalva in all cases. Only one patient had more than "trace" aortic incompetence.

Preoperative anticipation of this abnormality helps the surgeon correct the configuration and symmetry of the entire aortic root, rather than merely incise the valve commissures. Good functional results were obtained. Intrinsic valve abnormalities do not preclude satisfactory hemodynamic performance if symmetric reconstruction of the valve and aortic root structures is carried out.

▶ This innovative technique recognizes the significance of the supravalvular area as a component of aortic stenosis in certain patients and includes a spiral incision into the left coronary sinus with insertion of a patch to enlarge this area. The mean gradient was 28 mm Hg postoperatively, which is similar to results obtained in more routine aortic valvotomies. The great potential danger of this technique is obstruction of the orifice of the left main coronary artery. Whether exposure to this potential danger is justified in this subgroup of patients with aortic stenosis requires further clinical experience.—Hillel Laks, M.D.

Tetralogy of Fallot With Absent Pulmonary Valve: Early and Late Results of Surgical Treatment
B. C. McCaughan, Gordon K. Danielson, David J. Driscoll, and Dwight C. McGoon (Mayo Clinic and Found.)
J. Thorac. Cardiovasc. Surg. 00:200 207, February 1985   5–32

Thirty-five patients with tetralogy of Fallot and absent pulmonary valve underwent repair between 1957 and 1983. The 20 males and 15 females had a mean age of 8 years at operation. Twenty-one patients had minimal symptoms or none before operation; the other 14 were markedly symptomatic. The mean peak systolic right ventricle-pulmonary artery pressure gradients were 60 mm Hg in the minimally symptomatic group and 52 mm Hg in the markedly symptomatic patients. Right ventricular hypertrophy and pulmonary annular stenosis were present in all patients, and true pulmonary valve leaflets were absent. The ventricular septal defect was closed by direct suturing or with a patch, and the right ventricle-pulmonary artery pressure gradient was relieved. A tissue valve was used in nine patients. Five patients also had partial resection or plication, or both, of aneurysmal pulmonary arteries.

The mean peak systolic right ventricle-pulmonary artery gradient was reduced from 58 mm Hg to 23 mm Hg after operation. Operative mortalities were 5% in the minimally symptomatic group and 36% in the group with marked symptoms. One patient in the former group died later of complete heart block; all survivors were asymptomatic. Three of four late deaths in the markedly symptomatic group were related to cardiopulmonary insufficiency.

Minimally symptomatic patients with tetralogy and absent pulmonary valve should have elective repair in childhood. Markedly symptomatic neonates and infants should have intensive medical care, and if symptoms are refractory, should undergo corrective operation including patch closure of the ventricular septal defect, insertion of a valve or valved conduit in the right ventricular outflow tract, and partial resection or plication, or both, of the aneurysmal pulmonary arteries.

▶ The indications for insertion of a valve in the right ventricular outflow tract for this condition should also include consideration of pulmonary vascular resistance, presence of both pulmonary arteries, left ventricular function, right ventricular function, and tricuspid regurgitation. With the improved hemodynamics and longevity of pulmonary and aortic homografts, more extensive use of valves as part of the repair seems justified.—Hillel Laks, M.D.

Improved Right Ventricular Function After Intra-Atrial Repair of Transposition of the Great Arteries
Thomas P. Graham, Jr., Judith Burger, Harvey W. Bender, John W. Hammon, Robert J. Boucek, Jr., and Scott Appleton (Vanderbilt Univ.)
Circulation (Suppl.2)72:II-45–II-51, September 1985   5–33

The Senning operation was used for intra-atrial repair in 32 children with transposition of the great arteries who were operated on between 1978 and 1984 and followed up for 6–18 months. The results were compared with those in 26 patients having the Mustard operation between 1971 and 1978. None of the study patients was taking digitalis or diuretics at the time of postoperative catheterization, and all were clinically asymptomatic. All of the Senning operations and most of the Mustard operations were done under deep hypothermia and circulatory arrest.

The postoperative right ventricular ejection fraction was below normal in half of the Senning group, averaging 0.48. Those undergoing the Mustard procedure were older when operated on and had lower preoperative right ventricular ejection fractions. Systemic ventricular work-function curves during afterload stress showed a normal slope of systemic ventricular work vs. end-diastolic pressure in two of eight Senning patients. Both Mustard patients studied had abnormal findings.

Patients in both operative groups have done better in recent years, presumably because of a younger age at operation, better preoperative function, and, possibly, improved intraoperative myocardial protection. Early repair and minimal preoperative hypoxemia can be expected to optimize the outcome of intra-atrial repair of transposition of the great arteries.

▶ Long-term function of the right ventricle (RV) is a critical issue in choosing between the early arterial switch procedure and the delayed Senning operation.

This excellent study demonstrates that RV function in patients undergoing the Senning operation in the current era is better than previously described. This may be the result of earlier age at surgery, avoidance of prolonged hypoxia, and better myocardial protection. Further long-term follow-up studies are clearly needed to answer this important question.—Hillel Laks, M.D.

Decision Making in the Definitive Repair of the Heart With a Small Right Ventricle
M. de Leval, C. Bull, R. Hopkins, P. Rees, J. Deanfield, J. F. N. Taylor, W. Gersony, J. Stark, and F. J. Macartney (The Hosp. for Sick Children, London)
Circulation (Suppl.2)72:II-52–II-59, September 1985   5–34

The presence of right ventricular cavitary hypoplasia in conjunction with other congenital cardiac defects raises the question of how small a diminutive ventricle can be usefully and safely incorporated into a repair. The results of definitive repair were reviewed in 51 consecutive patients with pulmonary atresia and intact ventricular septum and, in 14 patients with virtual pulmonary atresia who were operated on between 1971 and 1984. Twenty-nine patients had complete repair with relief of right ventricular outflow tract obstruction and closure of intracardiac and extracardiac shunts. Eleven patients were palliated; 11 had complete separation of the systemic and pulmonary circulations by the Fontan operation.

Mortality was 34% in the patients having complete repair. All but 3 of 19 with an adequate tricuspid valve diameter survived. Eight of ten patients with a tricuspid valve diameter of less than the lower 99% confidence limit of the normal mean died. All patients who had a palliative operation had valves of small diameter. All ten survivors have had some systemic arterial desaturation and exercise intolerance. Seven patients survived the Fontan operation. Two of three with a two-portion right ventricle that was incorporated in the repair died.

A tripartite right ventricle with a tricuspid valve diameter above the lower 99% confidence limit of the normal mean can safely be incorporated in a complete repair of pulmonary atresia. Neonates without a trabecular portion should not have definitive repair, but relief of outflow tract obstruction and closure of shunts may be possible later. If distorted pulmonary arteries are present after palliation, or there is significant left ventricular dysfunction contraindicating the Fontan operation, an atrial communication and an extracardiac shunt should be left in place.

▶ This is an important paper describing the options available for definitive repair of pulmonary atresia with an intact ventricular septum. This is the first paper that we are aware of that has made an effort to define the acceptable degree of tricuspid valve and right ventricular (RV) hypoplasia that will allow a complete repair with closure of the atrial septal defect and relief of the RV outflow tract obstruction. The figure in the article showing the mean normal valve size and the lower 99% confidence limits for the tricuspid valve is a valuable aid and should probably be kept in the operating room as a ready reference.—Hillel Laks, M.D.

Surgical Repair of Ebstein's Anomaly: Selection of Patients and Early and Late Operative Results

Douglas D. Mair, James B. Seward, David J. Driscoll, and Gordon K. Danielson (Mayo Clinic and Found.)

Circulation (Suppl. 2) 72:II-70–II-76, September 1985   5–35

Seventy-two patients with Ebstein's malformation underwent repair between 1972 and 1984 because of progressive symptoms to New York Heart Association (NYHA) class III or beyond, increasing cyanosis, paradoxic emboli, or tachyarrhythmia from an accessory conduction path. Twenty-seven patients were aged 20 or older at the time of operation. Fifty-eight underwent plication and annuloplasty. Eleven had plication and insertion of a prosthesis, usually a Hancock porcine valve, and three patients with a previous Glenn shunt had plication and a Fontan operation.

All nine patients with a free wall accessory conduction pathway had it mapped and interrupted without complete heart block resulting. The hospital mortality was 7%, and there were three late deaths. Of the survivors, 87% were in NYHA functional class I or class II after a mean follow-up period of about 5 years. Five women had uneventful pregnancies. Exercise studies in recently treated patients indicate substantial improvement in exercise performance and in maximal oxygen consumption postoperatively.

Surgery for Ebstein's malformation presently is recommended when NYHA class III symptoms are present. Elective operation can be performed in less symptomatic patients if the cardiothoracic ratio reaches 0.65 or significant cyanosis and polycythemia develop as a result of right-to-left shunting through an atrial septal defect. The operation should include reconstruction of the tricuspid valve in addition to closure of the atrial septal defect.

▶ This is probably the largest reported series on repair of Ebstein's anomaly, with excellent results. The technique of tricuspid valve reconstruction for this lesion is well described. In view of its success, we agree with the authors' conclusion that this procedure should be undertaken earlier in the course of these patients, before massive cardiomegaly develops, even in the relatively asymptomatic patient. More routine mapping and the division of aberrant tracts might reduce further the incidence of postoperative arrhythmias and sudden death.—Hillel Laks, M.D.

Right Heart Assist by Intermittent Abdominal Compression After Surgery for Congenital Heart Disease

Robert A. Guyton, Susan C. Davis, Richard E. Michalik, Willis H. Williams, and Charles R. Hatcher, Jr. (Henrietta Egleston Hosp. for Children, Atlanta, and Emory Univ.)

Circulation (Suppl. 2) 72:II-97–II-100, September 1985   5–36

Right heart failure may be a serious problem after various congenital cardiac procedures such as the Fontan operation. Abdominal compression has been performed using a ventilator reservoir bag connected to a volume ventilator and placed on the child's abdomen. Fourteen children were so treated between 1981 and 1983. Pressures of 40–50 cm of water are produced within the bag at a rate of 10–20 inflations per minute. Right atrial pressures generally are elevated by 3–5 mm Hg when compression begins. Five patients had the Fontan operation, and four had repair of an atrioventricular canal defect.

Intermittent abdominal compression was part of unsuccessful resuscitation in three instances. In other cases the right atrial pressure was increased by 4 mm Hg on average, with a rise in mean arterial pressure of 10 mm Hg. Urine output improved in nearly all children. Compression was used for an average of 16 hours. The net fluid balance in the first 12 hours of compression in 11 children was negative 154 ml. The effects of abdominal compression were especially evident after the Fontan operation.

Right heart failure after surgery for congenital heart disease can produce massive volume overload, ascites, and pleural effusion. Intermittent abdominal compression has greatly reduced the need for volume infusion and can produce a negative fluid balance. Intermittent abdominal compression is especially useful after the Fontan operation, wherein the highest right atrial pressures are present after operation. Hematuria may occur transiently during the procedure; hemoglobinuria has not been noted.

▶ The authors describe the use of intermittent abdominal compression in the treatment of right heart failure after the Fontan procedure and other operations. Their use of a ventilator reservoir bag is innovative but may not have advantages over a simple blood pressure cuff placed around the abdomen and inflated with an intermittent inflation pump. The authors describe the management of these patients and use of the device in excellent detail. An additional caution is to avoid weaning the patient from the ventilator while on the venous assist device.—Hillel Laks, M.D.

Heart and Heart-Lung Transplantation

Infectious Complications in Heart-Lung Transplant Recipients

Robert G. Brooks, Jesse M. Hofflin, Stuart W. Jamieson, Edward B. Stinson, and Jack S. Remington (Palo Alto Med. Found. and Stanford Univ.)
Am. J. Med. 79:412–422, October 1985   5–37

Infectious complications were reviewed in 14 patients having heart-lung transplantation between 1981 and 1983 who survived for more than 3 days after operation. The 10 male and 4 female patients had a mean age of 33 years. Seven patients had ventricular septal defect with Eisenmenger's syndrome, six had primary pulmonary hypertension, and one had transposition of the great vessels. The mean follow-up period was 1 year. Cefamandole was given perioperatively for at least 2 days. Immunosuppression was with orally administered cyclosporine, methylprednisolone intravenously, rabbit antithymocyte globulin, and azathioprine orally.

A total of 29 infections occurred in 12 patients. Eighteen infections in 10 patients were bacterial, and 17 involved the lower respiratory tract. Four episodes of pneumonia were confirmed microbiologically. Nine donor tracheas were culture-positive. Nine viral infections occurred in seven patients. Six patients had cytomegalovirus infection, and three had herpes simplex virus infection. Two patients were found to have invasive candidiasis at autopsy. The patients with pneumonia generally responded to empirical broad-spectrum antibiotic therapy. Cytomegalovirus and *Candida albicans* contributed to one death, and herpes simplex virus to another. Thus, of 14 patients undergoing heart-lung transplantation, 12 contracted infections that contributed to death in 2 of the 3 patients who died.

Pulmonary infection is a prominent cause of morbidity in heart-lung transplant recipients. Most of the present patients had bacterial pulmonary infections, half of which occurred in the first 2 weeks. Treatment usually included antibiotics effective against anaerobic and gram-negative and gram-positive aerobic bacteria. None of the patients died of bacterial infection. Infectious complications, while prominent, are not a barrier to prolonged survival after heart-lung transplantation.

▶ This is a valuable experience with carefully studied patients undergoing heart-lung transplantation. Despite the high incidence of pneumonia (71%), most infections, particularly bacterial, responded to broad-spectrum antibiotic therapy. The authors discuss the difficulties of making a specific diagnosis in these patients and compare the infections with those seen in persons receiving heart transplants. This is an important report for those involved with heart-lung transplantation.—Hillel Laks, M.D.

Targeted Blood Levels of Cyclosporine for Cardiac Transplantation
Bartley P. Griffith, Robert L. Hardesty, Alfredo Trento, Ann Lee, and Henry R. Bahnson (Univ. of Pittsburgh)
J. Thorac. Cardiovasc. Surg. 88:952–957, December 1984   5–38

Since 1982, 57 cardiac transplant recipients have received cyclosporine as well as low maintenance doses of prednisone and rabbit antithymocyte globulin for immunosuppression. Cyclosporine was given in an initial dose of 10–17.5 mg/kg and subsequently in a dose of 5 mg/kg every 12 hours. The dose was adjusted three to five times weekly by targeting it to a whole-blood level of 1,000 ng/ml, determined by radioimmunoassay. A level as high as 1,500 ng/ml was accepted in case of rejection unless there was renal or hepatic toxicity.

An average cyclosporine dose of 8 mg/kg daily resulted in a blood level of 1,089 ng/ml in the first 6 postoperative weeks. Lower doses were required at 6 months. Forty-nine patients given targeted treatment had 12-month and 21-month cumulative survival rates of 79% and 71%, respectively. Three deaths were related to rejection. Neither nephrotoxicity nor hepatic toxicity was related to whole-blood cyclosporine levels, but patients were not repeatedly exposed to excessively high blood levels. Hepatic toxicity declined over time as the serum bilirubin level decreased.

Cyclosporine dosage is not related to whole-blood drug levels, and monitoring is necessary to ensure that a significant level of circulating drug is present. Renal and hepatic toxicity have occurred at all blood cyclosporine levels and are not interdependent. However, monitoring is necessary to determine whether acute perioperative renal failure is the result of cyclosporine toxicity.

▶ Despite the acknowledged effectiveness of cyclosporine, it is apparent that much remains to be learned about the optimal dosage for the individual patient. It remains to be seen whether there is an effective blood level for the individual patient that will provide adequate immunosuppression and also avoid the early and late side effects, most importantly, its nephrotoxicity and hypertension. The authors also allude to the worrisome problem of accelerated graft atherosclerosis that continues to occur even as early as 1–2 years post transplant despite what appears to be effective immunosuppression with cyclosporine.— Hillel Laks, M.D.

Long-Term Prolongation of Cardiac Allografts by Subtherapeutic Levels of Cyclosporine in Rats Conditioned With Pretransplant Blood Transfusions and Cyclosporine
G. P. Martinelli, R. Chung-Loy, L. Sher, D. Racelis, C. M. Miller, and H. Schanzer (Mt. Sinai Med. Ctr., New York)
Transplantation 39:1–5, January 1985   5–39

Cyclosporine (CsA) is becoming the mainstay of clinical immunosuppression, but the nephrotoxicity associated with this drug is a significant problem. An attempt was made to determine whether long-term cardiac graft survival is possible with short-term CsA therapy, or with the use of subtherapeutic doses, in rats conditioned with blood transfusions. Previous studies indicated that donor-specific transfusions interact with a short course of CsA, resulting in considerable prolongation of ACI and BUF rat grafts in LEW hosts.

Donor-specific depression of alloreactivity was confirmed by a depression in mixed lymphocyte reaction and in humoral antidonor responses in animals conditioned with blood transfusions and CsA. No effect of transfusions was apparent in animals prepared with CsA in a dose of 20 mg/kg daily for 5 days, but transfusions were helpful in hosts prepared with 10 mg/kg of CsA daily. Administration of 2.5 mg/kg of CsA daily for 30 days led to long-term prolongation of grafts in a large proportion of host animals, whereas in most control animals conditioned with CsA alone, or with CsA and nonspecific transfusions, graft rejection occurred within 3 weeks.

The successful results obtained with donor-specific transfusions and concomitant azathioprine therapy suggest that treatment with specific transfusions and CsA may be clinically applicable. Cyclosporine has a more discriminant immunosuppressive effect than azathioprine has and may allow the development of an immunosuppressive state leading to operational donor-specific tolerance.

▶ This interesting study explores the possibility of pretreatment of cardiac transplant recipients with donor-specific transfusions combined with low doses of cyclosporine. This combination inhibited cellular reactivity, as evidenced by depression of mixed lymphocyte reactivity and prolongation of graft survival, and also inhibited the hormonal response. Post transplant it was found that smaller doses of cyclosporine could be used effectively. The authors postulate that pretransplant donor-specific blood transfusion results in recruitment of donor-specific immune cells that can then be acted upon by the concomitantly administered cyclosporine. Although the logistics of clinical pretreatment of cardiac recipients are daunting, a further understanding of this phenomenon is clearly important.—Hillel Laks, M.D.

A Prospective Randomized Trial of Pretransfusion/Azathioprine/Prednisone Versus Cyclosporine/Prednisone Immunosuppression in Cardiac Transplant Recipients: Preliminary Results
Glenn R. Barnhart, Andrea Hastillo, Mitchell H. Goldman, Szabolcs Szentpetery, Timothy C. Wolfgang, Thalachallour Mohanakumar, Marc R. Katz, Sheelah Rider, Josephine Hanrahan, Richard R. Lower, and Michael L. Hess (Med. College of Virginia and McGuire VA Med. Ctr., Richmond)
Circulation 72 (Suppl. 2):II-227–II-230, September 1985   5–40

Twenty-five patients who underwent cardiac transplants in 1983 and 1984 were randomly assigned to receive immunosuppression either with azathioprine, antithymocyte globulin, prednisone, and pretransplant transfusion (PAAP) or with cyclosporine and prednisone (CyA). The 11 in the PAAP group had a mean age of 41 years and those given CyA had a mean age of 38 years. Pretransplant transfusion consisted of five to ten 50-ml units of random donor red blood cells or buffy coat. Cyclosporine was given orally to produce serum levels of 200–400 ng/ml in the immediate postoperative period; maintenance doses were reduced to achieve serum levels of 200 ng/ml.

No difference in early mortality was apparent, but serious infections were more frequent in the PAAP group. Acute cell-mediated allograft rejection was similar in the two treatment groups. More CyA-treated patients required antihypertensive therapy; pericardial effusion also was more frequent in this group, as was renal dysfunction. Two patients in the CyA group required dialysis, and four CyA-treated patients had seizures.

Cyclosporine therapy appears to reduce the risk of serious infection and the severity of rejection in cardiac allograft recipients, but some degree of renal functional impairment can be expected. Hypertension also is a problem with cyclosporine immunosuppression. It is not clear whether survival will be prolonged, but the adverse effects of cyclosporine may lessen the earlier benefits described with the use of this agent.

▶ This is a valuable preliminary report comparing the currently popular cyclosporine therapy with previously standard immunotherapy in a randomized fashion. The numbers are too small to show a difference in 1-year survival. The conclusions, which are similar to those reported in nonrandomized studies, still favor the use of cyclosporine despite its side effects, at least for the first year post transplant.—Hillel Laks, M.D.

Surgery for Arrhythmia

Experience With 118 Consecutive Patients Undergoing Operation for the Wolff-Parkinson-White Syndrome
James L. Cox, John J. Gallagher, and Michael E. Cain (Washington Univ.)
J. Thorac. Cardiovasc. Surg. 90:490–501, October 1985   5–41

Surgery was performed to correct the Wolff-Parkinson-White (WPW) syndrome in 118 patients between 1980 and 1985. The mean age was 28 years. Medical refractoriness or drug intolerance had led to surgical treatment in 60% of the patients and previous cardiac arrest in 14%. Other arrhythmias were present in one third of the patients. Two patients previously were operated on elsewhere for WPW syndrome.

One fifth of the patients had 2–4 accessory pathways, and 149 pathways

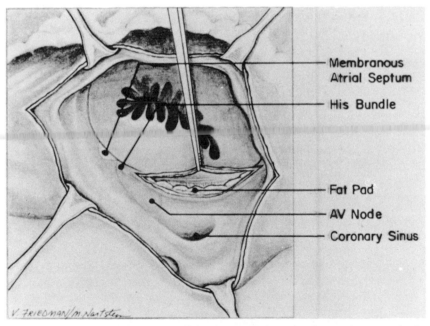

Fig 5–9.—Initial dissection for division of posterior septal accessory pathways. The patient's head is to the left. A standard right atriotomy is performed and the His bundle is identified with a hand-held electrode in its position immediately posterior to the membranous portion of the atrial septum. A supraannular incision is placed posterior to the His bundle and 2 mm above the tricuspid valve anulus to expose the fat pad overlying the posterior ventricular septum. (Courtesy of Cox, J.L., et al.: J. Thorac. Cardiovasc. Surg. 90:490–501, October 1985.)

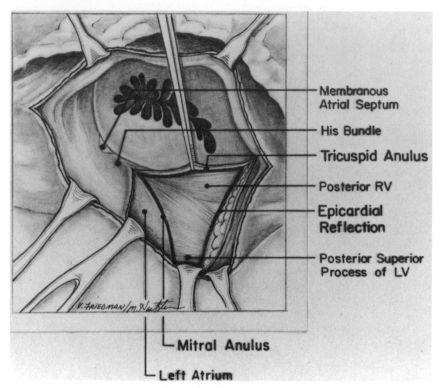

— Membranous
Atrial Septum

— His Bundle

— Tricuspid Anulus

— Posterior RV

Epicardial
Reflection

— Posterior Superior
Process of LV

└─ Mitral Anulus

└─ Left Atrium

Fig 5–10.—Completed dissection of the posterior septal space that is bounded by the tricuspid valve anulus, the mitral valve anulus, and the epicardial reflection. The mitral valve anulus and epicardial reflection are dissected to the left to expose the posterior superior process of the left ventricle (LV), which represents the beginning of the left posterior free wall. (Courtesy of Cox, J.L., et al.: J. Thorac. Cardiovasc. Surg. 90:490–501, October 1985.)

were present overall. Nearly 60% of accessory pathways were in the left free wall, and 25% were in the posterior septal region. Of the 149 accessory pathways, 148 were successfully divided. There have been no failures since the routine adoption of 2.5 × optical magnification, exclusive use of the endocardial approach under cardioplegic arrest, and the use of wider margins of surgical dissection. In addition, the valve anulus is sharply dissected, and only the ventricular insertion of the accessory pathway is divided. See Figures 5–9 and 5–10. Postcardiotomy syndrome developed in 7% of the patients. There have been no late recurrences of WPW syndrome.

Surgery is an effective approach to management of the WPW syndrome. Virtually all accessory paths now are divided at the initial attempt. Mortality is less than 1% for patients having elective operations who do not have associated anomalies. Surgery is viewed as a conservative alternative to lifetime medical treatment in young, otherwise healthy patients.

▶ This is a superb report of patients undergoing surgery for division of accessory pathways. These excellent results indicate that it can be performed safely and successfully. The procedure should not be reserved only for the failure of medical therapy; rather, it should be the preferred treatment for younger patients otherwise dependent on permanent drug treatment. The technical aspects are well described and should be studied by those undertaking this type of surgery.—Hillel Laks, M.D.

Cryosurgical Ablation of Left Parietal Wall Accessory Atrioventricular Connections Through the Coronary Sinus Without the Use of Extracorporeal Circulation
Jurgis Bredikis and Audrius Bredikis (Kaunas Med. Inst., Kaunas, Lithuania)
J. Thorac. Cardiovasc. Surg. 90:199–205, August 1985   5–42

A method was developed for cryodestruction of left parietal accessory atrioventricular connections (AAVC) of the Kent bundle type at the level of the atrioventricular fibrous ring. The accessory bundles are ablated by local cryothermia using a special cryoinstrument that is introduced into the coronary sinus through the right atrial wall. The procedure can be performed via a right or bilateral thoracotomy, but a median sternotomy is recommended. The probe in the coronary sinus is pressed against the left fibrous ring with its tip at the point indicated by the intraoperative mapping.

Signs of preexcitations and paroxysms of tachycardia resolved in all but 2 of the 21 patients having cryodestruction of AAVC without cardiotomy or cardiopulmonary bypass. Two patients required coronary sinus ligation. In the other patients patency of the coronary sinus was preserved, and there were no surgical complications. Cryoablation was performed more than once in 15 patients. No coronary angiographic changes were detected up to 6 months after the procedure. Electrophysiologic data confirmed the absence of AAVC function in 12 serially studied patients.

Cryoablation via the coronary sinus is a safe and comparatively simple means of destroying left parietal AAVC of the Kent bundle type. Mapping can be performed before and after the procedure, and cardiopulmonary bypass is not required.

▶ The authors describe a method of ablating accessory pathways using a cryoprobe introduced via the coronary sinus. It has the advantage of not requiring cardiopulmonary bypass, but it does require a median sternotomy and can result in perforation of the coronary sinus. This method appears to be an advance over the technique of cryoablation reported by Guiraudon and associates (*Ann. Thorac. Surg.* 37:67–71, 1984), which involves dissection of the perivascular fat in the atrioventricular groove. This has the disadvantage of usually requiring cardiopulmonary bypass. Most interesting in this report was the demonstration in six patients that cryoablation via the coronary sinus did not cause occlusion of adjacent coronary arteries or of the coronary sinus within 3–6 months after surgery. This technique seems to hold promise for left free wall tracts, particularly in patients in whom cardiopulmonary bypass is best avoided.—Hillel Laks, M.D.

Myomectomy and Endocardial Resection

Resection of the Interventricular Septum for Hypertrophic Obstructive Cardiomyopathy: Long-Term Results in 33 Patients

E. von der Lohe, C. Müller-Haake, C. Minale, R. von Essen, S. Effert, and B. J. Messmer (Rhine-Westphalia Technical Univ., Aachen, Germany)
Dtsch. Med. Wochenschr. 109:1749–1753, Nov. 16, 1984   5–43

Interventricular septal resection by the Morrow approach was undertaken in 33 patients with hypertrophic obstructive cardiomyopathy. The 24 males and 9 females had an average age of 48 years. Twenty-seven patients had typical hypertrophic cardiomyopathy, five had fibromuscular subaortic stenosis, and one patient had aortic valve stenosis with marked subvalvular hypertrophy. The most frequent indications for surgery were a high resting pressure gradient and severe symptoms despite chronic, high-dose drug treatment.

There was one postoperative death. Twenty patients had repeat cardiac catheterization within 1–16 months after operation. The mean resting pressure gradient fell significantly from 67 mm Hg to 7 mm Hg. Of the 25 patients reexamined within an average of 30 months after operation, 18 exhibited definite symptomatic improvement. Five others had partial improvement, and two reported no change in symptoms.

The low postoperative mortality of 3% makes resection of the interventricular septum the preferred treatment for symptomatic patients with hypertrophic cardiomyopathy. All patients in the present series who presented with syncope were free of it after surgical treatment.

▶ This excellent clinical experience with myomectomy for hypertrophic obstructive cardiomyopathy again demonstrates that, in experienced hands, the procedure can be performed with a low early mortality. Previous reports have shown that the yearly mortality of survivors of myomectomy is lower than that reported for nonsurgically treated patients. Results such as these support the continued use of myomectomy in patients with significant gradients not responsive to medical therapy.—Hillel Laks, M.D.

The Surgical Treatment of Endomyocardial Fibrosis: Results in 55 Patients

Dominique Metras, André O. Coulibaly, and Kouamé Ouattara (Abidjan, Ivory Coast)
Circulation (Suppl. 2) 72:II-274–II-279, September 1985   5–44

The surgical management of endomyocardial fibrosis (EMF) was reviewed in a series of 55 patients operated on between 1978 and 1983. Thirty-one male and 24 female patients had a mean age of 13 years. All were functionally disabled at the time of operation, and about half the patients were in poor general health. Most patients had both right and left ventricular involvement. A transatrial approach was used for valve replacement, valvuloplasty, and endocardiectomy as required. As little myocardial tissue as possible was removed, and tissue near the conduction pathways was preserved. Eight patients, seven with predominant left ventricular EMF, had conservative valve operations. Two patients had pericardiectomy for chronic effusion and calcified pericarditis.

The operative mortality was 16%; low cardiac output was the most common cause. The mean follow-up observation of surviving patients was 32 months. All patients were symptomatically improved, but more than half continue to take cardiac medications. Nearly all late survivors of left ventricular EMF surgery had normal physical findings. Postoperative angiograms showed nearly normal contours in the left ventricle and improved right ventricular contours. Four of six late deaths were valve related. There was no gross autopsy evidence of recurrent EMF in any instance.

This surgical procedure can be recommended in nearly all patients with EMF because of the favorable long-term results obtained. Surgery is best performed before there is irreversible liver or heart damage. Conservative valve surgery is worth an attempt, despite technical difficulties. The question of recurrent fibrosis remains open, but no definite evidence of recurrent EMF was obtained in the present series.

▶ This is an extensive experience with a lesion rarely seen in the United States. In the advanced stage some of these patients may be candidates for transplantation. The long-term results of survivors is impressive, and the early results might be improved with earlier surgery.—Hillel Laks, M.D.

Cardiac Assist Devices

Long-Term Follow-Up of Postcardiotomy Patients With Profound Cardiogenic Shock Treated With Ventricular Assist Devices

D. Glenn Pennington, William F. Bernhard, Leonard R. Golding, Robert L. Berger, Shukri F. Khuri, and John T. Watson (St. Louis Univ.; Boston Children's Hosp. Med. Ctr.; Boston Univ.; West Roxburg VA Hosp., Boston, and the Cleveland Clinic)
Circulation (Suppl. 2) 72:II-216–II-225, September 1985   5–45

In a small number of patients, postoperative cardiogenic shock is refractory to drugs and balloon pump support; these patients require more complete circulatory support to survive. The sequelae of ventricular assist were examined in 15 surviving patients at four centers who were followed up for a mean of 35 months after discharge. The patients, whose mean age was 53 years, were treated for postcardiotomy shock that in four instances was related to perioperative infarction. A Medtronic centrifugal pump ventricular assist device was used in five patients, a Pierce-Donachy pulsatile sac-type device in seven, and a paracorporeal axisymmetric device with xenograft valves in three. Thirteen patients had the device inserted so that they could be weaned from cardiopulmonary bypass.

The mean peak device flow was 2.4 L/minute/sq m, and the mean perfusion time was 94 hours. Bleeding was frequent. Three patients with normal ventricular function before operation remained normal; five others improved, five were unchanged, and two became worse. One patient died 6 months after operation of cardiomyopathy. Another patient was moderately disabled at follow-up examination. Thirteen patients were in New York Heart Association functional classes I and II after operation.

A survivor of postcardiotomy ventricular failure who is treated with a ventricular assist device has an excellent chance of returning to an active life; some of these patients may have normal ventricular function. Continued efforts to develop more effective and safer temporary ventricular assist devices are warranted.

▶ This is an important study of the potential for recovery after the use of a ventricular assist device in management of postoperative cardiogenic shock. Surprisingly, there is generally excellent cardiac and functional recovery in the long-term survivors. These findings are similar to those described in a group of patients who required intra-aortic balloon counterpulsation for weaning from cardiopulmonary bypass in whom it was found that the mean ejection fraction was similar preoperatively and postoperatively. This report therefore confirms that, in some patients, much of the perioperative injury resulting in cardiogenic shock is reversible. Otherwise viable patients undergoing cardiac surgery who sustain cardiogenic shock deserve the effort that the use of cardiac assist devices requires to achieve survival.—Hillel Laks, M.D.

The Pennsylvania State University Paracorporeal Ventricular Assist Pump: Optimal Methods of Use
Wayne E. Gaines, William S. Pierce, James H. Donachy, Gerson Rosenberg, Donald L. Landis, Wayne E. Richenbacher, and John A. Waldhausen (Pennsylvania State Univ. and Univ. of Maryland)
World J. Surg. 9:47–53, February 1985   5–46

A paracorporeal short-term ventricular assist device (VAD) has been used clinically since 1976 to wean patients from cardiopulmonary bypass when conventional methods are ineffective. The device uses a paracorporeally placed pneumatic pump of a polyurethane blood sac enclosed within a polysulfone case. Patients who cannot be weaned from cardiopulmonary bypass by conventional means, with a cardiac index of less than 1.8 L/minute/sq m and a systolic aortic pressure of less than 90 mm Hg, are candidates for a left VAD. Right ventricular failure often is present but not immediately apparent. Patients with significant complicating illness have not been treated with the VAD.

Since 1980, patients have received VAD support after cardiac surgery. Eleven patients had left VAD placement, eight were weaned, and six were discharged from the hospital. One patient was weaned from an isolated right VAD and discharged. None of four patients was weaned from biventricular VAD support. Five survivors are in New York Heart Association functional class I or class II. Two discharged patients died of unrelated or unknown causes.

Half of the deaths in this series appear to have been related to inadequate myocardial recovery. Thus, paracorporeal VAD can result in survival in selected patients. The condition of the patient at the time of VAD insertion, the time spent on cardiopulmonary bypass, and right ventricular function all should be taken into account, as should the extent of left ventricular necrosis. The factors that influenced survival included the patient's condition at the time of VAD insertion, the duration of cardiopulmonary bypass, right ventricular function and its ability to provide forward flow to the left heart, and the extent of permanent left ventricular necrosis. In more than 40% of the patients, permanent left ventricular necrosis resulted in dependency on the VAD.

▶ The VAD described in this large experience was effective in supporting the circulation and allowing ventricular recovery. A major advantage is the avoidance of heparinization. The device requires positioning outside the chest, with tunnels required for the large atrial and aortic cannulas. This is a potential disadvantage for patients whose ventricular function does not recover and who might require cardiac transplantation, increasing their chance for infection. In view of the cost of the equipment and the need for special training in its use, one might question whether similar results can be achieved with the use of the centrifugal pump combined with intra-aortic balloon counterpulsation.—Hillel Laks, M.D.

Use of a Centrifugal Pump Without Anticoagulants for Postoperative Left Ventricular Assist
George J. Magovern, Sang B. Park, and Thomas D. Maher (Allegheny Gen. Hosp., Pittsburgh)
World J. Surg. 9:25–36, February 1985   5–47

The Bic-Medicus Bio-Pump was designed for use as a left heart assist device without the need for heparinization. The vortex pump was evaluated in dogs and lambs for up to 3 weeks without anticoagulation. Dogs consistently survived 24-hour left ventricular assist by left ventricle-to-femoral artery bypass at flow rates of 1.8–3.2 L/minute. No adverse sequelae developed, wounds did not bleed excessively, and no thromboembolism occurred. Ovine studies over the longer term showed minimal thromboembolism. A graft was sutured to the descending thoracic aorta for arterial return in this model. Serum hemoglobin levels remained low.

The Bio-Pump was used in 21 patients who required prolonged left heart assist after cardiopulmonary bypass. Decompression was via a cannula placed through the right pulmonary vein into the left ventricle, and arterial return was via a Sarnsaortic arch cannula. The sternum remained open, but the skin was approximated. The activated clotting time was kept at 140, but anticoagulation was not routinely used. There were five long-term survivors, and four patients are still alive after 21–42 months. Five other patients were weaned from the pump but died in the hospital. The longest assist was 144 hours.

The Bio-Pump is especially useful in young patients with intractable arrhythmia and reversible damage after cardiac surgery. Essentially, mean nonpulsatile flow appeared to preserve renal, hepatic, and cerebral function for a period of days. Prolonged perfusion is possible without heparinization. Minimal doses of heparin are used as needed to maintain the activated clotting time at 140 seconds.

▶ This is an extensive experience with use of the centrifugal pump as a left ventricular assist device with minimal or no heparinization. Five of the 21 patients were long-term survivors and an additional five were weaned from the device but subsequently expired in the hospital. Many of the deaths were related to the development of right ventricular failure. Consideration should be given to more frequent use of biventricular assistance with two centrifugal pumps, as was used in one of the patients. There has been little experience with more prolonged use of this device and as a bridge to transplantation. Its ready availability and cost, however, make it an attractive alternative to the pneumatic sac type pumps. It is not clear whether cannulation of the left ventricle across the mitral valve, as used by the authors, is necessary in all cases as it makes weaning from the assist device difficult to assess.—Hillel Laks, M.D.

Myocardial Protection

The Role of Cardioplegic Solution Buffering in Myocardial Protection: A Biochemical and Histopathological Assessment
Pedro J. del Nido, Gregory J. Wilson, Donald A. G. Mickle, Bradley G. Bush, Ivan M. Rebeyka, Peter Klement, Reginald Harding, and Gordon A. Tait (Toronto Gen. Hosp., The Hosp. for Sick Children, and Univ. of Toronto)
J. Thorac. Cardiovasc. Surg. 89:689–699, May 1985   5–48

Preservation of high-energy phosphate in the myocardium is particularly important in the presence of coronary artery disease or valvular heart disease, when prearrest levels may be low. Myocardial protection by administration of two crystalloid cardioplegic solutions of low sodium content (27 mEq/L) was compared. The solutions, buffered with histidine to values observed in blood, had a potassium content of 10 mEq/L or 30 mEq/L. Unbuffered preparations of Roe's solution also were evaluated in a canine model of multidose cardioplegic arrest. A 4½-hour period of arrest was followed by 1 hour of reperfusion.

Use of unbuffered solution led to a fall in the myocardial adenosine triphosphate (ATP) concentration from 29 mM/kg to 8 mM/kg during arrest. The ATP levels remained at baseline in both buffered groups, and the myocardial glycogen concentration followed a similar pattern. Lactate production was much elevated in all groups during arrest. Intraventricular isovolumic developed pressure measurements showed better postarrest function in the buffered low-potassium group than in the other groups. Triphenyl tetrazolium staining and electron microscopy showed minimal myocardial necrosis in the buffered low-potassium group. Necrosis was most marked in the buffered high-potassium group, in which a third of the biventricular mass was irreversibly damaged.

Buffering capacity similar to that of blood can enhance preservation of myocardial ATP stores when crystalloid cardioplegia is used. Postarrest contractile function is improved, and reperfusion myocardial necrosis is minimized. The best results have been obtained using a low-potassium buffered solution.

► This interesting paper studies the interrelationship between buffering capacity and the potassium concentration in crystalloid cardioplegic solutions. The authors conclude that the lower amount of potassium (10 mEq/L) combined with the naturally occurring buffer histidine gives optimal protection, whereas the alkaline (pH 7.8) nonbuffered solution with a potassium concentration of 30 mEq/L results in poor recovery. The authors postulate that the absence of calcium combined with high KCl and high pH may result in deleterious consequences of the calcium paradox. It should be pointed out that blood cardioplegia contains histidine, the naturally occurring blood buffer.—Hillel Laks, M.D.

Improved Myocardial Recovery After Cardioplegic Arrest With An Oxygenated Crystalloid Solution

Robert A. Guyton, Lynne M. A. Dorsey, Joseph M. Craver, David K. Bone, Ellis L. Jones, Douglas A. Murphy, and Charles R. Hatcher, Jr. (Crawford W. Long Mem. Hosp., Atlanta, and Emory Univ.)
J. Thorac. Cardiovasc. Surg. 89:877–887, June 1985   5–49

The value of adding oxygen to cardioplegic solution was studied in a canine model in which 15 minutes of global ischemia was followed by heterogeneous delivery of solution during 1 hour. Very cold crystalloid hyperkalemic solution was used, with or without 100% oxygen. A prospective study of the metabolic effects of oxygenated and control cardioplegia was performed in 12 coronary bypass patients, using a blind prospective design. Perioperative changes in the ECG and levels of creatine kinase isoenzymes were reviewed in 151 coronary bypass patients. Ninety-four were protected with oxygenated solution.

In the canine study, oxygenation of cardioplegic solution was associated with better recovery in the left anterior descending circumflex regions. In the prospective clinical study, no significant differences were found between oxygenated and control solutions with respect to levels of creatine kinase, myoglobin, and lactate; coronary sinus flow; or oxygen consumption. Cardiac work 1 hour after cross-clamping also was similar in the two groups. In the retrospective series, 12-hour creatine kinase levels were similar when the cross-clamp time was 28 minutes or less, but, with a longer arrest time, creatine kinase-MB levels were more than twice as high in the nonoxygenated than in the oxygenated group. A significant difference persisted at 24 hours.

Oxygenated crystalloid cardioplegia appears to be advantageous with regard to both nonoxygenated solutions and blood cardioplegia. Simple systems can be used to deliver this form of protection. Up to 3 L of oxygenated crystalloid cardioplegic solution have been used in lengthy operations, scavenging the coronary sinus efflux to prevent systemic hyperkalemia.

▶ This interesting experimental and clinical study demonstrates convincingly that oxygenation of crystalloid cardioplegia improves myocardial protection.—Hillel Laks, M.D.

Intraoperative Myocardial Protection: A Comparison of Blood and Asanguineous Cardioplegia
J. E. Codd, H. B. Barner, D. G. Pennington, J. P. Merjavy, G. C. Kaiser, J. E. Devine, and V. L. Willman (St. Louis Univ.)
Ann. Thorac. Surg. 39:125–133, February 1985   5–50

This study compares the results of myocardial protection with blood cardioplegia vs. crystalloid cardioplegia in patients undergoing elective coronary revascularization. Blood cardioplegia was used in 97 patients and asanguineous cardioplegia in 84. The two groups were comparable demographically and clinically. Systemic hypothermia to 26 degrees was used. The asanguineous cardioplegia administered was Plegisol, which has a potassium chloride (KCl) content of 15 mEq/L. A 400-ml volume of both Plegisol and oxygenated, hemodiluted blood with 25 mEq of KCl per liter was used for induction of arrest. Repeat doses of 300 ml of blood cardioplegia were given every 20–25 minutes with KCl, 12 mEq/L.

Mean total pump times and cross-clamp times were similar in the two groups. Three patients receiving blood cardioplegia and five given asanguineous cardioplegia required balloon counterpulsation at the end of bypass. No ultrastructural abnormalities were found in either group. The ECG changes did not differ significantly. More patients given asanguineous cardioplegia required inotropic support for up to 24 hours postoperatively. Infarct size was significantly greater in the asanguineous cardioplegia group, as assessed from creatine kinase-MB release.

These findings suggest that blood cardioplegia provides better cellular protection than asanguineous cardioplegia does during aortic cross-clamping in elective cardiac surgery. The search for an ideal vehicle to deliver cold chemical cardioplegia should continue.

▶ This important report makes an objective effort to compare blood and crystalloid cardioplegia. Although excellent results were obtained with both methods, blood cardioplegia resulted in improved postoperative function and reduced creatine kinase-MB enzyme release. It is interesting that this blood cardioplegia solution consisted only of cold blood with KCl, 25 mEq/L or 12 mEq/L, with no other additives.—Hillel Laks, M.D.

Particle-Induced Coronary Vasoconstriction During Cardioplegic Infusion: Characterization and Possible Mechanisms

David J. Hearse, Cetin Erol, Lary A. Robinson, Miles P. Maxwell, and Mark V. Braimbridge (St. Thomas' Hosp., London, and Univ. of Nebraska)
J. Thorac. Cardiovasc. Surg. 89:428–438, March 1985   5–51

Permissible levels of contaminant particles in commercial intravenous solutions can lead to impaired coronary flow when infused intra-arterially in the isolated rat heart. Adverse effects on the infusion characteristics of crystalloid cardioplegic solution can be prevented by filtering the solution through a 0.8-μm filter just before use. The vasoconstrictor effect of particles in solution was studied in an isolated rat heart preparation. A commercially available intravenous solution was modified to produce the St. Thomas Hospital cardioplegic solution. The cumulative cardioplegic infusion time during a 3-hour period of global ischemia at 20 C was 19 minutes.

Baseline infusion of cardioplegic solution led to a 46% reduction in coronary flow. Flow impairment was only 13% after an 0.8-μm in-line filter was incorporated in the system, and the effect was reversed within 1 minute. Studies with filters of varying porosity indicated that the phenomenon is attributable to relatively small numbers of particles more than 10 μm in diameter. Hearts subjected to 3 hours of hypothermic ischemic arrest recovered almost completely on reperfusion with filtered solution, but not when unfiltered solution was used. The vasoconstrictor effect was prevented by administration of procaine, nifedipine, and adenosine triphosphate, and ameliorated by lidocaine and dipyridamole. Treatment with verapamil and isosorbide dinitrate was not effective.

Impaired coronary perfusion after infusion of cardioplegic solution is ascribed to repeated episodes of transient vasoconstriction, probably occurring at a small vessel level. The problem can be avoided by in-line filtration removing particles of 10 μm or larger. Inclusion of vasoactive agents (e.g., procaine or nifedipine) also may be helpful. Limits of purity for solutions should be revised for intra-arterial applications.

▶ The coronary vasoconstriction secondary to large particles in crystalloid cardioplegia is a fascinating phenomenon not previously described. The relief afforded by vasodilators would support their more routine use as components of cardioplegic solutions. As the authors point out, however, it has not yet been demonstrated whether this phenomenon occurs in man.—Hillel Laks, M.D.

Myocardial Recovery After Hypothermic Arrest: A Comparison of Oxygenated Crystalloid to Blood Cardioplegia. The Role of Calcium

Richard F. Heitmiller, Lawrence W. V. DeBoer, Gillian A. Geffin, Kyle W. Toal, John T. Fallon, Lambertus J. Drop, Richard S. Teplick, Dennis D. O'Keefe, and Willard M. Daggett, with the technical assistance of James Titus and Brian Redonnet (Massachusetts Gen. Hosp. and Harvard Univ.)
Circulation 72 (Suppl. 2):II-241–II-253, September 1985   5–52

Improved myocardial protection has been obtained during hypothermic arrest by using fully oxygenated multidose hyperkalemic crystalloid cardioplegic solution at 4 C. An attempt was made to determine whether the addition of red blood cells before oxygenation would provide further protection. The efficacy of cardioplegic solutions having a nominal hematocrit of 0, 10, or 30 was examined in canine hearts subjected to 5 hours of arrest at 10 C. Calcium ion was added to crystalloid solution to match that present in blood.

The coronary arteriovenous oxygen difference was greatest in the hematocrit-30 group. No substantial differences in percent adenosine triphosphate at 2 hours of reperfusion were noted. Left ventricular function declined most markedly in the crystalloid and hematocrit-10 groups; function remained stable in crystalloid-treated animals when calcium ion was added. Perfusion of cardioplegic solution was best maintained in the hematocrit-30 group. No major ultrastructural differences were found among the various groups.

Calcium is necessary for sustained functional recovery when cardioplegic solution is delivered fully oxygenated at 4 C. Addition of red blood cells to crystalloid cardioplegic solution at a hematocrit of 30 helps to maintain perfusion of the posterior papillary muscle and improves oxygen delivery. No benefit from adding red blood cells is apparent in ventricular function assessment beyond the effect of calcium ion.

▶ This paper sheds light on the continued debate over the benefits of blood over crystalloid cardioplegia. It should be recognized that the model included ligation of the pulmonary hila to minimize noncoronary collateral flow, which allows some blood with calcium to enter the coronary circulation even if there is no calcium in the cardioplegic solution. Although there was no difference in functional recovery between the animals receiving oxygenated crystalloid cardioplegia solution with calcium and those given the oxygenated crystalloid with red blood cells added to a hematocrit of 30%, cardioplegia with red blood cells resulted in better papillary muscle perfusion as measured by microspheres and better coronary arteriovenous oxygen difference. One could conclude that, because blood cardioplegia is already oxygenated, has a hematocrit of 30%, and contains calcium, it is simpler to administer than is oxygenated crystalloid cardioplegia with added red blood cells and calcium.—Hillel Laks, M.D.

Cardiopulmonary Bypass

Alterations in Plasma-, Monocyte-, and Lymphocyte-Fibronectin During Cardiopulmonary Bypass Surgery
Gershon Keren, Philip A. Gordon, Siow-Fong Lee, Michael Stewart, and Elliot T. Gelfand (Univ. of Alberta)
J. Clin. Pathol. 83:629–633, May 1985   5–53

Decreased plasma fibronectin levels have been associated with reduced reticuloendothelial phagocyte activity in patients who sustain trauma or burn injury, as well as in postoperative patients. Cryoprecipitate, a rich source of plasma fibronectin, corrects opsonic deficiency in both septic and nonseptic injury patients. The effects of cardiopulmonary bypass surgery on plasma and peripheral blood monocyte and lymphocyte fibronectin levels were examined in 18 consecutive patients undergoing elective cardiac surgery, usually coronary bypass graft surgery. The mean age was 53 years. Three patients received platelet concentrate after bypass.

A rapid fall in the plasma fibronectin concentration was noted after the institution of bypass, and lowered levels persisted for 48 hours postoperatively. The fibronectin level fell proportionately more than the IgG level did. Fibronectin on the surface of lymphocytes decreased during bypass and remained reduced at 24 hours. The level of monocyte-associated fibronectin increased during bypass. Heparinization did not reduce plasma fibronectin levels in the short time before bypass was started.

Circulating fibronectin is reduced during and after cardiac surgery with cardiopulmonary bypass. A fall in lymphocyte-associated fibronectin presumably reflects nonspecific adsorption, whereas an increase in fibrinectin binding to monocytes may have significant functional implications. Fibronectin in cryoprecipitate is degraded and therefore may not be ideal for infusion. Clinical trials may depend on the development of a purified fibronectin concentrate.

▶ Fibronectin is a plasma glycoprotein that opsonizes bacterial particles and other debris (e.g., fibrin aggregates), assisting in their clearance by monocytes and macrophages. This interesting study documents the reduction in fibronectin that occurs with cardiopulmonary bypass and explores its importance in the reduced immune competence that occurs after cardiopulmonary bypass.—Hillel Laks, M.D.

Postoperative Care

Prostaglandin E₁: A New Therapy for Refractory Right Heart Failure and Pulmonary Hypertension After Mitral Valve Replacement

Michael N. D'Ambra, Paul J. LaRaia, Daniel M. Philbin, W. David Watkins, Alan D. Hilgenberg, and Mortimer J. Buckley (Massachusetts Gen. Hosp. and Harvard Univ.)
J. Thorac. Cardiovasc. Surg. 89:567–572, April 1985　　　　　　　　5–54

Life-threatening right heart failure can follow mitral valve replacement, especially in patients with severe pulmonary hypertension or congestive heart failure. Survival is poor despite that many treatments tried. Intense pulmonary vasoconstriction may be present, which can preclude recovery of right ventricular function. The effects of the vasodilator prostaglandin E_1 (PGE_1), which dilates pulmonary arterial smooth muscle, were assessed in five consecutive patients with refractory right heart failure and pulmonary hypertension after mitral valve replacement. The PGE_1 was infused intravenously at dose rates of 30–150 ng/kg/minute in conjunction with infusion of norepinephrine into the left atrium at rates up to 1 μg/kg/minute.

The pulmonary vascular resistance rose to a mean of 55 Wood units after operation. Pulmonary artery pressures approached systemic levels, and left ventricular filling pressures were low. The mean cardiac index was 0.7 ml/minute/sq m. Pulmonary vascular resistance fell nearly to normal within an hour of PGE_1 therapy. The mean cardiac index rose to 2.4 ml/minute/sq m. Urine flow was maintained in all cases. All five patients recovered good right ventricular function, which continued on long-term follow-up observation.

Prostaglandin E_1 was helpful in these patients with right heart failure and pulmonary hypertension after mitral valve replacement, in conjunction with norepinephrine administration. All patients had rapid pulmonary vasodilator responses. None had right ventricular infarction or chronic right heart failure postoperatively.

▶ This is an important combination of pharmacologic agents to have at one's disposal when operating on patients with mitral valve disease and severe pulmonary hypertension. We have successfully used nitroglycerin or nitroprusside infusions in a similar fashion with norepinephrine infusion into the left atrium to combat the systemic vasodilator effects of these agents, but we have also come across patients in whom these agents were not effective.—Hillel Laks, M.D.

Comparison Between Antibiotic Irrigation and Mobilization of Pectoral Muscle Flaps in Treatment of Deep Sternal Infections
Hugh E. Scully, Yves Leclerc, Raymond D. Martin, Cathy P. Tong, B. S. Goldman, Richard D. Weisel, Lynda L. Mickleborough, and Ronald J. Baird (Toronto Gen. Hosp. and Univ. of Toronto)
J. Thorac. Cardiovasc. Surg. 90:523–531, October 1985   5–55

Data on 41 patients who contracted deep sternal infection with mediastinitis after cardiac surgery were reviewed. This group represented 1% of patients having median sternotomy between 1978 and 1983. Twenty-six patients had aortocoronary bypass surgery only, and 12 had valve surgery. Two patients had combined operations, and one had repair of a congenital cardiac defect. Nineteen patients treated between 1978 and 1981 underwent resternotomy with extensive debridement of nonviable tissue and primary closure of the wound. The mediastinum was irrigated with 0.5% povidone-iodine solution postoperatively. The 22 patients treated between 1982 and 1983 had similar debridement surgery, but the wounds were packed open and delayed closure was done with pectoral muscle flap mobilization, preserving the thoracoacromial pedicles and pectoral humoral attachments with their blood supply.

Staphylococcus aureus was the most frequent infecting organism in both treatment groups. Three patients in each group died in the hospital, one in each group because of infection. The length of stay in the intensive care unit was greater in the second group of patients undergoing delayed closure with pectoral muscle flaps. One patient in each group had recurrent or residual infection. Both patients have had satisfactory functional and cosmetic results after reoperation.

Although both methods gave similar early and late results, hospitalization was more prolonged in the delayed closure group. The authors have had experience with eight patients undergoing one-stage debridement and closure with pectoralis muscle flap reconstruction. Satisfactory cosmetic and functional results were obtained at reduced cost, and a second anesthetic was avoided.

▶ In most reports, the incidence of residual infection following débridement and primary closure with mediastinal irrigation has been somewhat higher than the authors' rates except for certain selected patients who had more localized infection and with adequate well-vascularized residual sternum for primary closure. In most patients with mediastinal infection, excellent results can be obtained by débridement with primary closure, using the pectoral muscle flaps. It is surprising how small the functional and cosmetic deficits are after this procedure. The authors conclude that this is the method of choice for a one-stage procedure —Hillel Laks, M.D.

6 Hypertension

Epidemiology

Duffy Antigens and Hypertension in a Black Population

Joseph M. Miller and John M. Miller (Provident Hosp., Baltimore)
Am. J. Public Health 75:558–559, May 1985   6–1

The reasons for the greater frequency and severity of hypertension in American blacks than in Caucasians remain unclear. An attempt was made to find an association between the presence of Duffy blood proteins, the best measure of "whiteness," and the prevalence of hypertension in a black population. Caucasians always have a positive phenotype for Duffy red cell antigen, but African blacks have only a small positive rate.

Sera from 722 patients at Provident Hospital were examined for antibodies to Fy^a and Fy^b, the positive Duffy antigens. A positive phenotype was found in 74 of 209 men and in 182 of 513 women. Hypertension was diagnosed in a total of 146 patients. Sixteen of 51 hypertensive men and 41 of 95 hypertensive women had positive Duffy proteins. The approximate relative risk for hypertension in the presence of positive Duffy proteins was only 1.2. After controls were applied for sex and age, the relative risk was 1.06.

In this study no positive association was found between hypertension and the presence of Duffy blood proteins. The findings fail to support a genetic relationship between the degree of "blackness" and the presence of elevated blood pressure, which is in contrast to results of past studies that were based on a visual or light-reflectance classification of color. Social class was not considered in the present study.

▶ The use of Duffy antigen analysis to determine the racial admixture in population studies is an interesting development. The greater severity and frequency of hypertension in American blacks is a matter of great concern. There is certainly reason to suspect that social and nutritional factors may play a role, but to date they do not explain the observation to the satisfaction of most observers. The application of more sophisticated studies, such as genetic ones, should help exclude nonenvironmental causes.—Walter M. Kirkendall, M.D.

Prevalence, Detection, and Control of Hypertension in a Biethnic Community: The San Antonio Heart Study

Laercio J. Franco, Michael P. Stern, Marc Rosenthal, Steven M. Haffner, Helen P. Hazuda, and Paul J. Comeaux (Paulista School of Medicine, Sao Paulo, Brazil, and Univ. of Texas at San Antonio)
Am. J. Epidemiol. 121:684–696, October 1985   6–2

Improvement in control of hypertension has been obtained in both blacks and Caucasians in recent years, but less is known of the diagnosis and treatment of hypertension in Mexican-Americans, the largest Hispanic subgroup in the United States.

Data from the San Antonio Heart study were obtained on 1,288 Mexican-Americans and 929 Anglos who were living in 3 socially distinct neighborhoods in San Antonio—a low-, a middle-, and a high-income area. (In the southwestern part of the United States, the term Anglos is commonly used to refer to non-Hispanic Caucasians.) A random sample of households was studied in each area to determine the prevalence of hypertension, which was defined as a diastolic pressure of 95 mm Hg or the current use of antihypertensive medication, in men and nonpregnant women aged 25–64 years.

The overall age-adjusted prevalence of hypertension for Mexican-American and Anglo men was 10% and 9.8%, respectively, and for women, 7.8% and 9.7%, respectively. After adjustment was made for obesity, Mexican-Americans exhibited a tendency toward lower rates of hypertension than Anglos at the same socioeconomic level. Only in women did the prevalence of hypertension decline with increasing socioeconomic status. Mexican-Americans had a higher proportion of newly diagnosed hypertension. Among patients with previously diagnosed hypertension, fewer Mexican-Americans were on antihypertensive medication.

The prevalence rates of hypertension that were found in this study are among the highest reported in the United States at the community level. Mexican-Americans nevertheless still lag behind Anglos at the same socioeconomic level in treatment and degree of control of hypertension, suggesting a role for sociocultural barriers to adequate medical care. There is evidence that Mexican-Americans respond at least as well as Anglos to community-based health education efforts.

▶ This information on hypertension among Mexican-Americans is valuable because it examines the prevalence and treatment of hypertensives in a major southwestern community and provides comparisons with a matched group of Caucasian hypertensives in the same location. The prevalence in both Mexican-Americans and Anglos was high. In the case of the Mexican-Americans, many hypertensives had not been detected or treated.

Studies of the Mexican-American population, particularly in regard to cardiovascular disease, are badly needed. Up until this time, despite the very large community of Mexican-Americans in the Southwest, little is known about vascular problems in the group of people or about their need for therapy.—Walter M. Kirkendall, M.D.

Alcohol, Nutrient Intake, and Hypertension in US Adults
Harvey W. Gruchow, Kathleen A. Sobocinski, and Joseph J. Barboriak (Med. College of Wisconsin, Milwaukee, and VA Med. Ctr., Wood, Wisc.)
JAMA 253:1567–1570, March 15, 1985   6–3

Increased intakes of both sodium and alcohol have been associated with elevated blood pressure. Multivariate techniques were used to analyze data from the first Health and Nutrition Examination Survey, to assess any contribution of alcohol to hypertension, and to determine the role of nutrient variables, compared with that of other established risk factors. Patients aged 18 to 74 years were included in the 9,553 subjects.

The importance of intakes of alcohol and sodium on blood pressure was confirmed. Intakes of both alcohol and sodium were correlated directly with systolic blood pressure among drinkers. Caloric intake, body mass index, and age also were correlated strongly with blood pressure. Gender was not a significant predictor of systolic blood pressure. Intake of potassium was correlated inversely with higher systolic blood, and intake of phosphorus was correlated directly. Intake of calcium was related to systolic pressure in non-Caucasian men only; it was not a significant predictor of systolic pressure overall.

These findings reaffirm the importance of intakes of alcohol and sodium on blood pressure in adults in the United States. Age, race, and obesity are paramount determinants of hypertension. Intake of nutrients is comparatively less important.

The independent relation between body mass index and systolic blood pressure, however, suggests that long-term dietary factors which may not be adequately assessed in dietary recall surveys probably contribute more substantially to elevated blood pressure. Further study of dietary factors in hypertension is warranted because they are more amenable to intervention than nondietary factors.

▶ This analysis of information from the first national Health and Nutrition Examination survey makes several observations that run contrary to previous studies. Although McCarron et al. (*Science* 224:1392–1398, 1984) and Harlan et al. (*Am. J. Epidemiology* 120:17–28, 1984) found that calcium intake was indirectly related to blood pressure, the present study found this to be true only for systolic blood pressure in non-Caucasian men. Interestingly, high alcohol, sodium, and phosphorus intakes were identified as important nutritional predictors of higher systolic blood pressure. Potassium intake was related inversely to the systolic blood pressure.

These analyses with different conclusions based on essentially the same information emphasize the complexity of interpreting retrospective nutritional data. The analysis must be looked upon as relatively soft information.—Walter M. Kirkendall, M.D.

Alcohol Consumption and Blood Pressure in a New Zealand Community Study

J. M. Paulin, F. O. Simpson, and H. J. Waal-Manning (Univ. of Otago, Dunedin, New Zealand)
N.Z. Med. J. 98:425–428, June 1985   6–4

Several epidemiologic studies have shown alcohol consumption to be associated with increased blood pressure. Such an association was examined in 901 adults who participated in a multiphasic health survey in 1981. Those who were using oral contraceptives or drugs that can lower blood pressure were excluded. The study population included 78% of eligible adults living in a town near Dunedin. Some alcohol was used at least once a month by 85% of men and 52% of women. Mean reported weekly intake was 171 gm for men and 56 gm for women. Alcohol use was most prevalent in men aged 20–29 years.

The 24-hour output of urinary sodium was negatively related to alcohol intake in women, but not in men. The output of urinary potassium was unrelated to alcohol intake in both sexes. Psychometric scores for anger, anxiety, and depression could not be related to alcohol intake. Mean systolic and diastolic blood pressures, which were adjusted for age and body mass index, increased significantly with increasing alcohol consumption in men, but no such association was apparent for women.

These findings support a positive association between alcohol intake and blood pressure in men and are generally consistent with findings in England, Denmark, United States, and Australia. A similar relationship has been described for women but was not found in the present study. If a causal relationship exists between alcohol consumption and hypertension, reduced intake of alcohol could decrease the mean blood pressure level and thereby the prevalence of hypertension in the community.

▶ These observations support several other studies suggesting that there is a linear, positive relationship between ingestion of alcohol and elevated blood pressure. Among those who took over 300 gm of alcohol per week (approximately 14 cans of beer), there was a 9/9 mm Hg increase in blood pressure over that seen among nondrinkers.

Information on the women did not suggest a relationship between blood pressure and alcohol consumption. Relatively few of the women drank alcohol and only three were labeled as heavy consumers of spirits.

The message seems to be that if you drink alcohol, don't drink much. Clearly, alcohol in large amounts is associated with elevated blood pressure, at least among men.—Walter M. Kirkendall, M.D.

An Epidemiological Approach to Describing Risk Associated With Blood Pressure Levels: Final Report of the Working Group on Risk and High Blood Pressure
Working Group on Risk and High Blood Pressure (Natl. Inst. of Health, Bethesda, Md.)
Hypertension 7:641–651, July–August 1985   6–5

Blood pressure-related risks increase in an essentially continuous manner, and points of demarcation are arbitrary, even though they are desirable for distinguishing among ranges of risk. Risks can be predicted from single blood pressure measurements, but the effects of treatment are known only in relation to levels of blood pressure that are recorded on two or more occasions before treatment.

Diastolic blood pressure has primacy, but systolic pressure should not be disregarded. An intermediate-risk diastolic pressure of 80–89 mm Hg is specified on initial measurement, and of below 90 mm Hg on repeat measurement. If the initial diastolic pressure is below 90 mm Hg but the systolic pressure is 160 mm Hg or above, rescreening is indicated, and 160 mm Hg is used as a systolic criterion on the second occasion.

In recent years several sources have questioned the diastolic criteria of 95, or even 90 mm Hg, or have proposed new ones. The Working Group proposes that minimal, intermediate, and higher risks be distinguished on the basis of an intermediate risk range of 80–89 mm Hg. All persons with an initial diastolic pressure of 90 mm Hg or above should be promptly rescreened, and those with persistent elevations should be regarded as having confirmed high blood pressure and a reducible risk. Persons at minimal risk should be checked annually or whenever medical care is given.

A favorable risk status is well defined by a diastolic blood pressure below 80 mm Hg, and this can be accepted as a desirable health attribute. The risk level of 80–89 mm Hg represents a potentially important group from a preventive standpoint. Persons initially at higher risk but without confirmed high blood pressure after the second measurement should be considered to have intermediate risk blood pressure. Blood pressure-related risk is identifiable at an early stage, and is remediable to a great extent.

▶ This study demonstrates that the risk from cardiovascular disease is a continuous one from relatively low blood pressure levels (80 mm Hg diastolic) up into the hypertensive range. Individuals with blood pressures in the 80–89 mm Hg diastolic range are very numerous in our society. It is from this group that the majority of persons with heart attacks come. By identifying this group with intermediate risk, physicians might consider opportunities for nondrug treatment to reduce cardiovascular risk factors. It should be emphasized that there is no support in this review or elsewhere for lowering of blood pressure with drugs in individuals with blood pressure below the 90-mm Hg diastolic range.

This report also standardizes the nomenclature concerning blood pressure levels and suggests certain follow-up criteria based on the level of the blood pressure.—Walter M. Kirkendall, M.D.

Basic Research

Increased Susceptibility to Osmotic Disruption of the Blood-Brain Barrier in Chronic Hypertension

Kinya Tamaki, Seizo Sadoshima, and Donald D. Heistad (Univ. of Iowa)
Hypertension 6:633–638, September–October 1984   6–6

Disruption of the blood-brain barrier has been implicated in the development of hypertensive encephalopathy. Susceptibility of the blood-brain barrier to disruption by administration of a hyperosmolar solution was examined in normotensive Wistar-Kyoto rats, stroke-prone spontaneously hypertensive rats (SHRSPs), and spontaneously hypertensive rats (SHRs) not prone to stroke. Permeability of the blood-brain barrier was estimated by the ratio of ^{125}I-albumin in brain and blood. The blood-brain barrier was disrupted with an intracarotid injection of 1.6 M arabinose in saline.

Permeability of the blood-brain barrier was less than 0.4% with the barrier intact. After arabinose injection, the mean degree of permeability was 18% in SHRSPs, 21% in SHRs, and 10% in Wistar-Kyoto rats. A reduction in blood pressure after nitroprusside administration in SHRSPs did not reduce permeability to albumin. Survival was significantly less in SHRSPs than in Wistar-Kyoto rats after disruption of the blood-brain barrier, but survival was better in SHRSPs given nitroprusside.

Increased susceptibility of the blood-brain barrier in SHRs and SHRSPs is masked by vascular hypertrophy, which produces augmented autoregulatory vasoconstriction during acutely increased arterial pressure and protects the barrier. Hypertensive encephalopathy in SHRSPs may be related to disruption of the blood-brain barrier. A reduction in arterial pressure may help to reduce edema formation when the barrier is disrupted, even if permeability to albumin is not decreased.

▶ The authors used a hyperosmolar solution injected into the cerebral circulation to demonstrate that the circulations of spontaneously hypertensive rats and stroke-prone rats were more susceptible to disruption by this stimulus than were the circulations of the control animals. Without the osmotic stimulus, permeability of the labeled albumin was much the same. In the absence of an acute rise in arterial pressure, the authors believe that vascular hypertrophy during chronic hypertension promotes greater autoregulatory vasoconstriction and protects the brain against cerebral edema from increases in pressure.

In the spontaneously hypertensive rats, they were also able to demonstrate that the reduction of pressure with nitroprusside reduced the tendency to increase permeability in these brain vessels.

The study was not designed to demonstrate differences in permeability in various parts of the brain. It would be of interest to know whether small vessels in various areas of the brain are either more or less protected against osmotic and blood pressure disruption. It would also be of interest to know whether drugs can reduce the disruption of the blood-brain barrier in specific areas of the brain selectively.—Walter M. Kirkendall, M.D.

A New Mechanism in One-Kidney, One Clip Hypertension
Leonard T. Skeggs, Jr., Frederic E. Dorer, Kenneth E. Lentz, Joseph R. Kahn, and Steven N. Emancipator (VA Med. Ctr., Cleveland, Case Western Reserve Univ.)
Hypertension 7:72–80, January–February 1985   6–7

The renin-angiotensin system does not appear to be responsible for maintenance of elevated blood pressure in experimental one-kidney, one-clip (1K1C) hypertension. The hog kidney contains a nonrenin substance, designated antigen M, that elicits a cross-reacting antibody in hypertensive

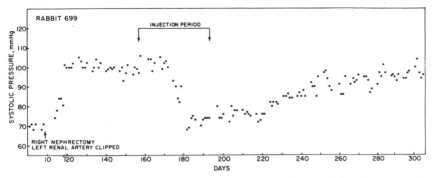

Fig 6–1.—Blood pressure response to direct immunization in a rabbit model of one-kidney, one-clip hypertension. Purified hog kidney renin was the antigen. (Courtesy of Skeggs, L.T., Jr., et al.: Hypertension 7:72–80, January–February 1985. By permission of the American Heart Association, Inc.)

rabbits and produces a blood pressure reduction. An attempt was made to isolate antigen M from the hog kidney.

Hog kidney renin was purified with immobilized monoclonal antirenin. Immunization of 1K1C hypertensive rabbits with the purified renin lowered the blood pressure to normal. A blood pressure-lowering antibody that is not antirenin was isolated from these rabbits and shown immunocytochemically to be localized in arterial and arteriolar smooth muscle tissue sections in both normal and hypertensive rabbits. The blood pressure response to direct immunization of a rabbit with 1K1C hypertension with purified hog kidney renin is shown in Figure 6–1. Antibody stained the cytoplasm of smooth muscle and other cells in sections of the kidney, aorta, carotid artery, heart, liver, pancreas, adrenal gland, and small bowel from normal and hypertensive rabbits.

Renin appears to be converted to a form present most obviously in arterial and arteriolar smooth muscle, where it presumably produces vasoconstriction. Its neutralization by specific antibody lowers blood pressure in the 1K1C hypertensive rabbit. Both exogenous renin and endogenous renin are converted in vivo to an antigen M substance.

▶ As demonstrated in the preceding paper, the mechanism for production of hypertension in the one-kidney, one-clip experimental model is not understood. This group believes that renin, although not high in the blood, is lodged in arteriolar and arterial smooth muscle cells, where it produces vasoconstriction. The authors were able to neutralize the effect of renin by use of a specific antibody.

There is still a body of evidence that suggests that some renal factor other than renin is responsible for inducing some of the blood pressure elevation in this model of hypertension.—Walter M. Kirkendall, M.D.

Sodium and Volume Depletion Activates Neurogenic Mechanisms in Renal Hypertensive Dogs

William D. Sweet, Ronald H. Freeman, James O. Davis, and Daniel Villarreal (Univ. of Missouri)

Hypertension 7:39–46, January–February 1985   6–8

It remains unclear how a presumed sodium/volume excess maintains chronic one-kidney, one-clip (1K1C) renal hypertension when the angiotensin-pressor component is normal, but both the central and peripheral sympathetic nervous systems may participate. The roles of the sympathetic and renin-angiotensin systems were assessed in conscious, sodium-replete and sodium depleted dogs with established 1K1C hypertension. Sodium-replete 1K1C hypertensive dogs also were studied after renal artery stenosis was produced, when the plasma renin activity was elevated and sodium and water balances were positive. Hemodynamic responses to pharmacologic block of ganglionic transmission with hexamethonium and to block off the renin-angiotensin system with captopril were examined.

All experimental groups had elevated blood pressure compared with findings in control animals, and there were no significant differences in baseline plasma catecholamine levels among the three hypertensive groups. Ganglionic blockade produced a greater fall in blood pressure in sodium/volume-depleted dogs than in the other groups. Captopril administration decreased blood pressure markedly in the high-renin sodium/volume-depleted animals, and also in high-renin animals studied 3 days after clipping. Captopril had a smaller depressor effect in the normal-renin groups.

Sodium/volume depletion activates both adrenergic-dependent and angiotensin-dependent mechanisms to maintain blood pressure at hypertensive levels in conscious dogs with established 1K1C renal hypertension. The adrenergic system does not appear to have an important role in the early, high-renin phase of benign 1K1C hypertension. Accelerated renovascular hypertension seems to be mediated primarily by the renin-angiotensin system.

▶ Elevation of blood pressure in the one-kidney, one-clip hypertensive experimental animal or its counterpart in man has been a subject of considerable debate. Because plasma renin activity is generally not elevated beyond the first few days of hypertension in experimental animals, it has been assumed that an increase in plasma volume, neurogenic mechanisms, or other centrally acting events such as release of vasopressin may contribute to the blood pressure elevation. In this study, renin and the neurogenic mechanisms were involved when the animals were sodium depleted. In the sodium-replete animal, both acutely and chronically, use of the converting enzyme inhibitor captopril lowered blood pressure, but not to control levels. When ganglionic blockade as well as converting enzyme inhibition were employed in the sodium-depleted hypertensive animal, blood pressure fell to normal ranges.

When the counterpart of one-kidney, one-clip hypertension occurs in man, these observations support the use of diuretics, sympathetic blocking drugs, and when necessary, converting enzyme inhibitors as treatment.—Walter M. Kirkendall, M.D.

Control of Glomerular Hypertension Limits Glomerular Injury in Rats With Reduced Renal Mass
Sharon Anderson, Timothy W. Meyer, Helmut G. Rennke, and Barry M. Brenner, with the technical assistance of J. L. Troy, R. L. DeGraphenried, J. L. Noddin, A. W. Nunn, and D. Sandstrom (Brigham and Women's Hosp., Boston, and Harvard Univ.)
J. Clin. Invest. 76:612–619, August 1985   6–9

Adaptation to a reduction of renal mass in the rat includes hyperfiltration in the remaining nephrons secondary to an elevated glomerular capillary plasma flow rate and hydraulic pressure. Injury to remaining glomeruli might result from these changes, leading to progressive azotemia and eventual glomerular sclerosis. The effects of controlling systemic blood pressure pharmacologically after renal ablation on the adaptive rise in glomerular capillary hydraulic pressure were studied in Munich-Wistar rats. A 5/6 renal ablation was obtained by removing one kidney and infarcting renal artery branches to the other. Blood pressure was monitored weekly, and micropuncture studies were carried out.

The development of systemic hypertension after renal ablation was prevented by enalapril therapy. The mean glomerular transcapillary hydraulic pressure gradient was maintained nearly at normal, without significant compromise in the single nephron glomerular filtration rate or the glomerular capillary plasma flow rate. Glomerular structural lesions, including segmental sclerosis, developed in untreated rats. Glomerular injury was much less evident in enalapril-treated animals.

Control of glomerular hypertension limits glomerular injury in this rat model of renal ablation. The findings support a role for glomerular hemodynamic changes in mediating progressive renal injury when the number of nephrons is reduced. Control of hypertension appears to slow the progression of renal disease in diabetics, and early, aggressive control of blood pressure also seems indicated in hypertensive patients with renal disease.

▶ This article is well worth reading since it brings together information bearing on glomerular hyperperfusion and progressive renal disease. The authors have demonstrated that with reduction of renal mass, progressive renal glomerular damage results from the glomerular hyperperfusion. Their study indicated that the use of the converting enzyme inhibitor enalapril retarded glomerular damage and proteinuria. Whether all programs to reduce glomerular filtration pressure are equally successful in reducing glomerular damage is not yet known. It may be that the unique effect of converting enzyme inhibitors on efferent glomerular constriction makes these drugs unusually effective.

If the observations concerning glomerular hyperperfusion either from protein feeding or hypertension can be applied to man, as initial reports suggest, they have far-reaching implications. The concept has been applied already to protein restriction in patients with renal insufficiency. Diabetics with hypertension have been treated with captopril with apparent benefit. One can invision many other areas, including the treatment of patients with hypertension, symptoms of aging, and solitary kidneys, in which it would be prudent to examine methods to reduce glomerular hyperperfusion to prevent glomerular sclerosis.—Walter M. Kirkendall, M.D.

Renal Adaptation to Potassium in the Adrenalectomized Rabbit: Role of Distal Tubular Sodium-Potassium Adenosine Triphosphatase

Lal C. Garg and Neelam Narang (Univ. of Florida)
J. Clin. Invest. 76:1065–1070, September 1985   6–10

The increase in renal sodium-potassium adenosine triphosphatase (Na-K-ATPase) activity with increased potassium intake is considered an adaptive mechanism for excreting more potassium ion. Certain mineralocorticoids (e.g., aldosterone) also increase Na-K-ATPase activity selectively in the late distal tubule and collecting duct. The effect of dietary potassium intake on Na-K-ATPase activity in the distal nephron was studied in adrenalectomized rabbits to determine whether renal adaptation to K^+ can occur independently of mineralocorticoids. Enzyme activity was determined by a fluorometric microassay in the distal convoluted tubule, connecting tubule, cortical collecting duct, and outer medullary collecting duct. Dietary K^+ was 100 mEq/kg, 300 mEq/kg, 500 mEq/kg, or 700 mEq/kg.

An increase of more than 200% in Na-K-ATPase activity occurred in the cortical collecting duct of adrenalectomized animals as the dietary K^+ intake increased. Enzyme activity in this segment correlated linearly with K^+ excretion. A 50% increase in Na-K-ATPase activity occurred in the connecting tubule, but no significant change in activity occurred in the distal convoluted tubule or in the medullary collecting duct as dietary K^+ increased. No significant changes in levels of plasma or urinary sodium or in magnesium-ATPase activity were observed.

Potassium loading leads to increased Na-K-ATPase activity in the connecting tubule and cortical collecting duct in the adrenalectomized rabbit. The effect is independent of any priming action of adrenal steroids. The findings may explain how tolerance to a moderate K^+ load develops in patients with uncomplicated adrenal insufficiency who are maintained by means of high salt intake.

▶ This paper gives a bit more information concerning the renal handling of potassium. The ability of man to increase the excretion of potassium when faced with a gradually increasing load of this cation has long been of interest. There is no question that an increase in the excretion of aldosterone plays a major role in this process, and indeed potassium is one of the more potent stimuli for the production of aldosterone. This study demonstrates that sodium-potassium ATPase activity rises sharply in the distal collecting tubule and the connecting tubule of the kidney when the organism is faced with a potassium challenge even when adrenal cortical hormones are absent. The authors did not prove the relative importance of aldosterone-related and aldosterone-independent rises in renal ATPase activity. It is reasonable to speculate, however, that when the body is faced with a surfeit of potassium, both mechanisms operate additively or synergistically.—Walter M. Kirkendall, M.D.

A Conformationally Constrained Vasopressin Analog With Antidiuretic Antagonistic Activity

Gerald Skala, Clark W. Smith, Catherine J. Taylor, and James H. Ludens (Upjohn Co., Kalamazoo, Mich.)
Science 226:443–445, Oct. 26, 1984   6–11

A working model of the biologically active conformation of the neurohypophyseal hormones arginine vasopressin and lysine vasopressin was used to design a bicyclic vasopressin analogue that acts as an antagonist of the antidiuretic activity of vasopressin. The analogue is [5,8-cyclo-(1-β-mercaptopropionic acid,2-phenylalanine,5-aspartic acid,8-lysine)] vasopressin, or bicyclic MPA-LVP.

Model data were derived from a three-dimensional structure of vasopressin bound to its antidiuretic receptor. The model suggested that the carboxamide group of asparagine in position 5 is a key element in determining intrinsic activity; the basic moiety on the side chain of the residue in position 8 also is an active element, the two working together for maximum efficacy. The protected peptide intermediate was synthesized on a poly-N-acrylylpyrrolidine resin. When the antidiuretic potency was tested in rats, the antagonistic activity of bicyclic MPA-LVP could not be ascribed to diuretic activity itself. Highly variable responses were obtained in a pressor assay; only partial agonistic and antagonistic activity was evident.

Bicyclic MPA-LVP may be the first example of predictive design of an inhibitory peptide analogue based on data derived from a hypothetical biologically active conformation. This approach should reduce the work needed to find peptide hormone antagonists. When there is an adequate hypothesis for the relationship between conformation and biologic activity of a peptide, both inhibitory analogues and highly potent, specific agonists can be designed.

▶ Although the vasopressin analogue developed antagonized antidiuretic activity of the pituitary reference standard quite effectively, the compound gave highly variable responses when tested against the pressor activity of vasopressin. The authors believe that there is only partial activity against the pressor activity of vasopressin.

Of more importance is that the development of analogues of vasopressin should give eventually the ability to investigate its mode of action and ensure that more effective antagonists will be developed. It is also likely that the major functions of vasopressin will be better demonstrated and studied by the use of appropriate analogues.

Indeed, already such an analogue has been used to study the hypertension caused by nucleus tractus solitarius lesions in rats (Sned et al.: *Hypertension* 7:262–267, 1985).—Walter M. Kirkendall, M.D.

Atrial Natriuretic Factor: A Circulating Hormone Stimulated by Volume Loading
R. E. Lang, H. Thölken, D. Ganten, F. C. Luft, H. Ruskoaho, and Th. Unger (Univ. of Heidelberg)
Nature 314:264–266, March 21, 1985   6–12

Cardiocytes of mammalian atria contain granules in numbers related to salt loading and blood volume. Crude extracts of rat atria and granules have potent natriuretic and diuretic effects that are mediated by peptides identified as atrial natriuretic factor (ANF). There is indirect evidence that at least some of these peptides may be released into the blood and act as hormones. Volume-loading studies were done using a sensitive, specific radioimmunoassay for ANF and 3 rat synthetic peptides, atriopeptins I, II, and III. Antibody was obtained in rabbits using atriopeptin II.

Several immunoreactive peaks were found when analyzing atrial extracts by high-pressure liquid chromatography. A rise in right atrial pressure in perfused hearts led to much greater release of ANF-like material into the perfusate. This material was also found in rat plasma. Plasma concentrations were increased by volume expansion. Radioimmunoassay of plasma after blood volume expansion showed a major peak between atriopeptin II and atriopeptin III, corresponding to the major peptide in the cardiac perfusate.

This is the first demonstration of ANF in the blood. More ANF peptides are needed as reference substances to elucidate the nature of circulating ANF. Most ANF-like immunoreactive material in atrial extracts probably represents storage forms of ANF serving as biosynthetic precursors for ANF released into the blood. Most plasma ANF probably is formed in cardiac tissue. Stretching atrial cardiocytes with volume expansion may result in secretion of the natriuretic and diuretic peptides. Whether high brain centers are involved via neuronal reflex arcs remains to be determined.

▶ There is much indirect evidence that an atrial natriuretic factor is transported to the kidney or influences renal activity by a neurogenic mechanism. The demonstration of the hormone in blood is important and gives credance to the general idea that atrial natriuretic factor(s) are important in the regulation of blood pressure, renal function, and extracellular volume. A purified factor has been demonstrated to cause, in experimental animals, an increase in glomerular filtration rate, diuresis, and natriuresis; a reduction of blood pressure; and a reduction of plasma renin and plasma aldosterone levels (Maack et al.: *Am. J. Med.* 77:1069–1075, 1984).—Walter M. Kirkendall, M.D.

Clinical Investigation

Blood Pressure in the "Low-Pressure System" and Cardiac Performance in Essential Hypertension

Gerard M. London, Michael E. Safar, Anne L. Safar, and Alain Ch. Simon (Broussais Hosp., Paris)
J. Hypertension 3:337–342, August 1985   6–13

Central venous pressure has been found to be elevated in patients with sustained essential hypertension, even in the absence of heart failure. The mechanism of this effect was examined in men with sustained, uncomplicated essential hypertension who received rapid infusions of dextran.

Forty-nine hypertensive men and 27 age-matched normotensive men with comparable body weight were studied. All treatment was discontinued at least 1 weeks before the study, and a diet that contained 100 mEq of sodium daily was given in hospital for 6 days before hemodynamic studies were carried out in the fasting state. Subjects then received an infusion of 500 ml of 6% dextran within 4 minutes via a peripheral vein.

The increase in central venous pressure (CVP) averaged 5.6 mm Hg in hypertensive patients and 3.7 mm Hg in controls. Respective mean pulmonary wedge pressures were 12.6 and 8.9 mm Hg. Cardiac output and heart rate were similar in the two groups. Total peripheral resistance was significantly increased in hypertensive patients, and total blood volume was significantly reduced.

The cardiac output-CVP relation was normal after rapid volume expansion, but the slope of the curve that related blood volume to CVP was significantly reduced. In hypertensive patients CVP correlated significantly with age, even for a constant arterial blood pressure. The correlation between arterial blood pressure and CVP was significant even for a constant age.

Central venous pressure is increased in men with essential hypertension, apart from any change in cardiac pump function or hypovolemia. Reduced compliance of the venous bed or the left ventricle, or both, appears to be responsible. The strong correlation between age and venous disorder is similar to that found in arterial circulation. Long-term longitudinal studies that start in childhood will help elucidate the role of the venous system in essential hypertension.

▶ This article makes several points. One of major importance is that the venous system is stiff in hypertensives and becomes less compliant with age. This mimics what is seen in the arterial circulation in older hypertensives. The authors believe that the changes in the venous component of the circulation have been overlooked because of relatively small increases in pressure and difficulties in studying the low-pressure system.

The concept that primary hypertension contributes importantly to pressure in the venous circulation is one that has not yet been exploited from a diagnostic or therapeutic standpoint. One might be able to classify hypertensives in a more logical fashion by measuring venous compliance, and one might be able to better treat such patients with drugs having a primary effect on large-capacitance vessels.—Walter M. Kirkendall, M.D.

Atriopeptins as Cardiac Hormones

Philip Needleman, Steven P. Adams, Barbara R. Cole, Mark G. Currie, David M. Geller, Marshall L. Michener, Clifford B. Saper, David Schwartz, and David G. Standaert (Washington Univ.; Monsanto Research Labs., St. Louis; and Med. Univ. of South Carolina)
Hypertension 7:469–482, July–August 1985   6–14

The atrial peptide is a potential hormonal mediator of change in composition of body fluid, extracellular volume, and systemic blood pressure. The atria are sites of low-pressure baroreceptors that are involved in regulating the volume of plasma. Stimulation of these receptors by distention leads to diuresis, bradycardia, hypotension, and decreased systemic vascular resistance. A variety of atrial peptides has been isolated from rat and human tissues.

Many studies have demonstrated natriuretic and diuretic properties in atrial extracts. Atrial peptide-induced natriuresis probably is a result of factors other than increased glomerular filtration rate. Direct tubular actions seem to occur. Atrial peptides may especially affect secretions of renin and aldosterone when baseline levels are elevated.

A single class of atriopeptin-specific binding sites has been described in membranes of the rabbit aorta. Little is known of the physiologic stimuli for atriopeptin release. Atriopeptin immunoreactive neurons have been found in rat brain. Their function remains to be determined, but the anteroventral periventricular nucleus likely is involved.

Abnormalities in levels of atrial peptides may be associated with states of fluid imbalance, altered vascular tone, or cardiac degeneration. Clinical trials of atrial peptides are feasible unless unforeseen toxicity problems arise. Analogues can readily be synthesized. Serum assays will help characterize the kinetics of atriopeptin release in such disorders as hypertension, renal disease, and congestive heart failure.

▶ This is a good review of atrial peptides and their impact on cardiovascular function as of early 1985. An atrial peptide or a class of them is almost certainly a central factor in volume regulation in the low-pressure areas of the circulation. They clearly have an effect on the renal handling of sodium and water and on vasomotor tone and probably on the secretion of hormones such as aldosterone and vasopressin.

With better methods of characterization and analysis of the peptides now available, it is certain that we will have an explosion of knowledge in this field.—Walter M. Kirkendall, M.D.

Reactivity to Norepinephrine and Effect of Sodium on Blood Pressure During Weight Loss

Björn Fagerberg, Ove K. Andersson, Bengt Persson, and Thomas Hedner (Univ. of Göteborg, Sweden)
Hypertension 7:586–592, July–August 1985   6–15

The means by which weight-reducing diets tend to lower blood pressure in obese hypertensive subjects are uncertain, but a change in sympathetic outflow has been proposed. The effects of a moderate weight-reducing diet on the regulation of blood pressure and activity of the sympathetic nervous sytem were examined in 18 middle-aged men with untreated hypertension who weighed 20% to 40% above normal and had supine diastolic blood pressure of 94–105 mm Hg, but were otherwise healthy.

Ten subjects received an energy-restricted diet with constant sodium intake, which was designed to produce a weight loss of 1 kg per week. In 8 other subjects an attempt was made to lower excretion of urinary sodium to below 100 mM daily. The diets were followed for 9–11 weeks.

Mean body mass fell by 9 kg in the group with constant sodium intake, but mean intra-arterial pressure did not change significantly. Urinary excretion of norepinephrine decreased, but plasma concentration did not. When sodium intake was restricted so that the mean 24-hour excretion was 95 mM, body mass decreased by 9 kg on average, and mean arterial pressure fell by 4–19 mm Hg. Plasma concentration of norepinephrine decreased significantly, but urinary excretion did not. The pressor response to infusion of norepinephrine was increased in the constant-sodium group but was unchanged in the sodium-restricted group.

Moderate energy restriction alone reduces sympathetic neural outflow with concomitant increased reactivity to norepinephrine, probably due to up-regulation of α-adrenergic receptors. There is no substantial net effect on arterial pressure. The blood pressure declines when energy restriction is combined with a lowered intake of sodium, which prevents up-regulation of reactivity to norepinephrine, thereby permitting the lowered sympathetic outflow to reduce the blood pressure.

▶ There has been controversy about whether concomitant sodium restriction is necessary for blood pressure reduction in hypertensive patients on a calorie-reducing diet. These authors observed that reduction of sodium chloride added to weight loss lowers blood pressure, perhaps by its effects on blood vessel reactivity to norepinephrine. Others have reached opposite conclusions, namely, that the blood pressure reduction noted in obese patients on a reducing diet is not salt related.

It is well known, however, from this and other studies that a low-sodium diet will reduce the pressor response to infused norepinephrine, and it is probably reasonable to assume the same response to endogenously produced catecholamines. This study is flawed because there were few patients tested and they were not characterized in regard to salt sensitivity. The study was carried out with outpatients, and so assuring compliance with salt restriction and specimen collection was difficult. In this regard, although sodium levels in the patients in the salt-restricted group dropped to half what they were before treatment, the levels of urinary potassium also fell—a somewhat disquieting observation.

The literature on the topic of weight loss in the obese hypertensive suggests that salt restriction may help weight loss lower blood pressure, but that blood pressure reduction occurs in the absence of salt restriction in many subjects.—Walter M. Kirkendall, M.D.

Acute and Chronic Effects of the Converting Enzyme Inhibitors Enalapril and Lisinopril on Reflex Control of Heart Rate in Normotensive Man

Adesuyi A. Ajayi, Brian C. Campbell, Catherine A. Howie, and John L. Reid (Stobhill Gen. Hosp., Glasgow, Scotland)
J. Hypertension 3:47–53, February 1985   6–16

Increased parasympathetic tone has been described in both hypertensive and normotensive subjects after receiving captopril. The effects of acute and chronic administration of the newer converting enzyme inhibitors enalapril and lisinopril on sympathetic and parasympathetic reflex control of heart rate were examined in 10 normotensive, sodium-replete male subjects aged 19–39 years. A Valsalva maneuver, cold pressor test, and diving test were repeated 4–6 hours after administration of 10 mg of enalapril, 10 mg of lisinopril, or placebo. Subjects also received atropine, 0.04 mg/kg, and 10 mg of edrophonium intravenously.

Both enalapril and lisinopril impaired the vagally mediated early cardiac acceleration that was associated with lying down in the standing to lying test. Blood pressure fell with no change in heart rate after acute dosing and after 7 days of treatment. Bradycardia that was induced by facial immersion was significantly attenuated by lisinopril and by edrophonium. Neither enalapril nor lisinopril altered the heart rate or blood pressure response to the Valsalva maneuver or cold pressor testing. Levels of plasma noradrenaline were unchanged.

Converting enzyme inhibition by enalapril and lisinopril produces modest reductions in arterial pressure without reflex tachycardia in normotensive subjects. Increased parasympathetic activity, either centrally or peripherally, may explain these effects. Baroreflexes and sympathetic function are not impaired.

▶ This report extends observations with other converting enzyme inhibitors that are known to lower blood pressure and yet not cause reflex tachycardia. This study indicates that these drugs in some fashion increase parasympathetic activity to prevent the increase in heart rate.

The authors examined the possibility that sympathetic activity might be reduced by these compounds largely because of angiotensin II withdrawal. However, they found no attenuation of blood pressure change following the cold pressor test and demonstrated that both captopril and enalapril had effects that closely resembled those following edrophonium, a parasympathetic agonist.—Walter M. Kirkendall, M.D.

How Free Care Reduced Hypertension in the Health Insurance Experiment

Emmett B. Keeler, Robert H. Brook, George A. Goldberg, Caren J. Kamberg, and Joseph P. Newhouse (Rand Corp., Santa Monica, and Univ. of California at Los Angeles)

JAMA 254:1926–1931, Oct. 11, 1985   6–17

Previous observations have indicated slightly lower average diastolic blood pressures with free care than with cost-sharing plans in the Rand Health Insurance Experiment, a randomized, controlled trial of cost sharing in the general United States population. The outcomes now have been assessed for subgroups of hypertensive patients, and the effects of cost sharing on the process and quality of care received by hypertensive patients have been examined. The study included 3,958 subjects aged 14 to 61 years from 2,005 families. Seventy percent of subjects participated for 3 years, and 30% participated for 5 years.

Eleven percent of subjects met at least one criterion for hypertension at exit from the study; 14% met at least two criterion at entry. The average adult had significantly lower diastolic blood pressure at the end of the study with free care than with cost sharing. The difference for all clinically defined hypertensives averaged 1.9 mm Hg, and for the low-income subjects the difference was 3.5 mm Hg. Differences were similar for blacks and whites. Additional contact with the physician was responsible, leading to better detection and treatment of hypertensives who were not initially under care. Free care also was associated with better compliance with dietary and smoking recommendations, and with more use of medication by those who required it.

This process and quality-of-care analysis of hypertensive patients supports the reported beneficial effect of free care on control of blood pressure. Free care for all is, however, an expensive and indirect means of helping a relative few. Screening examinations with notification of the personal physician is responsible for more than half of the gain in control of blood pressure that has occurred with free care at low cost.

▶ It is probably not surprising that blood pressure is lowered to a greater degree in patients who receive totally free care as opposed to those who had cost-sharing plans. The reduction of blood pressure was associated with additional contacts with physicians, and greater compliance with restrictions on diet and smoking and instructions on the use of medications. Nevertheless, even with the free plan, compliance with many treatment recommendations was poor. In addition, many patients in this group had uncontrolled blood pressure or anxiety about their blood pressure.

It seems to me that this study is a more eloquent plea for better education of patients concerning hypertension and the need for treatment than for free care for the hypertensive population.—Walter M. Kirkendall, M.D.

Alcohol Stimulation of Renin Release in Man: Its Relation to the Hemodynamic, Electrolyte, and Sympatho-adrenal Responses to Drinking

I. B. Puddey, R. Vandongen, L. J. Beilin, and I. L. Rouse (Royal Perth Hosp., Western Australia)

J. Clin. Endocrinol. Metab. 61:37–42, July 1985   6–18

Regular moderate alcohol consumption has been associated with increased blood pressure, but the mechanism of this pressor effect is uncertain. The elevated plasma renin activity (PRA) in moderate drinkers suggests that the renin-angiotensin system may be involved. The acute effects of alcohol ingestion on renin secretion were studied in 20 normal males

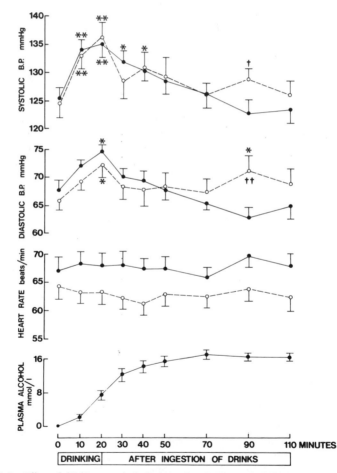

Fig 6–2.—Effect of drinking nonalcoholic beer (O--O) or nonalcoholic beer with alcohol added (●——●) on systolic and diastolic blood pressure (B.P.), heart rate, and plasma alcohol concentration in 20 men. Differences were significant between the treatment groups: †, $P < .05$; ††, $P < .01$. The significance of difference within the treatment groups from values at 0 minutes: *, $P < .05$; **, $P < .01$. (Courtesy of Puddey, I.B., et al.: J. Clin. Endocrinol. Metab. 61:37–42, July 1985. Copyright by the Endocrine Society.)

aged 20–24 years who were mild to moderate drinkers and did not smoke. Studies were done at least 5 days apart using beer, both nonalcoholic and with ethanol, 1 ml/kg, added.

The PRA rose significantly 70 minutes after alcohol ingestion and was about double the baseline value at 110 minutes. The fall in the plasma epinephrine concentration seen in control studies did not occur after alcohol ingestion, and the rise in the plasma norepinephrine level was blunted. A 30% greater diuresis occurred after alcohol ingestion. Potassium excretion was reduced, but sodium excretion was similar in the control and alcohol studies. The plasma glucose level rose significantly in both studies. A later fall in diastolic blood pressure was seen after alcohol ingestion (Fig 6–2). Heart rates were consistently higher in the alcohol study.

Alcohol ingestion produced acute stimulation of renin secretion at a peak plasma alcohol level of 17 mM/L in these normal males. Contributing factors may include an acute fall in the plasma potassium level, plasma volume contraction after diuresis, or a fall in diastolic blood pressure. A direct effect of alcohol on the juxtaglomerular cell or on neuronal control of renin release remains possible, but it is unlikely that repeated activation of the renin-angiotensin system mediates the pressor effect of regular moderate alcohol consumption.

▶ There is substantial evidence that moderate to high levels of alcohol consumption are associated with increased blood pressure. This study is an attempt to explain the acute rise in blood pressure that occurs with alcohol consumption. The authors did not believe that the increase in plasma renin activity was responsible, although plasma renin activity went up slowly some time after the acute pressor rise. Plasma norepinephrine levels correlated somewhat better with the acute rise in blood pressure, but the rise was seen also in the control population.

Alcohol is a potent stimulus to the hormonal and cardiovascular system in man. The exact mechanism(s) by which these changes occur are still unknown.—Walter M. Kirkendall, M.D.

The Role of Plasma Osmolality, Angiotensin II and Dopamine in Vasopressin Release in Man

J. J. Morton, J. M. C. Connell, M. J. Hughes, G. C. Inglis, and E. C. H. Wallace (Western Infirmary, Glasgow, Scotland)
Clin. Endocrinol. (Oxf.)23:129–138, August 1985   6–19

The influence of angiotensin II on vasopressin release from the posterior pituitary is uncertain, as is the role of dopamine in vasopressin release. A sensitive, specific radioimmunoassay for arginine vasopressin was used to evaluate the effects of plasma osmolality, angiotensin II, and dopamine in the release of arginine vasopressin (AVP) in 12 normal persons. Studies were done after overnight fasting, some in conjunction with fluid restriction for 24 hours. Sodium restriction for 3–5 days also was carried out, and

6 normal men received a 1-hour infusion of dopamine at a rate of 1 μg/kg/minute.

Water loading lowered plasma AVP levels to below the limit of detectability. The plasma AVP level correlated significantly with both plasma osmolality and the serum sodium level. Receptor thresholds differed substantially among individuals for both osmolality and sodium level. Sodium restriction did not alter the serum sodium level significantly. The circulating angiotensin II activity increased by more than fivefold, but no effect on plasma AVP activity was evident. Dopamine infusion also failed to change the plasma AVP level. Neither intervention altered the blood pressure.

These findings confirm the importance of the osmoregulatory mechanism regulating AVP secretion in man, but no effect of either circulating angiotensin II or dopamine on the resting plasma AVP level was observed. The latter factors would seem to have no significant role in controlling AVP release from the posterior pituitary under physiologic conditions.

▶ This study suggests that if angiotensin II and dopamine have any role in vasopressin release, it is in the nonresting subject under circumstances not measured in their study. I was impressed by the precision of the vasopressin assay and by the extreme sensitivity of vasopressin release to minor changes in serum sodium and osmolality. The authors indicated that an increase in osmolality of 1 mOsm per kilogram will increase the concentration of vasopressin in the plasma 0.12 pmole/L, and increase urine concentration by almost 300 mOsm/kg. The gain in the system is impressive.—Walter M. Kirkendall, M.D.

Direct and Indirect Blood Pressure During Exercise
Paul H. Rasmussen, Bruce A. Staats, David J. Driscoll, Kenneth C. Beck, H. William Bonekat, and W. Dean Wilcox (Mayo Clinic and Found.)
Chest 87:743–748, June 1985   6–20

Modern monitoring equipment was used to compare direct radial artery blood pressure with indirect cuff pressure at rest and on graded exercise in 27 individuals without apparent atherosclerosis or heart disease. The chief indication for testing was dyspnea of unknown origin. The series included 10 females with a mean age of 33 years and 17 males with a mean age of 32 years. The radial artery was catheterized, and simultaneous pressures were obtained by auscultating the brachial artery during cycle ergometer exercise to exhaustion.

Catheter blood pressure measurements generally exceeded cuff measurements both at rest and with exercise. The overall correlation coefficient was greater for systolic pressure than for diastolic pressure (0.84 vs. 0.67). The coefficient of variation was greater for diastolic comparisons, especially during exercise. Systolic catheter and cuff blood pressures increased with the work level, but the catheter-cuff systolic pressure difference declined. Differences in catheter-cuff diastolic pressure did not change as the work level increased.

Both the direct and cuff methods of measuring blood pressure have advantages for making observations during exercise. Normality is best assessed by the indirect method, whereas beat-by-beat trends are best evaluated by direct intra-arterial pressure measurement. It is hazardous to add an "average" catheter-cuff pressure difference to the cuff pressure to obtain an "expected" direct blood pressure.

▶ This is the first article I have seen comparing direct radial artery blood pressure and indirect diastolic pressure taken at rest and during exercise. The indirect diastolic blood pressure measurement was made at the fourth phase, but on occasion, because of indistinctness of sound, the disappearance of sound was used for the diastolic pressure. This might have contributed to the poor correlation between intra-arterial and indirect diastolic blood pressure measurements.

In general, higher pressures were recorded intra-arterially both at rest and during exercise in this relatively young group. One might suspect that the differences during exercise would be even greater in an older population, primarily because of stiffness in the brachial vessels.—Walter M. Kirkendall, M.D.

Arterial Blood Pressure Response to Heavy Resistance Exercise
J. D. MacDougall, D. Tuxen, D. G. Sale, J. R. Moroz, and J. R. Sutton (McMaster Univ.)
J. Appl. Physiol. 58:785–790, March 1985   6–21

Marked blood pressure elevation has been associated with submaximal static exercise. Blood pressure changes during maximal dynamic contractions were studied in experienced body builders during a typical weight-training session. Five healthy men aged 22–28 years participated. Blood pressure was recorded by a capacitance transducer connected with a brachial artery catheter. The single-arm curl, overhead press, and double-leg and single-leg presses were performed to failure at 80%, 90%, 95%, and 100% of maximum.

Extreme elevation of both systolic and diastolic blood pressure occurred at initiation of each lift and persisted for the 2–3 seconds needed for the lift. A rapid fall toward baseline accompanied lowering of the weight. Higher pressures occurred with repetitions. Mean peak pressures with different exercises are shown in Figure 6–3. Obvious Valsalva maneuvers were not performed in most instances, and mouth pressures never exceeded 70 mm Hg. A purposeful Valsalva maneuver producing a mean mouth pressure of 130 mm Hg led to a mean blood pressure elevation from 135/90 to 190/170 mm Hg.

Lifting heavy weights can produce a fourfold rise in systolic and diastolic blood pressure. Mechanical compression of blood vessels with each contraction apparently combines with a potent pressor response and a Valsalva response to produce these extreme pressure elevations, even when a relatively small muscle mass is used. Few injuries are known to have resulted

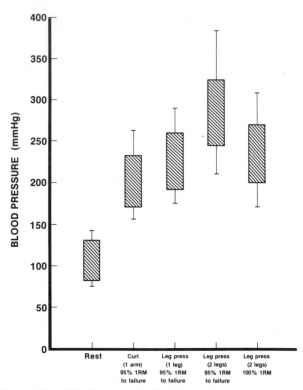

Fig 6–3.—Mean ± SD peak blood pressure for all individuals during performance of various exercises at 95% and 100% of their single maximum lift (1 RM). (Courtesy of MacDougall, J.D., et al.: J. Appl. Physiol. 58:785–790, March 1985.)

from excessive elevations in blood pressure in weight lifters, although brain stem ischemia and subarachnoid hemorrhage have occurred.

▶ The striking increase in blood pressure seen with weight lifting and similar muscle training was recorded with intra-arterial monitors. The authors have considered the mechanisms by which these rises in blood pressure occur. They believe that the blood pressure rises are largely the result of contraction of muscle mass and body tissue supplemented by force from a submaximal Valsalva maneuver.

Of greater interest is why these extraordinarily high pressures don't cause acute vascular damage. Other studies (Hamilton et al.: *Am. J. Physiol.* 141:40–50, 1944) have demonstrated that similar rises in pressure are immediately transferred to the cerebrospinal fluid as well. It is possible that by reducing transmural pressure across cerebral vessels, the enormous intra-arterial rises are blunted. Nevertheless, one wonders whether such pressures may contribute to blood vessel rupture and, particularly, lesions such as Charcot-Bouchard aneurisms.—Walter M. Kirkendall, M.D.

Renovascular Hypertension

Osler's Maneuver and Pseudohypertension

Franz H. Messerli, Hector O. Ventura, and Celso Amodeo (Ochsner Clinic and Alton Ochsner Med. Found., New Orleans)
N. Engl. J. Med. 312:1548–1551, June 13, 1985   6–22

Osler described a condition of "pseudohypertension" in which cuff pressure is inappropriately high compared with intra-arterial pressure due to excessive athcromatosis. A higher cuff pressure presumably is necessary to compress a sclerotic, calcified vessel. Discrepancies as great as 64 mm Hg have been found in elderly patients. Consequent overestimates of arterial pressure can have important clinical implications. Osler's maneuver, performed by assessing the palpability of the pulseless radial or brachial artery distal to a point of occlusion, was conducted in 24 hypertensive patients older than age 65 years. A clearly palpable artery that was pulseless was considered to be Osler positive. Hypertension was designated when cuff readings were consistently higher than 160/95 mm Hg.

Average cuff pressures were consistently higher in the 13 Osler-positive patients than in the 11 negative patients. Differences in the former between cuff and intra-arterial pressures ranged from 10 to 54 mm Hg and averaged more than 15 mm Hg for both systolic and diastolic readings. Intra-arterial systolic pressure exceeded cuff systolic pressure in 2 Osler-positive patients. Indices of arterial compliance were lower in the Osler-positive patients. Systemic hemodynamics were comparable in the two patient groups. The difference between mean cuff and intra-arterial systolic pressures correlated well with the pulse wave velocity in all patients, and diastolic correlation was also evident.

Reduced arterial compliance in pseudohypertension appears to result from risk factors other than arterial pressure. Osler's maneuver can be used to distinguish true hypertension from pseudohypertension, but the presence of the latter does not rule out true hypertension.

▶ The possibility of "pseudohypertension," particularly in older patients, is a clinical worry. Intra-arterial blood pressure measurements are clearly inappropriate in an outpatient setting because they are invasive, expensive, and impractical in most clinics involved in the care of older patients.

Osler's maneuver as described in this article is an interesting attempt to identify those patients with pseudohypertension. The technique may be quite good in the hands of the authors of this report, but my own observations suggest that there should be a more objective way of measuring palpability of the pulseless radial or brachial artery. Once an objective method is found and quantitated, it may be much easier to classify these individuals and to test the hypothesis. Osler's maneuver may be capable of identifying the patient with abnormally high indirect blood pressure measurements.—Walter M. Kirkendall, M.D.

Neural Circulatory Control in the Hyperdynamic Circulatory State Syndrome

David S. Goldstein and Harry R. Keiser (Natl. Heart, Lung, and Blood Inst., Bethesda, Md.)

Am. Heart J. 109:387–390, February 1985   6–23

Patients with hyperdynamic circulatory state syndrome exhibit tachycardia at rest, labile hypertension, and an accentuated tachycardiac response to isoproterenol, with marked amelioration by propranolol. In one male patient there was evidence of altered neural control that was not attributable to an abnormal response to β-adrenoceptors.

Man, 22, had had episodes of "pounding" of the heart, flushing of the neck and chest, palmar sweating, tremulousness, and marked hypertension and tachycardia, both spontaneously and with threatening environmental situations. Blood pressure ranged from 125/70 to more than 170/100 mm Hg at rest, and the pulse rate varied from below 60 to 130 beats/minute. The resting cardiac index, measured on 4 different days, averaged 4.4 L/minute/sq m, compared with an age-controlled mean of 2.5 L/minute/sq m. A hyperdynamic apical impulse and a 3/6 systolic ejection murmur were noted. Pheochromocytoma was ruled out.

The venous plasma level of norepinephrine was 528 pg/ml. Averaged baroreflex-cardiac sensitivity was low. Intravenous administration of diazepam to the point of sedation decreased the level of venous norepinephrine and improved baroreflex-cardiac sensitivity. An excessive rise in systolic pressure followed administration of phenylephrine. Heart rate responses to isoproterenol were excessive. Both isoproterenol and yohimbine produced marked anxiety, systolic hypertension, tachycardia, flushing, and tremulousness; diazepam attenuated the response to yohimbine.

This patient had simultaneous parasympathetic inhibition and sympathetic stimulation that were associated with his hypertension and tachycardia. The hyperdynamic circulatory state appears to have been caused by an abnormality of central neural circulatory control, which was most marked during anxiety responses. In some cases of hyperdynamic circulatory state syndrome a functional derangement that involves baroreceptor pathways through the nucleus tractus solitarius of the medulla may produce simultaneous sympathetic arousal and parasympathetic inhibition, thus permitting paroxysmal hypertensive, tachycardiac responses to conditional environmental stimuli.

▶ These authors believe that there is evidence of both sympathetic and parasympathetic impairment in this disorder and that a central lesion is responsible. Because a similar state can be seen in experimental animals after lesions in the nucleus tractus solitarius, the investigators believe that this may be the locus of the problem in patients such as this. With increasingly sophisticated diagnostic tools such as positron emission tomography and magnetic resonance, we soon may be able to test, by visual means, for lesions in the nucleus solitarius tract.—Walter M. Kirkendall, M.D.

Renal Artery Angioplasty: Technical Considerations and Results
S. Kadir, R. Patterson Russell, S. L. Kaufman, G. Melville Williams, J. F. Burdick, R. I. White, Jr., and Karen Soya-Grimm (Johns Hopkins Med. Inst.)
Fortschr. Geb. Rontgenstr. Nuklearmed. Erganzungsband 141:378–383, October 1985   6–24

Nonoperative management of renovascular hypertension by percutaneous transluminal angioplasty (PTA) offers an alternative to surgery in selected cases. Between November 1978 and April 1982 PTA was attempted in 34 patients with 38 affected renal arteries. Two patients had bilateral procedures, and 2 had repeat procedures. Mean age of the 21 female and 13 male subjects was 44 years. Thirty-one patients had hypertension that was refractory to medical treatment. Three patients were treated to preserve or restore renal function. Heparin was given intra-arterially during the procedure. The femoral approach was used in 27 patients and the axillary approach was used in 7. Angioplasty was performed with a 5F or 7F catheter. Both polyvinyl chloride and polyethylene balloon catheters were used.

Angioplasty was technically successful in 32 of 38 (84%) attempts. Five patients required renovascular bypass surgery. Twenty-four patients with 26 lesions were followed up for a mean of 15 months. Hypertension was cured in 5 patients, and 15 others had lasting improvement. Four patients had recurrent symptoms. Mean diastolic brachial pressure fell significantly from 98 to 84 mm Hg after PTA.

Four patients had major complications, and 3 of them required surgery. There were no procedure-related deaths.

Hypertension was cured or improved in 75% of patients in this series. Most cures were in patients with fibromuscular dysplasia. Patients with atherosclerotic disease were not cured, but 87% had improved blood pressure after PTA. This study showed that relief of a pressure gradient alone will not suffice. An anatomical lumen should be restored by using the 7F catheter system with a larger angioplasty balloon.

▶ We continue to learn more about the technical details of renal artery angioplasty. It clearly is useful in many patients with fibromuscular dysplasia and in some with atherosclerotic renal artery disease. As the procedure has evolved, despite improvement in technique, we still have little comparative information concerning the value of the angioplasty and its dangers relative to other treatment modalities. I fear also that if more data are not obtained concerning the use of this technique, it will be employed inappropriately. It is tempting to use a treatment like this in relatively innocuous renal artery narrowing, which may have no clinical significance. Because of the potential for loss of kidney function or even more severe problems with the use of this procedure, it should be mandatory that the significance of the renal artery lesion be demonstrated to objective observers before the procedure is done.—Walter M. Kirkendall, M.D.

Screening for Renovascular Hypertension: Is Renal Digital-Subtraction Angiography the Preferred Noninvasive Test?

Robert J. Havey, Frank Krumlovsky, Francisco delGreco, and Helen Gartner Martin (Northwestern Univ.)
JAMA 254:388–393, July 19, 1985   6–25

Controversy persists about which noninvasive study, such as radionuclide renography, intravenous pyelography (IVP), or renal digital subtraction angiography (DSA), is preferred in screening for renovascular hypertension. To resolve this controversy, a critical review was undertaken of the available published data concerning the use of these tests in screening for renovascular hypertension.

Radionuclide renograms have been employed to detect renal artery stenosis (RAS) in hypertensive patients for over 2 decades. The newer sequential renal scanning techniques offer higher accuracy than the ^{131}I-iodohippurate sodium renogram. In screening for RAS, the renogram is primarily used in the iodinated contrast-sensitive patient; however, high cost limits its widespread use despite its promising results. The rapid-sequence IVP has been more widely evaluated and carefully scrutinized than any other noninvasive screening test for renovascular hypertension. It is not a perfect test, but when used in conjunction with a careful history and physical examination, it still has a major role in the diagnosis of renovascular hypertension. It has a proved record of safety, is widely available, and is easily interpreted. It provides acceptable levels of sensitivity and specificity when used in selected, moderate- to high-risk patients. In a review of data on 2,040 patients with arteriographically documented RAS, the IVP in hypertensives had a sensitivity of 74.5% and a specificity of 86.2%. Although renal DSA has become the preferred test to detect RSA in many centers, the literature review indicates that it offers no diagnostic advantage over carefully performed and interpreted rapid-sequence IVP. Among 406 hypertensive patients who had both renal DSA and conventional renal arteriograms, the overall sensitivity and specificity of renal DSA were 87.6% and 89.5%, respectively. However, 7.4% of all renal DSAs performed are uninterpretable. Hence, although renal DSA appears to have greater sensitivity, its high rate of technically unsatisfactory examinations lessens or even negates that advantage, eliminating any practical difference between the hypertensive IVP and the renal DSA. Further, renal DSA involves greater invasiveness, greater cost (2.7 times more than IVP), and potentially greater risk of contrast medium-induced renal failure. Overall, the positive and negative predictive values of the IVP are 84% and 77%, respectively, and for DSA, they are 89% and 88%, respectively, but since over 7% of all DSAs provide nondiagnostic information, the actual predictive values of the DSA are lower.

The rapid-sequence IVP remains the preferred noninvasive test in screening for renovascular hypertension.

▶ This study indicates that intravenous pyelography is the preferred screen for renal artery hypertension. Our group has moved in the other direction. Because

7% to 10% of DSAs provide nondiagnostic information, when I am faced with the reasonable possibility that a patient has renal artery stenosis, I suggest renal angiography. Although invasive, the angiogram is diagnostic in a high percentage of instances. It avoids the need for either IVP or DSA. Obviously, it should only be done when a skillful angiographer is available.—Walter M. Kirkendall, M.D.

Therapeutic Effect of Calcium Channel Blockade in Primary Aldosteronism
J. L. Nadler, W. Hsueh, and R. Horton (Univ. of Southern California)
J. Clin. Endocrinol. Metab. 60:896–899, May 1985   6–26

Calcium ion has an important role in aldosterone synthesis and secretion and in the regulation of vascular tone. Extracellular Ca^{2+} is necessary for the effects of both angiotensin II and potassium ion on calcium uptake and flux in zona glomerulosa cells. The effects of nifedipine, a calcium entry blocker, were assessed in ten hypertensive patients (seven women) with a diagnosis of primary aldosteronism, aged 35 to 66 years. Five patients had an aldosterone-producing adenoma, and five had idiopathic hyperaldosteronism. Studies were done with a sublingual dose of 20 mg of nifedipine when patients were taking an 80-mEq sodium, 80- to 100-mEq potassium diet. Six patients then received 30 to 50 mg of nifedipine daily in capsule form and were restudied after 3 to 4 weeks.

Acute nifedipine administration reduced the blood pressure to normal within 1 hour without severe hypotension. The pulse rate did not change significantly. Plasma cortisol, potassium, and the suppressed plasma renin concentrations were unchanged. The plasma aldosterone concentration was markedly reduced by nifedipine in both patient groups. Clinical treatment suppressed plasma aldosterone concentrations. Serum potassium concentrations became normal without supplementation, and the blood pressure remained normal. Side effects were minimal; body weight was unchanged.

Calcium channel blockers may represent a new medical approach to primary aldosteronism. Nifedipine therapy controlled blood pressure and reduced aldosterone concentrations in patients with both idiopathic hyperaldosteronism and aldosterone-producing adenoma in this study. The effects persisted over a month of treatment, and serious side effects did not occur.

▶ This therapy is based on the calcium dependence of angiotensin II and potassium in aldosterone production. Nifedipine has lowered blood pressure in this group of patients and, in addition, lowered plasma aldosterone. It is of interest that improvement was seen in patients with either primary aldosteronism or idiopathic (bilateral hyperplasia) hyperaldosteronism. This is an extremly interesting observation, not only from the standpoint of therapy, but also because it suggests the mechanisms by which these disorders develop.— Walter M. Kirkendall, M.D.

The Sympathetic Nervous System and Hypertension in Primary Aldosteronism

Emmanuel L. Bravo, Robert C. Tarazi, Harriet P. Dustan, and Fetnat M. Fouad (Cleveland Clinic Found.)
Hypertension 7:90–96, January–February 1985   6–27

The sympathetic nervous system has been implicated in the development and maintenance of hypertension that is induced by electrolyte-active steroids. This relationship was examined in 13 women and 11 men with a solitary aldosterone-producing adenoma. Mean age of the 24 was 47 years. Twenty-seven patients with essential hypertension were evaluated for comparison. Neither group had evidence of renal dysfunction or cardiac decompensation. Basal levels of plasma catecholamines and responses to head-up tilt and manipulation of the level of dietary sodium were examined. Seven study patients received propranolol intravenously, and hemodynamic measurements were repeated. Five study patients also received phentolamine by infusion.

Levels of plasma catecholamines were comparable in the two groups of hypertensive patients, as were the responses to head-up tilting. Both groups had significant declines in arterial pressure and volume of plasma on sodium deprivation. Responses to acute β-blockade were similar in patients with aldosteronoma and those with essential hypertension. Combined α- and β-adrenergic blockade reduced mean arterial pressure by 10 mm Hg in study patients.

The sympathetic nervous system has no significant role in maintaining elevated arterial pressure in patients with primary aldosteronism. The findings, along with the known sensitivity of these patients to salt and water depletion, suggest that mineralocorticoid hypertension can be explained by the combined effects of sodium overload and peripheral alteration of membranes. The permeability of altered membrane may lead to abnormal cation turnover, thus enhancing vasoconstriction. An increase in intracellular sodium due to inhibition of the sodium pump can lead to increased levels of intracellular calcium and, in turn, increased vascular tone.

▶ There has been speculation and some experimental evidence to support the concept that the sympathetic nervous system is enhanced in patients with primary aldosteronism. This paper uses direct evidence to refute that view.

Because of evidence from many studies that constriction of resistance and capacitance of vessels in response to norepinephrine is potentiated by treatment with salt-retaining hormones, I had believed that there was a possibility that the sympathetic nervous system did play a role in the hypertension of primary aldosteronism. Indeed, if one accepts the experimental observations, one could hypothesize that evidence of sympathetic activity should be depressed in patients with primary aldosteronism if the sympathetic nervous system is not involved. The experiments in the present investigation tend to negate any major role for the sympathetic nervous system. Phentolamine given in quite adequate doses had very little effect on blood pressure.

On the basis of the authors' idea of mechanisms for blood pressure elevation in primary aldosteronism, calcium channel blocking agents might be uniquely effective in lowering the blood pressure in this disorder (see the next digest).— Walter M. Kirkendall, M.D.

Diagnosis and Treatment of Renin-Secreting Tumors: Report of Three Cases

Dominique Baruch, Pierre Corvol, François Alhenc-Gelas, Marie-Anne Dufloux, Tam T. Guyenne, Jean-Claude Gaux, Alain Raynaud, Jean-Marie Brisset, Jean-Marc Duclos, and Joel Menard (Natl. Inst. of Health and Med. Research and St. Joseph's Hosp., Paris)

Hypertension 6:760–766, September–October 1984   6–28

Three cases of renin-secreting renal juxtaglomerular cell tumors were encountered at a hypertension clinic in the past decade. The two women and one man were aged 21 to 69 years. Only 20 such cases have been reported since 1967.

In these three patients severe hypertension was associated with hypokalemia and increased activity of plasma renin and plasma aldosterone. One patient was followed up for 4 years and one was followed up for 5 years without correct diagnosis before surgery. Renin blockade by β-blockers and angiotensin II antagonists was unreliable, and measurements of venous renin failed to adequately localize the tumor. Direct radioimmunoassay showed total plasma renin was markedly elevated. Renal arteriography showed an avascular area that corresponded to the tumor in all three cases. All three patients were cured of hypertension and hypokalemia after removal of the tumor.

Diagnostic failure may help explain the seeming rarity of juxtaglomerular cell tumors. The many factors which influence the secretion of renin by these tumors make the results of studies that involve pharmacologic blockade unreliable.

The tumors in the present cases were not consistently localized by renal venous sampling. At arteriography oblique views should be obtained, and the study should be repeated if a renin-secreting tumor is strongly suspected. Renin measurement by radioimmunoassay also is helpful in establishing the diagnosis. Attempts to diagnose renin-secreting tumors should be systematically pursued in patients with severe, or even moderate hypertension and apparently unexplained secondary hyperaldosteronism.

▶ These tumors seem to be extremely rare. The appearance of three patients with such tumors in one clinic suggests that some of them may be overlooked. The tumors appear in the context of severe secondary aldosteronism in patients with normal renal arteries. Oblique films of the kidney during radiologic examinations seem to be helpful in finding these relatively small masses. Although renal vein renins should be able to localize the tumor, in this series in only one situation did the renal vein sampling correctly localize the tumor. This could be because of unusual renins produced by the tumor or because of the secretion of large amounts of inactive renin.—Walter M. Kirkendall, M.D.

Pheochromocytoma: Diagnosis, Localization and Management
Emmanuel L. Bravo and Ray W. Gifford, Jr. (Cleveland Clinic Found.)
N. Engl. J. Med. 311:1298–1303, Nov. 15, 1984   6–29

Early diagnosis of pheochromocytoma offers the possibility of curing hypertension and may prevent some deaths. Most patients are symptomatic, some dramatically, and marked fluctuations of blood pressure are a characteristic finding. Most often secretion of urinary catecholamines and catecholamine metabolites is measured, and the diagnosis most often can be confirmed or excluded from a 24-hour urine specimen. The results may, however, be misleading, and the collection process may be difficult.

Both the glucagon stimulation test and a clonidine suppression test have been useful in diagnosing pheochromocytoma. Recent experience with the clonidine test is shown in Figure 6–4. Computed tomography (CT) is the most useful localizing procedure, and it should eliminate the need for angiography in nearly all instances. Selective caval sampling is required only when an extra-adrenal tumor is suspected. Adrenergic tumor can be demonstrated by scintigraphy with ^{131}I-metaiodobenzylguanidine.

Pheochromocytoma is cured by surgical removal, and morbidity can be minimized by volume expansion before operation and generous replacement of the blood that is lost during the procedure. An α-adrenergic blocker

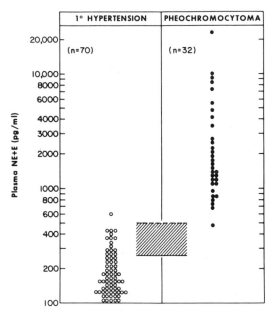

Fig 6–4.—Effect of oral clonidine (0.3 mg) on values of plasma catecholamines in patients with essential hypertension or pheochromocytoma. Values shown represent lowest levels reached (at either 2 or 3 hours) after administration of clonidine. Cross-hatched area represents mean +2 SD of basal values in normotensive control subjects. All but one patient with pheochromocytoma had values above 500 pg/ml after receiving clonidine. One patient with essential hypertension had a value above 500 pg/ml. NE + E, norepinephrine plus epinephrine. (Courtesy of Bravo, E.L., and Gifford, R.W., Jr.: N. Engl. J. Med. 311:1298–1303, Nov. 15, 1984. Reprinted by permission of The New England Journal of Medicine.)

such as phenoxybenzamine or prazosin will help control hypertension and minimize fluctuations in blood pressure during induction of anesthesia and throughout surgery. If the site of tumor is in doubt, however, or multiple tumors are suspected, α-adrenergic blockade should be avoided. Propranolol can be given during surgery if arrhythmia becomes a problem. Hypertensive crises are managed with phentolamine and sodium nitroprusside, and postresection hypotension is managed with extra fluid. Inoperable malignant pheochromocytoma sometimes is radiosensitive. Other patients can be treated by α- or β-adrenergic blockade or by blocking the synthesis of catecholamines with metyrosine.

▶ This is a comprehensive article that provides much valuable information and merits reading. The authors emphasize the specificity and sensitivity of the measurement of plasma catecholamines for the detection of patients with pheochromocytoma. They give valuable information on both the glucagon stimulation and clonidine suppression tests for diagnosing patients with pheochromocytoma.

There is no universal agreement that for diagnosis of pheochromocytoma measurement of plasma catecholamines is superior to 24-hour urine determination of catecholamines and their metabolites. Both methods apparently will detect the vast majority of patients with this condition if they are properly utilized.

The authors do not strongly recommend that α-adrenergic blockade by instituted before operation for pheochromocytoma. In our patients, the use of phenoxybenzamine prior to surgery has been an extremely important measure that has helped prevent the wide blood pressure fluctuations and cardiovascular instability during removal seen before this drug was employed.—Walter M. Kirkendall, M.D.

Extra-Adrenal and Metastatic Pheochromocytoma: The Role of ^{131}I Meta-Iodobenzylguanidine (^{131}I MIBG) in Localization and Management
Norman W. Thompson, Maria D. Allo, Brahm Shapiro, James C. Sisson, and William Beierwaltes (Univ. of Michigan)
World J. Surg. 8:605–611, August 1984   6–30

Experience with the use of ^{131}I-MIBG in scintiscanning to detect pheochromocytomas from June 1980 to August 1983 was reviewed. A total of 353 patients with suspected pheochromocytomas were screened, and 95 proved cases were found in patients aged 9 to 69 years. Eighteen patients had familial disease.

In these studies ^{131}I-MIBG, 0.5 mCi/1.7 sq m (not to exceed a total dose of 0.5 mCi) was used in conjunction with Lugol's iodine. Ten patients with inoperable primary pheochromocytoma or unresectable metastases that showed uptake of activity were given therapeutic doses of ^{131}I-MIBG, with approximately 100 mCi as the initial dose. Presently an initial dose of 200 mCi is used, and most patients have received 2 or 3 doses, with a maximum of 600 mCi.

All but 10 of the 95 pheochromocytomas were visualized by ^{131}I-MIBG scintigraphy. No false positive results were obtained. All but 1 of 19 intra-adrenal sporadic tumors were localized by scintiscanning, as were 15 of 18 extra-adrenal pheochromocytomas; 6 of the 18 were in intra-abdominal sites. Eight of 9 mediastinal tumors were discovered by scintiscanning. Forty-four patients in all had malignant pheochromocytoma.

Five of 10 treated patients showed objective responses to ^{131}I-MIBG, with a decrease in tumor size to less than 50% of baseline or a significant fall in the level of urinary catecholamines, or both.

Scintiscanning with ^{131}I-MIBG is a safe, noninvasive means of diagnosing and localizing pheochromocytomas, and it also may be useful therapeutically. Most extra-adrenal metastatic lesions have been visualized. The specificity and sensitivity of the test make it ideal for total body screening. Cystic lesions may be difficult to visualize. Although MIBG labeled with ^{123}I may visualize some of these lesions, this radionuclide has a short half-life, is more expensive, and is not practical for routine use.

▶ These investigators from the University of Michigan have had extensive experience with the use of the ^{131}I meta-iodobenzylguanidine. This material, like guanethidene, enters edernergic granules and reliably identifies pheochromocytomas and their metastases. The authors have also used the compound as therapy for patients with inoperable primary pheochromocytomas and for the treatment of nonresectable metastases.

It is of considerable interest that the ^{131}I-MIBG scans were not falsely positive in any case. Falsely negative scans occurred in 10% of the 95 patients and were generally associated with cystic lesions.

Because this isotope is picked up in the adrenergic granule and has no effect on receptors, one can continue to administer α-blockers such as phenoxybenzamine while evaluation or treatment with ^{131}I-MIBG is under way.—Walter M. Kirkendall, M.D.

Oncologic Aspects of Pheochromocytoma: The Importance of Follow-up
H. William Scott, Jr., and Susan A. Halter (Vanderbilt Univ.)
Surgery 96:1061–1066, December 1984   6–31

Data on 69 patients with pheochromoyctoma seen between 1950 and 1983 were reviewed. Nine (13%) had malignant lesions. Ten were younger than age 30 years. Five patients had bilateral adrenal tumors, and 17 had extra-adrenal tumors, 1 with an adrenal pheochromocytoma as well. Four patients had multiple endocrine neoplasia type 2. Fifty-eight patients had tumor removal or biopsy, with 1 hospital death (1.7%). Two patients found to have extensive metastases underwent biopsy only. Five patients initially though to have benign lesions were found to have malignancy when recurrent or metastatic disease, or both, developed. Eight of the nine malignancies produced excessive catecholamines. Six of the 9 patients had had symptoms of pheochromocytoma for 3 to 30 years. Five malignancies were of extra-adrenal origin. In most malignant cases initially diagnosed as benign the morphological features were no different from those of most biologically benign pheochromocytomas.

Seventeen patients died during follow-up, 7 of recurrent malignant pheochromocytoma. One other patient died of hypertension and chronic pyelonephritis, and 1 with malignant hypertension died shortly after removal of a small pheochromocytoma. Four deaths were due to other malignancies. The overall incidence of malignancy in the 60 patients with benign pheochromocytoma was 23%. Nine patients (15%) had benign tumors other than pheochromocytoma; the most common was uterine leiomyoma.

Several biologically malignant pheochromocytomas in this series were initially thought to be benign by both the surgeon and the pathologist. Lifetime follow-up of patients with pheochromocytoma is necessary and is the responsibility of the primary operating surgeon.

▶ This study makes the point that if one follows patients with pheochromocytoma for up to 33 years as these investigators did, additional tumors will often be found either associated with the pheochromocytoma or in other tissues. Up to one third of the patients ultimately had a malignant neoplasm.—Walter M. Kirkendall, M.D.

Preoperative Diagnosis of Renovascular Hypertension: The Use of Acute Stimulation of Renin Secretion
Krister Delin, Mattias Aurell, and Göran Granerus (Univ. of Göteborg, Sweden)
Acta Med. Scand. 215:363–369, 1985   6–32

It has not been possible to define the levels of renal venous renin that permit reliable selection of patients with curable renovascular hypertension. Data were reviewed on 25 hypertensive patients with fibromuscular dysplasia (FMD) and 44 with arteriosclerotic (AS) renovascular disease to determine the predictive values of renin tests, including procedures to stimulate release of renin, in the preoperative investigation of these patients. Patients were hospitalized for 4–5 days before study, and drugs that suppress the secretion of renin were withdrawn. Presently, a sodium-restricted diet is given for 3 days.

Patients were stimulated by tilting them 45–60 degrees for 5–20 minutes, by slow-graded hemorrhage of 0.5 L, or by intravenous injection of furosemide or dihydralazine or infusion of trimethaphan to reduce the mean arterial pressure by 25%.

After operation hypertension was cured in 15 patients with FMD, and 3 others were improved. Three patients with AS were cured, and 13 others were improved at follow-up. Eight of 9 patients in the FMD group and 8 of 17 in the AS group who had renal venous renin ratios of 1.5 or above basally were improved after surgery. Nine of 14 with FMD and 7 of 24 with AS who had lower ratios were improved.

After acute stimulation of renin release 18 patients with FMD and 26 with AS had unilateral secretion of renin by the diseased kidneys, and 14 patients in each group were operated on successfully.

Stimulation of renin secretion led to a correct preoperative diagnosis in more than one third of the patients who were operated on successfully in this study. The predictive value of a negative test increased from 0.58 to 0.80. The findings support inappropriate activity of the renin-angiotensin system as a major factor in causing renovascular hypertension in man.

▶ The value of this paper is that it records a fairly large experience with patients with renal artery stenosis. The authors also demonstrate the usefulness of stimulating renal secretion when renal vein renin studies are done. Such stimulation is done in many clinics in this country, and the value of the maneuver has been commented on in several articles.

Although measurement of renal vein renins is an important maneuver in determining the significance of a renal artery lesion, results even with stimulation of renin do not always correctly predict operative success. Other factors must be considered before the decision to operate is made. These include, but are not limited to, the appearance of the lesion, the degree of poststenotic dilatation, the reduction in kidney mass, the hyperconcentration of contrast material on the involved side, and the appearance of collateral vessels to the kidney.—Walter M. Kirkendall, M.D.

Clinical Hypertension

MRC Trial of Treatment of Mild Hypertension: Principal Results
Medical Research Council Working Party
Br. Med. J. 291:97–104, July 13, 1985   6–33

In all, 17,354 patients with phase V diastolic pressures of 90–109 mm Hg were entered into a trial comparing bendrofluazide and propranolol. The single-blind study included men and women aged 35–64 years and accumulated more than 85,500 patient-years of observation. Daily doses of bendrofluazide, 10 mg, and propranolol, 240 mg, were given. The target diastolic pressure of less than 90 mm Hg was to be reached within 6 months of entry into the study.

The average blood pressure fell after entry into the trial in all treatment groups (Figs 6–5 through 6–8). The average postentry pressure was lower in bendrofluazide-treated patients than in the propranolol-treated group. In the latter group, pressure control was less evident in older patients. The stroke rate was reduced with active treatment, but overall rates of coronary events did not change significantly. Rates of all cardiovascular events were reduced with active treatment. Mortality from all causes was comparable in treated patients and in those given placebo. Mortality was reduced in actively treated men, but increased in treated women. Rates of coronary events and all cardiovascular events were reduced in nonsmokers taking propranolol. This difference from results with bendrofluazide therapy was sigificant.

Treatment of mild hypertension reduced the stroke rate, but did not

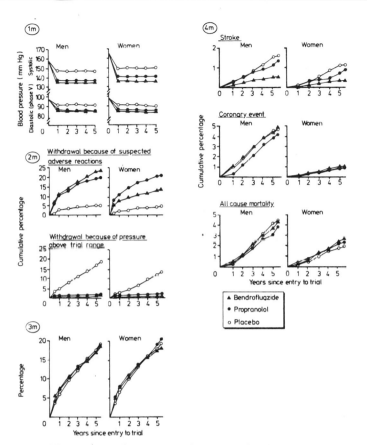

Fig 6–5 (upper left).—Mean blood pressure levels by gender and randomized treatment group.
Fig 6–6 (middle left).—Cumulative percentages of patients withdrawn from randomized treatment.
Fig 6–7 (bottom left).—Cumulative rates of patients lapsing from follow-up examination.
Fig 6–8 (right).—Cumulative percentages of patients with terminating events (stroke, coronary events, and all causes of mortality) by gender and randomized treatment group.
(Courtesy of the Medical Research Council Working Party: Br. Med. J. 291:97–104, July 13, 1985.)

seem to save lives or substantially alter the overall risk of coronary heart disease in this large trial. Bendrofluazide therapy may have been superior to propranolol therapy in preventing stroke, but the β-blocker may have prevented coronary events in nonsmoking patients. Nonsmokers had lower rates of all events than smokers had, and the difference in rates between smokers and nonsmokers was greater than the effect of drug treatment for stroke and for all cardiovascular events.

▶ These results have been long awaited. Over 17,000 patients were recruited over a 9-year period from 1973 to 1982. Population was largely from 176 general practice group practices distributed throughout England, Scotland, and Wales. The follow-up period was 5½ years. Our short summary of this paper cannot do justice to the mass of information it provides. Those interested in the treatment of mild hypertension should read this article not only to appreciate the results, but also to understand the problems in the design and execution of the trial.

In short, active treatment for hypertension was associated with reduction in stroke rate, but there was no clear overall effect on the incidence of coronary events. Active treatment had no effect on overall cause for mortality, but there was a beneficial effect in men and an adverse effect in women. Eleven hundred patients randomized to placebo treatment and 76 randomized to active drug treatment developed blood pressure above the diastolic range of 110 mm Hg. The patients were removed from the study and received active treatment.

Interestingly, there was no difference in cardiac mortality among patients treated with a diuretic or with the β-blocker. In a subgroup analysis, the authors stated that there was no firm evidence of an association between benzochlorothiazide and coronary death.

This study is unique because of the size and because some 190 locations were involved. Although it was placebo controlled, it was "single blinded" since the physician was aware of the treatment given. These factors may have been responsible for the relatively low morbid event rate, although the morbid event rates were similar to those seen in the Australian National Blood Pressure Trial. They were much lower, however, than in comparable patients observed in the Hypertension Detection and Follow-up Program carried out in the United States.

Direct treatment seems to be clearly beneficial among hypertensive men in this population, diuretic therapy being perhaps the more effective. In women, overall mortality was greater in drug-treated patients than in placebo-treated ones, although the numbers were small. The dangers to hypertensive patients who smoke were clearly defined.

Many interesting bits of additional information should be available when the data are subjected to closer scrutiny.—Walter M. Kirkendall, M.D.

Orthostatic Hypertension: Pathogenetic Studies
David H. P. Streeten, J. Howland Auchincloss, Jr., Gunnar H. Anderson, Jr., Robert L. Richardson, F. Deaver Thomas, and Jeffrey W. Miller (State Univ. of New York Upstate Med. Ctr., Syracuse)
Hypertension 7:196–203, March–April 1985   6–34

Diastolic hypertension on standing only was observed in 181 of 1,800 untreated referred patients. The diastolic criterion was 90 mm Hg. Initial studies of these patients indicated excessive orthostatic tachycardia and bluish discoloration of the legs on standing. The patients were intolerant of diuretic therapy. The possible role of excessive orthostatic pooling of blood was evaluated in 12 patients with orthostatic hypertension (table), 3 with persistent hypertension while recumbent, and 8 normotensive healthy controls. Pressure suit studies were preformed using medical antishock trousers. Intravascuar blood pooling was assessed with sodium pertechnetate-labeled blood cells.

The rise in diastolic pressure on standing was attenuated or almost

BLOOD PRESSURES AND HEART RATES IN PATIENTS
WITH ORTHOSTATIC HYPERTENSION

Patient	Sex	Age	Blood pressure (mm Hg)		Heart rate (beats/min)	
			Recumbent	Standing	Recumbent	Standing
1	F	37	106/80	108/92	84	102
2	F	70	134/72	164/106	88	92
3	F	53	128/74	130/102	76	144
4	F	36	118/80	122/108	68	112
5	F	46	144/76	132/102	56	68
6	F	27	132/88	142/100	66	124
7	F	56	162/88	158/104	104	120
8	M	18	134/78	130/106	92	124
9	M	48	148/86	160/118	52	68
10	M	33	124/80	122/118	88	116
11	M	36	134/90	128/104	64	104
12	M	34	128/82	142/102	64	88
Mean		41.2	133/81	137/105	68	105
SEM		—	4.0/1.6	4.7/2.0	7.1	6.4

(Courtesy of Streeten, D.H.P., et al.: Hypertension 7:196–203, March–
April 1985. By permission of the American Heart Association, Inc.)

eliminated by inflation of the pressure suit. The orthostatic reduction in cardiac output was more marked in patients with orthostatic hypertension than in the normal controls. The decline was less marked during pressure suit inflation. The orthostatic increase in intravascular pooling was significantly greater in study patients than in the normotensive controls. End-diastolic volume of the left ventricle declined more with orthostasis in the study patients. Standing, but not handgrip exercise, was associated with higher plasma norepinephrine levels in patients with orthostatic hypertension.

An orthostatic rise in diastolic blood pressure is associated with excessive venous pooling of blood in patients with orthostatic hypertension. Cardiac filling is reduced, stimulating a vigorous sympathetic discharge via the low-pressure cardiopulmonary receptors. Abnormally intense arteriolar constriction results, raising the diastolic blood pressure to more than 90 mm Hg in the upright position.

▶ The phenomenon of an increase in blood pressure with standing has long been known but has been inadequately studied. Streeten and associates' observations are of interest. This study suggests that the capacitance system is unusually distensible in this group, which implies that the disease should occur in younger hypertensives who have not achieved the stiffness of veins seen among older patients with high blood pressure. As the investigators indicate, there are a number of other possibilities for this reflex increase in blood pressure. I agree with them that the trigger, based on present evidence, is likely to be the patulous and poorly reactive venous system.—Walter M. Kirkendall, M.D.

Is Calcium More Important Than Sodium in the Pathogenesis of Essential Hypertension?
David A. McCarron (Oregon Health Sciences Univ.)
Hypertension 7:607–627, July–August 1985   6–35

Many workers remain skeptical as to whether sodium or a defect in sodium balance is the chief factor in essential hypertension. Data have accumulated rapidly suggesting that calcium may be an equally important factor. Biochemical and organ defects related to calcium metabolism have been associated with high blood pressure in human beings. In hypertensive persons, various defects in cellular calcium concentration, membrane binding, and transport kinetics are present in blood cells and adipocytes. Results of studies in experimental animals have been consistent with clinical observations. Recent investigations have questioned a relationship between sodium ingestion and development of high blood pressure in experimental models of essential hypertension. Well-designed trials of sodium restriction have brought into question the efficacy of lowering sodium intake to improve blood pressure control or prevent the emergence of high blood pressure in persons at increased risk.

A shift toward less calcium bound to calmodulin could occur on the basis of either available dietary calcium or altered binding affinity of calcium for its sites on calmodulin. This shift would reduce the activity of those intracellular processes that maintain total cellular calcium at some optimal higher level. Membrane leakiness to both sodium and calcium could follow, with increased intracellular sodium and calcium, reduced sarcoplasmic reticulum uptake of calcium, reduced endogenous cyclic adenosine monophosphate, and reduced Na,K-adenosine triphosphatase. Further work is needed to clarify any role for altered calcium homeostasis in the pathogenesis of human hypertension.

▶ Dr. McCarron's paper is one of two articles on the current subject that appeared in the July–August 1985 issue of *Hypertension*. The other is by Dr. Graham A. MacGregor on the topic "Sodium Is More Important Than Calcium in Essential Hypertension." Together the two articles summarize the issues as seen by these two proponents. They both represent scholarly opinions on the situation at the time of the presentations. They are well worth reading.

My view is that the calcium hypothesis is flawed by its reliance on information from the National Health and Nutritional Examination Survey of 1971 to 1974. Feinleib et al.'s (*Science* 226:384–386, 1984) analysis of the same data failed to duplicate McCarron's findings. The considerable speculation concerning absorption, movement of calcium to the metabolic pool of the body, its effect on membranes and intracellular processes, and finally its excretion is so great and the hard data so tenuous concerning the effect of calcium on blood pressure that I am not yet inclined to accept the indirect relationship between calcium consumption and blood pressure.—Walter M. Kirkendall, M.D.

Impaired Reticuloendothelial Function in Patients Treated With Methyldopa

John G. Kelton (McMaster Univ.)
N. Engl. J. Med. 313:596–600, Sept. 5, 1985   6–36

Red blood cell autoantibodies form in about 20% of patients given the antihypertensive drug methyldopa, possibly because of impairment of the ability of lymphocytes to suppress autoantibody formation. It is not clear why most patients with IgG autoantibodies do not have hemolysis. Because antibody-dependent reticuloendothelial function is an important factor in cell clearance, reticuloendothelial function was assessed in 9 patients who took 500–1,500 mg of methyldopa daily for longer than 1 year. The rate of clearance of radio-labeled autologous red blood cells sensitized by anti-D alloantibody was measured using ^{51}Cr-labeled cells. Autologous red blood cells were sensitized with about 2,000–4,000 molecules of IgG per cell.

Five of the 9 study patients had a positive direct antiglobulin test result, but only 1 had laboratory evidence of hemolysis. Reticuloendothelial clearance was impaired in those without hemolysis, but not in the patient with hemolysis. In 4 of the 8 patients without hemolysis significantly impaired clearance curves were found. Methyldopa-induced autoantibody did not prevent sensitization by anti-D alloantibody.

In patients with methyldopa-induced antired blood cell autoantibody, the lack of hemolysis is related to impaired Fc-dependent reticuloendothelial function. Abnormal reticuloendothelial function is also found in patients with normal levels of red blood cell IgG, suggesting that the drug itself is responsible for impaired reticuloendothelial function. It is not likely that this impaired function will have major adverse effects in these patients.

▶ This defect in reticuloendothelial function has not been observed to this time because the reticuloendothelial system and its role in cell clearance have only recently received experimental attention. It seems likely that the absence of hemolysis in patients treated with methyldopa who have a positive direct antiglobulin test may be explained by this impairment in the reticuloendothelial system.

The paper emphasizes once more the fascinating hematologic effects of methyldopa. These effects, along with the potential of methyldopa to cause liver disease on occasion, make it an antihypertensive that must be used with caution.—Walter M. Kirkendall, M.D.

Potassium Supplementation in Hypertensive Patients With Diuretic-Induced Hypokalemia

Norman M. Kaplan, Alfred Carnegie, Philip Raskin, Jo Ann Heller, and Marcia Simmons (Southwestern Med. School)

N. Engl. J. Med. 312:746–749, March 21, 1985   6–37

Animal studies have shown that hypokalemia has variable effects on blood pressure; however, administration of potassium supplements reportedly lowers the blood pressure in normokalemic hypertensive patients. In a randomized, crossover, double-blind study, 16 hypertensive patients who continued to receive a constant dosage of diuretic medication to maintain serum potassium levels below 3.5 mmole/L were given either potassium chloride, 60 mmole/day, or placebo tablets, each for 6 weeks, to determine the effects of potassium supplements on hypokalemic hypertension. Serum potassium determinations were obtained along with blood chemistry studies, lipid profile, and plasma renin and aldosterone determinations at the end of each phase of the study.

Systolic, diastolic, and mean blood pressure significantly fell progressively during the period of potassium supplementation. Mean blood pressure fell by an average of 5.5 mm Hg ($P = .004$), with a fall of at least 4 mm Hg observed in 9 patients (Fig 6–9). Serum and urinary potassium concentrations rose significantly in 15 patients; the correlation between the changes in mean blood pressure and the serum potassium concentration was 0.417 ($P = .11$). The fall in blood pressure was correlated with a fall in plasma renin activity ($r = .568$, $P = .043$), but not with changes in plasma aldosterone levels or other variables.

Short-term potassium supplementation that corrects diuretic-induced hypokalemia in hypertensive patients may cause a significant fall in blood pressure. This reduction may result in part from the fall in renin production; other possible mechanisms include natriuresis, direct neural effects, reduction of peripheral resistance, and antagonism of the effects of natriuretic hormone.

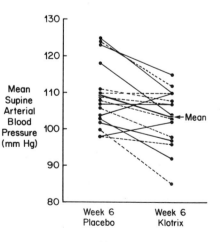

Fig 6–9.—Mean supine arterial blood pressure in each patient after 6 weeks of placebo and 6 weeks of potassium chloride therapy. *Broken lines* indicate patients who took the placebo first, and *solid lines* indicate those who took potassium chloride first. The mean level for all 16 patients is shown as the *heavy line*. (Courtesy of Kaplan, N.M., et al.: N. Engl. J. Med. 312:746–749, March 21, 1985. Reprinted by permission of The New England Journal of Medicine.)

▶ The hypokalemia that regularly develops after diuretic therapy has been a source of much study. There are proponents of the view that modest reductions in potassium after diuretic therapy are not harmful and that potassium replacement is unnecessary in most patients. There are others who believe that the hypokalemia may be responsible for a number of ill effects among diuretics, including the changes in carbohydrate metabolism and the rise in serum cholesterol levels that often accompany diuretic use. The possibility that hypokalemia may, in fact, sustain hypertension is suggested by this study. In normokalemic hypertensive patients, potassium administration has had a spotty record in lowering blood pressure, but the preponderance of evidence suggests that potassium does lower blood pressure to a limited degree.

This study indicates that potassium chloride supplementation lowered blood pressure significantly in at least 9 of the 16 patients observed. The study was a randomized placebo crossover and the consistency of the blood pressure-lowering effect of the potassium chloride was reasonably impressive in this small population. It should be noted, however, that some of the patients continued to have plasma potassium levels below 3.5 mmole/L. There was no observed effect on serum cholesterol, triglycerides, or glucose and insulin levels after oral glucose loading following potassium chloride administration. It would be interesting to know whether the small reductions in blood pressure reported to occur when a potassium-retaining diuretic (such as amiloride and triampterine) is added to hydrochlorothiazide are the result of increasing levels of potassium chloride in the body.—Walter M. Kirkendall, M.D.

Transdermal Clonidine Therapy in Hypertensive Patients: Effects on Office and Ambulatory Recorded Blood Pressure Values
Marie-Denise Schaller, Jürg Nussberger, Bernard Waeber, Marinette Porchet, and Hans R. Brunner (Centre Hospitalier Universitaire Vaudois, Lausanne, Switzerland)

JAMA 253.233–235, Jan. 11, 1985   6–38

A transdermal disk is available that releases clonidine at a constant rate for 1 week, leading to reduced blood pressure in hypertensive patients. This approach was assessed in four men and three women (mean age, 47 years) with uncomplicated essential hypertension. The baseline diastolic pressure with the patient seated exceeded 95 mm Hg. The disk delivers clonidine at a constant rate of 8.8 μg/hour. A second disk was added in five patients in whom diastolic pressure of more than 90 mm Hg persisted.

Blood pressure measured in the outpatient clinic fell from 162/102 to 147/96 mm Hg during 4 weeks of treatment, not a significant change. However, ambulatory pressure profiles indicated a reduction in systolic and diastolic pressures (Fig 6–10), and the overall average diastolic pressure, recorded with a portable recorder, fell significantly. Orthostatic hypotension did not occur, nor did body weight change during the study. Three patients had local skin irritation beneath the disk adhesive, but no patient had to withdraw from the trial because of side effects.

Transdermal clonidine application is an effective means of lowering

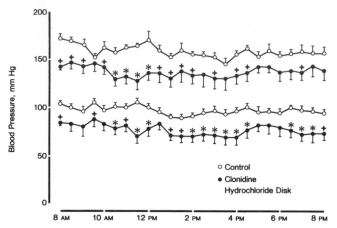

Fig 6–10.—Blood pressure profiles recorded using an ambulatory system before and after 4 weeks of transdermal treatment with clonidine hydrochloride in seven patients. Means are ± SEM. Asterisks indicate $P < .05$; crosses, $P < .01$. (Courtesy of Schaller, M.-D., et al.: JAMA 253:233–235, Jan. 11, 1985. Copyright 1985, American Medical Association.)

blood pressure in hypertensive patients, but localized skin reactions and other side effects may be a problem. Clonidine generally is assumed to reduce sympathetic outflow by activating α_2-adrenoceptors in brain areas involved in cardiovascular homeostasis.

▶ The transdermal application of clonidine has been demonstrated to provide a smooth plasma level of clonidine without the spikes one sees with twice daily oral administration. It has been hoped that clonidine administered in this fashion would cause fewer side effects than under oral administration. Some studies indicate that this is so. It is a particularly good form of the drug to use in patients who have absorptive problems and hypertension, particularly those with rapid bowel transit and diarrhea.

The major problem has been patch irritation, which occurs commonly, and patch sensitivity, which occurs less commonly but is very difficult to counter.—Walter M. Kirkendall, M.D.

Whole-Day BP Monitoring in Ambulatory Normotensive Men
Jan I. M. Drayer, Michael A. Weber, and William J. Hoeger (VA Med. Ctr., Long Beach, Calif., and Univ. of California at Irvine)
Arch. Intern. Med. 145:271–274, February 1985   6–39

A noninvasive, automated, ambulatory blood pressure monitoring system was used in 34 healthy normotensive men with casual pressures of less than 150/95 mm Hg. The men avoided excessive physical activity during the 24-hour monitoring period. Casual blood pressures were recorded in the seated position just before the start of monitoring. The age range was 23–60 years.

Average daytime blood pressures (128 mm Hg) were significantly higher

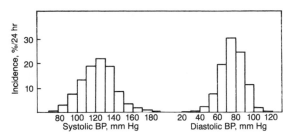

Fig 6–11.—Systolic and diastolic blood pressure readings obtained during 24-hour blood pressure monitoring in 34 healthy normotensive individuals. (Courtesy of Drayer, J.I.M., et al.: Arch. Intern. Med. 145:271–274, February 1985. Copyright 1985, American Medical Association.)

and nighttime pressures (109 mm Hg) were significantly lower than casual blood pressures were, the latter averaging 119 mm Hg. An average of 16% of readings in each tracing indicated a systolic pressure of more than 140 mm Hg (Fig 6–11). More than 25% of these elevations were in 6 men. The average incidence of diastolic pressure of more than 90 mm Hg was 14% in each monitoring period. It exceeded 25% in 6 individuals. Elevated pressures were not age related, but men with a family history of hypertension tended to have more systolic elevations than did those with no such history. Repeated casual pressure measurements after 32 days gave comparable results.

Casual blood pressure measurements in healthy normotensive men can predict the whole-day average blood pressure as well as future casual blood pressure. However, casual blood pressures obtained in hypertensive patients do not reliably predict whole-day average blood pressures.

▶ The investigators demonstrated once more that diurnal variation in blood pressures was similar to that found with invasive 24-hour-a-day monitoring. They also found that the high diastolic pressure for the day was seen early in the morning, while the high systolic pressure was in the afternoon. Additionally, normotensive individuals with a family history of hypertension had slightly higher daytime and nighttime systolic and diastolic blood pressures than did normotensive individuals with no family history of hypertension.

One of the problems in using noninvasive 24-hour-a-day blood pressure monitors has been how to deal with the numerous false measurements, which on occasion can represent 30% of the readings obtained. The authors did not give an estimate of the number of false readings, but they did indicate that their subjects had to have 75% of the readings valid during the 24 hours and that no data were lost for a period longer than 1 hour. They also asked the subjects to refrain from excessive physical activity during monitoring.

Despite the availability of equipment for 24-hour-a-day monitoring and its validation, there is much noise in the system and some difficulty in interpreting the results. In addition, before maximum use can be made of the equipment, we will need to know more about the 24-hour blood pressure in normals and in hypertensives, and we may even have to redefine our criteria for hypertension when such techniques are used. Casual, indirect blood pressure measurements taken precisely, repeatedly, and under the proper conditions are still the gold standard for diagnosis and management of hypertension.—Walter M. Kirkendall, M.D.

Comparison of Weight Reduction With Metoprolol in Treatment of Hypertension in Young Overweight Patients

Stephen W. MacMahon, Graham J. Macdonald, Leah Bernstein, Gavin Andrews, and Ralph B. Blacket (Prince Henry Hosp. and Univ. of New South Wales, Sydney, Australia)
Lancet 1:1233–1236, June 1, 1985   6–40

The effects of weight reduction and metoprolol therapy on blood pressure and plasma lipid levels were compared in a randomized trial in 56 overweight patients less than 55 years of age who had diastolic blood pressures of 90–109 mm Hg. Individualized dietary programs were prescribed to reduce the caloric intake by 1,000 calories daily. Metoprolol was given in a dose of 100 mg twice daily. Results in the patients were compared with those in a group given placebo in a double-blind design.

Weight declined by 7 kg on average in the weight-reduction group and rose slightly in the other groups. Body mass index decreased from 32.6 to

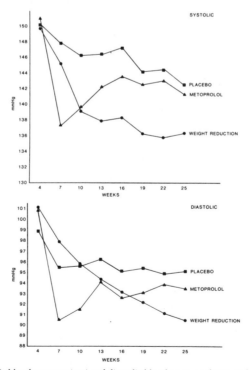

Fig 6–12.—Systolic blood pressure *(top)* and diastolic blood pressure *(bottom)* determined from weeks 4 to 25 in the various study groups. (Courtesy of MacMahon, S.W., et al.: Lancet 1:1233–1236, June 1, 1985.)

30.1 in the weight-reduction group. Systolic blood pressure fell significantly in all 3 groups during 25 weeks of observation. Diastolic pressure fell significantly only in the weight-reduction and metoprolol-treated groups (Fig 6–12). Changes in blood pressure correlated closely with weight change in the weight-reduction group. The total cholesterol:high-density lipoprotein cholesterol ratio decreased by 11% in the weight-reduction group and increased by 19% in the metoprolol group. The plasma triglyceride value rose by 56% in the metoprolol group.

Weight reduction leads to significant decreases in blood pressure in young overweight hypertensive patients, without occurrence of the adverse effects on plasma levels of lipids and lipoproteins that are seen with some first-line antihypertensive drugs. Whether comparable results can be obtained in community practice remains to be seen. Despite problems of attrition and noncompliance, however, weight reduction is a feasible approach to lowering blood pressure in mildly hypertensive individuals.

▶ This study of relatively young, overweight hypertensive patients is of interest because it extended over 5 months. Seventy percent of the patients randomized to the dietary program were able to adhere to the restrictions and complete the program. Sixty percent of those who lost 5 kg or more had normal blood pressure by the end of the follow-up. Interestingly, the authors did not report that sodium restriction was part of the dietary restriction.

The changes in lipids, which occurred with the various programs, were desirable in the diet restriction group and undesirable in the metoprolol-treated group. In all candor, however, despite the desirability of not worsening cholesterol or triglyceride markers, there is no evidence that these small drug-induced changes in lipids or in their metabolism have affected cardiovascular mortality or morbidity in long-term trials. The possibility that adverse effects will be obtained when HDL cholesterol levels are lowered and LDL cholesterol and triglycerides are elevated by drugs remains a pregnant possibility. Hard evidence is needed on the progression or nonprogression of atherosclerotic disease after treatment with these drugs.—Walter M. Kirkendall, M.D.

The Effect of Antihypertensive Drug Treatment on Mortality In the Presence of Resting Electrocardiographic Abnormalities at Baseline: The HDFT Experience
The Hypertension Detection and Follow-up Program Cooperative Research Group (Natl. Heart, Lung, and Blood Inst., Bethesda, Md.)
Circulation 70:996–1003, December 1984   6–41

The results of the Multiple Risk Factor Intervention Trial (MRFIT) indicated possibly increased mortality in hypertensive patients with abnormalities in the resting ECG. Hypertension Detection and Follow-up Program (HDFP) data were analyzed further to determine whether stepped-care drug therapy is associated with a similar outcome in patients who had a mean baseline diastolic pressure of 90–104 mm Hg and abnormalities in the resting ECG. Of 7,825 HDFP patients, 5,173 met MRFIT eligibility criteria and qualified for comparison with "mild" hypertensive patients in this trial. Resting ECG abnormalities were present in 1,963 patients at baseline.

When resting ECG abnormalities were absent, mortality rates for coronary disease, major cardiovascular diaseases, and all causes were consistently lower with stepped care than in a referred care group, as in the MRFIT. However, patients with abnormalities in the resting ECG also had lower mortality for major cardiovascular disease and all causes when given stepped care, in contrast to the MRFIT findings. For coronary heart disease, mortality was slightly higher with stepped care in whites and in black women. The HDFP patients with resting ECG abnormalities at baseline had higher mortality than occurred in those without such abnormalities.

The HDFP data fail to support the view that intensive diuretic therapy may increase mortality in hypertensive patients with resting ECG abnormalities at baseline. However, the findings do support the provision of optimal medical care, including sustained normalization of blood pressure, for persons with relatively mild hypertension and target organ damage or abnormalities in the ECG.

▶ This is a retrospective analysis of data from the Hypertension Detection and Follow-up Cooperative Program. It examines the same information that caused concern after a retrospective analysis of data in the Multiple Risk Factor Intervention Trial. The HDFP experience does not show an increase in cardiovascular morbidity for patients with resting EKG abnormalities if the patients were treated vigorously in the step-care clinics. This is in contrast to the MRFIT data.

There were other differences between the two trials. More patients in the HDFP study received chlorthalidone as the initial diuretic than in the MRFIT study. In the MRFIT study, the referred group of patients with EKG abnormalities at baseline had a better prognosis for cardiovascular disease than those with a normal EKG at baseline. This unexpected finding was not seen in the HDFP data, which indicated that patients with EKG abnormalities in the referred care group had a larger number of cardiovascular deaths than those with no EKG abnormalities in the same group.

The authors of this report, while recognizing the opportunity for mischief from any drug, come down very solidly on the side of lowering blood pressure in those individuals who are hypertensive by any appropriate means, drug or nondrug. The experience of the HDFP, in general, has supported the treatment of the mild to moderately severe hypertensive with drugs not only from the standpoint of lowering mortality, but also from the standpoint of preventing morbid events, including strokes, myocardial infarctions, and development of left ventricular hypertrophy.—Walter M. Kirkendall, M.D.

Dietary Therapy Slows the Return of Hypertension After Stopping Prolonged Medication
Herbert G. Langford, M. Donald Blaufox, Albert Oberman, C. Morton Hawkins, J. David Curb, Gary R. Cutter, Sylvia Wassertheil-Smoller, Sara Pressel,

Connie Babcock, John D. Abernethy, Jeanne Hotchkiss, and Myra Tyler (Univ. of Mississippi, Albert Einstein College of Medicine, Univ. of Texas at Houston, and Univ. of Alabama at Birmingham)
JAMA 253:657–664, Feb. 1, 1985   6–42

The efficacy of restricting sodium intake and advising weight loss for hypertensive individuals withdrawn from prolonged drug therapy was examined in a series of 496 patients who were normotensive while taking treatment. The patients were entered into the Hypertension Detection and Follow-up Program with a diastolic blood pressure of at least 90 mm Hg. Patients randomized to discontinue drug therapy were withdrawn from medication during a period of 2–8 weeks; they were placed in sodium restriction and weight reduction groups 1–2 weeks after the baseline visit. The goals were to reduce sodium intake to 70 mEq daily while increasing

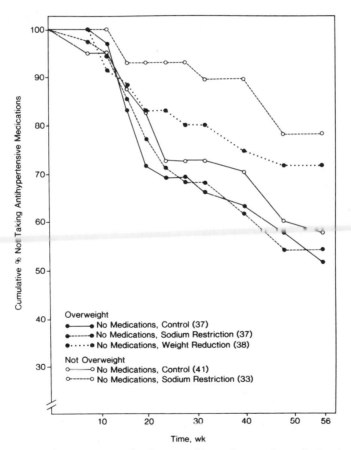

Fig 6–13.—Cumulative percentage of patients not taking antihypertensive medication shown by intervention group. All had mild hypertension. (Courtesy of Langford, H.G., et al.: JAMA 253:657–664, Feb. 1, 1985. Copyright 1985, American Medical Association.)

the potassium intake to 100 mEq daily, and to reduce body weight toward the desirable level, chiefly by reducing caloric consumption.

In overweight individuals, body weight fell by an average of 5%. Both these persons and the nonoverweight, sodium-restricted patients reduced their sodium output. All active intervention groups achieved increased drug-free proportions compared with no-medication controls. The highest success was obtained in the overweight weight-reduction group and the nonoverweight sodium-restriction group. Patients with mild hypertension did better than severely affected patients did in all groups (Fig 6–13). Logistic regression analysis showed that randomization to either the weight loss group, if overweight, or the sodium-restriction group was associated with a greater chance of remaining free of antihypertensive therapy.

Both weight loss and sodium restriction enhance the success of withdrawal from antihypertensive therapy after several years of treatment. Withdrawal should be considered for mildly hypertensive patients who have been controlled with single-drug treatment and are willing to cooperate with dietary modification and to remain under observation.

▶ This study looked at a phenomenon that has been frequently observed, namely, that some hypertensives maintain their normotensive state after stopping antihypertensive drugs. Several points deserve emphasis: (1) All patients had been on antihypertensive medications for many years. (2) The patients were followed and the observations were made for 56 weeks after the study began. (3) Clearly, those individuals who lost weight or reduced their sodium intake did better than their counterparts who did not in terms of maintaining the lowered blood pressure. (4) It is also important to recognize that the more severe the hypertension, the less likely it is that this salutary effect will be seen. (5) The authors emphasize, and I think that this is important, that normotensive individuals who discontinue hypertensive medication after they have had a confirmed diagnosis of hypertension are suspect of developing high blood pressure again. They should be observed on a more frequent schedule than other normotensive persons.

Other nondrug measures were not considered in this study. It is possible that the good results in the weight loss and salt restriction group simply identified patients who had less stressful life-styles or occupations not associated with a high risk of hypertension or some other factor not related to weight or salt.

This study is impressive because 500 patients were involved and were followed closely for a relatively long interval.—Walter M. Kirkendall, M.D.

Hypertension in Pregnancy

Antihypertensive Treatment in Pregnancy: Analysis of Different Responses to Oxprenolol and Methyldopa
E. D. M. Gallery, M. R. Ross, and A. Z. Gyory (Sydney Univ. and Royal North Shore Hosp., St. Leonards, Australia)
Br. Med. J. 291:563–566, Aug. 31, 1985   6–43

Hypertension in pregnancy remains the most frequent medical cause of maternal and perinatal morbidity and mortality; complications are reduced in incidence when hypertension is controlled. A total of 183 hypertensive pregnant women underwent treatment with oxprenolol or methyldopa when the sitting diastolic blood pressure exceeded 90 mm Hg on two occasions at least 24 hours apart, 95 mm Hg on two occasions at least 12 hours apart, or 100 mm Hg on two readings 8 hours apart. Oxprenolol was given to 96 women in an initial dose of 40 mg twice daily, and methyldopa to 87 women in a dose of 250 mg twice daily. To maintain a sitting diastolic pressure of 80 mm Hg, doses were adjusted up to 640 mg of oxprenolol or 3 gm of methyldopa daily. If necessary, hydralazine was added in a starting dose of 12.5 mg twice daily and a maximum dose of 300 mg daily.

Hypertension was adequately controlled in both treatment groups. Hydralazine was required in 35% of the patients, and 7% received all three drugs. Mean birth weights were normal in both groups. Overall, 19% of the infants were admitted to intensive care, usually because of prematurity or asphyxia.

Adequate control of hypertension in pregnancy can allow good fetal growth. Initial treatment with oxprenolol seems reasonable, because hypertension in pregnancy can accelerate in an unpredictable manner. This drug is recommended if there is no maternal contraindication to β-blockade. The long-term effects of treatment probably are similar to those in nonpregnant women, including some relief of vasoconstriction, some retention of salt and water, and plasma volume expansion.

▶ Oxprenolol is a nonselective β-blocker with mild to moderate intrinsic sympathomimetic effect. The authors speculate that the intrinsic sympathomimetic effect may be partially or wholly responsible for the increased birth weight of the babies given this drug for up to 10 weeks. They further speculate that the intrinsic sympathomimetic activity causes vasodilatation to achieve this result. Although this is an attractive hypothesis, there are very few data to support it.

There seems to be little question that lowering blood pressure in pregnant patients with hypertension achieves results that are superior to the previously described natural clinical course of this common complication of pregnancy. The evidence now supports the contention that β-blockers, particularly atenolol, oxprenolol, and probably a variety of others including labetolol, are safe and effective drugs to use at this critical time. To date, the Food and Drug Administration has not approved any of these agents for this indication. Methyldopa and hydralazine continue to be antihypertensive drugs commonly employed for pregnant patients in the United States.—Walter M. Kirkendall, M.D.

First Year of Life After the Use of Atenolol in Pregnancy Associated Hypertension

B. Reynolds, L. Butters, J. Evans, T. Adams, and P. C. Rubin (Stobhill Gen. Hosp., Glasgow, Scotland)
Arch. Dis. Child. 59:1061–1063, November 1984   6–44

There has been concern over adverse fetal and neonatal effects of β-blockers when used to treat hypertension in pregnancy. A placebo-controlled study of atenolol was carried out in 120 women with hypertension in the last trimester of pregnancy; pediatric follow-up observation was made to age 1 year. The patients, with blood pressures of 140–170/90–110 mm Hg, received atenolol in a peak dose of 200 mg daily. The average duration of treatment was 5 weeks. No other antihypertensive medication was prescribed.

There were no major congenital malformations. Respiratory distress syndrome requiring ventilation occurred in six infants born to women given placebo. All children in the atenolol group were graded normal on the Denver development screening test at all stages of follow-up examination. Three infants born to women in the placebo group had subnormal scores. Two were graded "doubtful" at age 8 months, but later were "normal," whereas the third infant was definitely abnormal and had spastic quadriparesis with severe pseudobulbar palsy.

These findings emphasize the importance of good blood pressure control in women who are hypertensive in pregnancy. The use of β-blockers in the last trimester is not likely to be associated with major fetal, neonatal, or pediatric side effects. Premature labor was the most prominent single factor in morbidity in the present series. It is not likely that a β_1-antagonist (e.g., atenolol) would directly influence uterine motility; poor blood pressure control probably was responsible for premature labor.

▶ Prospective, placebo-controlled studies of drug treatment of hypertension in pregnancy are as scarce as hen's teeth. Additionally, it is reassuring to have information concerning the babies for the first year after delivery.

The authors make a strong case for the control of hypertension during the last 3 months of pregnancy. All six babies requiring ventilation were born to mothers in the placebo group, who presumably had poorer blood pressure control than in the atenolol-treated population.—Walter M. Kirkendall, M.D.

Pregnancy in Women With Renal Disease and Moderate Renal Insufficiency
Susan H. Hou, Susan D. Grossman, and Nicolaos E. Madias (St. Margaret's Hosp. for Women, Dorchester, Mass.; Tufts Univ.; New Jersey Med. College; and College Hosp., Newark)
Am. J. Med. 78:185–194, February 1985   6–45

The overall impact of pregnancy on the course of renal disease remains uncertain. Data were reviewed concerning 25 pregnancies in 23 women having a prepregnancy serum creatinine level of at least 1.4 mg/dl. Pregnancies terminated by first-trimester abortion were excluded. Twelve women had primary glomerular disorders, 5 had interstitial diseases, and 6 had other renal diseases.

Seven women (30%) had a pregnancy-related decline in renal function. In one patient end-stage renal failure developed in the third trimester of pregnancy. Six women had primary glomerular diseases. None was severely hypertensive at the time of conception. Ten other women had a decline in renal function consistent with the natural course of renal disease. The rise in the glomerular filtration rate usually noted in pregnancy generally was not observed in these patients. Hypertension developed or worsened during pregnancy in 14 instances. Nine women had a diastolic pressure of at least 110 mm Hg in the third trimester. No women died, and 92% of pregnancies resulted in live births. Most of the life births were premature, often because of induction or section delivery. Two infants had congenital anomalies.

Renal function declines in a substantial number of women with moderate renal insufficiency who become pregnant, but fetal survival is much better than previously reported. Pregnancy may hasten the need for dialysis, especially in women with glomerular disease. The risk of prematurity is high, but the chance is good of a healthy infant being delivered. A women whose renal disease is rapidly becoming worse may choose to conceive before severe renal insufficiency develops.

▶ The impressive observation in this study was the very respectable fetal survival rate of 92%. The downside was the belief that the decline in renal function was accelerated in a number of these women. The authors point out that this risk may be acceptable to some patients who live in a society in which people survive for years with renal failure, but the adoption of children is virtually impossible for women with renal disease. This information may help some potential parents define the risks.—Walter M. Kirkendall, M.D.

Hypertension in Pregnancy
Marshall D. Lindheimer and Adrian I. Katz (Univ. of Chicago)
N. Engl. J. Med. 313:675–680, Sept. 12, 1985   6–46

Hypertensive disorders of pregnancy remain a major cause of maternal and fetal morbidity and mortality. Preeclampsia, which complicates up to 10% of all pregnancies, usually occurs in nulliparas near term. Most women with chronic hypertension have essential hypertension, but a few have renal artery stenosis, coarctation, pheochromocytoma, primary aldosteronism, or kidney disease. Some women become hypertensive without proteinuria in the last trimester or immediately after delivery, with a return to normal blood pressure within 10 days of delivery.

Vascular sensitivity is altered in preeclampsia, and the glomerular filtration rate is reduced. The therapeutic implications of the decrement in plasma volume remain uncertain. The genesis of eclamptic seizures remains to be determined. Hospitalization is indicated when preeclampsia is suspected. Induction generally is indicated near term, or if severe hypertension persists despite a trial of antihypertensive drug therapy. Antihypertensive drugs should be avoided if maternal blood pressure is only mildly elevated. Electronic fetal monitoring should be carried out. Hydralazine is administered parenterally when the diastolic pressure is 105 mm Hg or higher;

the use of diazoxide is limited to patients with resistant hypertension. Calcium-channel blockers may be effective. Most physicians do not administer diuretics to hypertensive pregnant patients. Plasma expansion has yielded impressive results, but carries a risk of cerebral or pulmonary edema, especially after delivery.

In patients with chronic hypertension, the fetal prognosis is guarded when the blood pressure does not decline by midpregnancy. Most workers withhold treatment unless the diastolic blood pressure exceeds 75–80 mm Hg in the second trimester, or 85–90 mm Hg in the third trimester. Methyldopa and hydralazine are effective and safe, and β-blockers are being used increasingly in this setting. Captopril therapy should be avoided. Diuretics may be given to patients with refractory disease, especially if the fetus is immature and termination of the pregnancy is the only alternative.

▶ This is an interesting state-of-the-art review concerning diagnosis and management of hypertension in pregnancy. The digest cannot do justice to the concentrated material in the article, and I would advise readers interested in the subject to read the article. The paper is well referenced, and I believe that its conclusions are appropriate.—Walter M. Kirkendall, M.D.

Low-Dose Oral Contraception and Blood Pressure in Women With a Past History of Elevated Blood Pressure
Charles C. Tsai, H. Oliver Williamson, Bonnie H. Kirkland, Judy O. Braun, and Chan F. Lam (Med. Univ. of South Carolina)
Am. J. Obstet. Gynecol. 151:28–32, Jan. 1, 1985   6–47

The dose of sex steroids in an oral contraceptive preparation is an important factor in blood pressure regulation and hypertension. Sixty-one women with a history of elevated blood pressure used a low-dose preparation containing 0.4 mg of norethindrone and 35 μg of ethinyl estradiol for 3–24 months. Seventeen women had hypertension of unknown cause, 17 were preeclamptic, and 27 had hypertension associated with oral contraceptive use. The mean peak past blood pressures were 141 mm Hg systolic and 98 mm Hg diastolic. Sixty-one other women without hypertension were matched with the study participants for age, race, initial weight, and duration of oral contraceptive use.

High-risk women had significantly higher blood pressures before and after oral contraceptive therapy than found in those at low risk, but mean systolic and diastolic blood pressures did not increase in the study group when compared with baseline blood pressures. Hypertension recurred in 5 high-risk women (8%), but blood pressures at the time of drug withdrawal were comparable to past peak pressures. Three of these women previously had hypertension of unknown etiology. No significant body weight changes accompanied treatment.

The renin-angiotensin-aldosterone system has been implicated in oral contraceptive-induced hypertension. Oral contraceptive preparations containing lower amounts of progestogen and estrogen are associated with less elevated blood pressure. The occasional recurrence of elevated blood pressure might be related to decreased feedback suppression of renin release, or to an increased plasma ethinyl estradiol level.

▶ Several studies have suggested that the dosage of sex steroids in oral contraceptive preparations is an important determinant of the elevation of blood pressure and the occurrence of hypertension among users. The majority of the studies have been done in patients with normal blood pressure. This study examines the response of blood pressure in individuals who have had elevated blood pressure from primary hypertension, preeclampsia, or previous oral contraceptive use. Of interest to me was the finding that 2 of the 61 normotensive patients in the control population of this study developed hypertension after 3 and 21 months of use. The observation on these normotensive women plus the elevation of blood pressure in 5 women who had previously had hypertension indicate the need for caution in the use of even this low dosage of steroid combination.

A better understanding of how oral contraceptives occasionally cause hypertension is definitely needed.—Walter M. Kirkendall, M.D.

Serial Plasma Oncotic Pressure Levels and Echoencephalography During and After Delivery in Severe Pre-eclampsia
Michael Zinaman, Jonathan Rubin, and Marshall D. Lindheimer (Univ. of Chicago)
Lancet 1:1245–1247, June 1, 1985   6–48

The reasons that seizures occur in preeclamptic gravidas are not well understood. The reduced plasma level of albumin in these patients suggests that cerebral edema is a factor. The effects of standard parenteral treatment on plasma oncotic pressure were studied in nine nulliparas with severe preeclampsia. Cerebroventricular width was monitored ultrasonographically. The patients, who had a diastolic blood pressure of more than 110 mm Hg and proteinuria of at least 2 +, received 5% dextrose in isosmotic Ringer's lactate during labor, as well as magnesium sulfate and hydralazine. Nine normotensive women matched with the patients for age, race, and parity served as controls.

The average total fluid intake by preeclamptic women from a mean of 16 hours before delivery to a mean of 21 hours afterward was about 7 L. Hourly infusate volumes averaged 191 ml, and the mean hourly output was 142 ml. Oncotic pressure decreased in both hypertensive and normotensive women, but values were consistently and significantly lower in the preeclamptic patients. The average pressure within 16–18 hours post partum was 14 mm Hg, compared with 16 mm Hg in controls. Cerebroventricular widths were comparable in both groups before, during, and after labor.

Plasma oncotic pressure is lower in preeclamptic patients than in normotensive parturients, and falls further during labor. Conventional treatment of severe preeclampsia apparently carries a risk of a dangerous reduction in plasma oncotic pressure, with resultant cerebral swelling or pulmonary edema. The use of intravenously administered crystalloid therapy should be minimized during labor in preeclamptic patients.

Hypotension

Vasopressin Secretion in Progressive Autonomic Failure: Evidence for Defective Afferent Cardiovascular Pathways

T. D. M. Williams, S. L. Lightman, and R. Bannister (Charing Cross and Westminster Med. School, Westminster Hosp., and St. Mary's Hosp., London)
J. Neurol. Neurosurg. Psychiatry 48:225–228, March 1985   6–49

The plasma arginine vasopressin (AVP) response to headup tilt is blunted in patients with progressive autonomic failure with multiple system atrophy. This could result from lesions at sites within ascending neural pathways from cardiovascular stretch receptors in the thorax, or from lesions affecting vasopressin-secreting cells within the hypothalamus. The AVP response to administration of hypertonic saline was examined in six patients with progressive autonomic failure; the three men and three women were aged 55–74 years. Six normal individuals also were studied. The patients had a blocked response to the Valsalva maneuver and marked postural hypotension. Three also had central neurologic features of multiple system atrophy.

Basal AVP levels were appropriate for plasma sodium and osmolality, and levels increased progressively during hypertonic saline infusion in all patients. The plasma sodium level and osmolality also increased. The mean blood pressure rose from 96 mm Hg to 112 mm Hg. Controls also had increases in plasma sodium level, osmolality, and AVP during saline infusion, but no change in mean blood pressure.

These findings suggest that loss of the AVP response to tiling in patients with progressive autonomic failure is secondary to lesions in ascending pathways from cardiovascular receptors. The rise in blood pressure during saline infusion may have been caused in part by increased circulating levels of AVP. There is evidence that a vasopressin-like peptide is present in sympathetic nerves, and a decrease in the peptide may account for increased sensitivity to exogenous vasopressin in patients with progressive autonomic failure.

▶ It has long been known that patients with progressive autonomic failure with multiple-system atrophy (Shy-Drager syndrome) have normal vasopressin levels at rest. This study neatly dissects the fact that patients with this disorder cannot respond with increased vasopressin levels to upright posture. Yet they do respond to intravenous administration of hypertonic saline.

Because of the importance of vasopressin in sustaining the blood pressure under certain circumstances, it is quite likely that the inability of these patients to respond to the upright posture with vasopressin release is important in their orthostatic hypotension. The vasopressin response to head-up tilt can serve as a test for the integrity of ascending cardiovascular neural pathways (Zerberl et al.: *Am. J. Med.* 74:265–271, 1983).—Walter M. Kirkendall, M.D.

Micturition Syncope: A Reappraisal

Wishwa N. Kapoor, Jacqueline R. Peterson, and Michael Karpf (Univ. of Pittsburgh)
JAMA 253:796–798, Feb. 8, 1985 6–50

Micturition syncope occasionally occurs in generally healthy young people who suddenly lose consciousness during or just after urinating in the early morning. Recovery is rapid, and recurrences are rare. A prospective study was made of 33 patients with this disorder, i.e., 8 healthy young persons and 25 older individuals; most of the latter were women. Subjects in the older groups had multiple medical problems and were taking several medications.

Certain predisposing factors (e.g., recent upper respiratory infection or alcohol intake) were identified in half of the younger patients. Nine of the 25 older patients had recurrent episodes, and 21 had micturition syncope after a prolonged period of recumbency or sleep. Orthostatic hypotension was present in all but 3 of the 25 older individuals. Fourteen of these patients had been taking diuretics. Several patients had abnormal ECG results, but these did not define the cause of syncope. In fact, ECG monitoring was diagnostic only in one patient with ventricular tachycardia. Management included blood or fluid administration, increased salt intake, and discontinuance of diuretic therapy. No recurrences developed in either group during a mean follow-up period of 15 months. Withdrawal of diuretic therapy was effective in a patient having more than 100 episodes of micturition syncope.

Most patients in this series were older and female and had multiple underlying illnesses. The mechanism of the disorder is unclear, both in these patients and in healthy young men, although most older patients have orthostatic hypotension. It was suggested that physiologic changes during sleep or micturition may lead to a decline in cerebral blood flow and resultant micturition syncope.

▶ These authors emphasize that the majority of subjects with this disorder were older women. They also demonstrated that the majority had many medical problems and were taking several drugs.

The several young patients who were generally thought to be healthy are the more spectacular victims of micturition syncope. Fortunately, this group generally had only one episode and in the majority of young patients there was no clear precipitating factor, except possibly alcohol consumption and fever.—Walter M. Kirkendall, M.D.

Intra-individual Variability in Postural Blood Pressure in the Elderly

Lewis A. Lipsitz, Helene A. Storch, Kenneth L. Minaker, and John W. Rowe (Hebrew Rehabilitation Ctr., Beth Israel Hosp., Brigham and Women's Hosp., Charles A. Dana Research Inst., Harvard Univ., and West Roxbury/Brockton VA Med. Ctr.)
Clin. Sci. 69:337–341, September 1985 6–51

Advancing age appears to be associated with abnormal blood pressure regulation, especially during postural stress. Up to 30% of persons aged at least 65 years have orthostatic hypotension. Variability in blood pressure and body weight was studied in 19 persons aged 73–98 years (mean age, 87 years) residing in a long-term care facility. They had many chronic physical and cognitive disabilities, but were ambulatory and clinically stable, and were not using cardiovascular drugs. Blood pressures were measured before and after standing on awakening on 12 or 13 days for a period of 2–4 weeks.

Wide day-to-day variation in postural blood pressure responses was noted. The mean postural change in systolic pressure was −3 mm Hg, with a coefficient of variation of 533%. Postural changes in systolic pressure correlated closely with the basal supine systolic blood pressure. A postural pressure decline was associated with a basal systolic pressure of more than 160 mm Hg. Postural change correlated negatively with basal supine systolic pressure in most patients. Body weights remained constant. Only 1 patient had a mean postural decline in systolic pressure exceeding 20 mm Hg, but nearly half of the patients had at least 1 decline of this magnitude during the study period.

Elderly persons with normal basal blood pressure have intact regulation of standing pressure. Postural hypotension is a variable phenomenon related to elevated basal systolic blood pressure. Orthostatic hypotension in the elderly is distinct from idiopathic orthostatic hypotension, which is associated with large daily fluctuations in body weight.

▶ This group of authors has been very active in examining the problems of orthostatic hypotension in older people. They were the first to describe postprandial orthostatic hypotension and have commented on the use of caffeine for treating this problem.

In this study, they emphasize that orthostatic hypotension in this group of patients is a variable phenomenon related to supine hypertension. They postulate that the mechanisms by which hypertension might influence orthostatic hypotension may be the impaired neural reflex sensitivity often seen in the hypertensive, as well as decreases in vascular compliance, and diminution of baroreceptor stretch and relaxation reflexes. The decline in baroreflex sensitivity could be responsible for the extreme lability of blood pressure seen in the elderly.

Clearly, measuring the upright blood pressure in the elderly hypertensive is a very important clinical maneuver.—Walter M. Kirkendall, M.D.

Decreased Sympathetic Neuronal Uptake in Idiopathic Orthostatic Hypotension
Ronald J. Polinsky, David S. Goldstein, Robert T. Brown, Harry R. Keiser, and Irwin J. Kopin (Natl. Inst. of Neurological and Communicative Disorders and Stroke and Natl. Heart, Lung, and Blood Inst., Bethesda, Md.)
Ann. Neurol. 18:48–53, July 1985   6–52

Differences in the disappearance rates of levo-norepinephrine (l-NE) and dextro-norepinephrine (d-NE) reflect stereospecificity in the vesicular uptake or metabolism of NE, whereas isoproterenol is not taken up by sympathetic neurons; thus, neuronal catecholamine uptake can be assessed by comparing the plasma disappearance rates of NE and isoproterenol. Rates of disappearance of intravenously administered l-NE, d-NE, and isoproterenol were determined in 12 normal persons, 6 patients with multiple system atrophy, and 11 with idiopathic orthostatic hypotension. None of the patients had evidence of peripheral neuropathy or signs suggestive of systemic disorder associated with autonomic dysfunction.

The NE isomers were removed at comparable rates in all groups. The NE isomers were cleared more rapidly than isoproterenol was in normal persons, but in patients with idiopathic orthostatic hypertension the initial disappearance of the NE isomers was slower than normal and similar to the rate of isoproterenol disappearance. The plasma NE level and NE clearance were lower in patients with idiopathic orthostatic hypertension than in normal persons. Norepinephrine clearance and the apparent NE secretion rate were normal in patients with multiple system atrophy. In those with orthostatic hypertension IOH, the apparent release rate of NE into plasma from sympathetic neurons was significantly lower than in normal persons.

Reduced clearance of NE accompanies sympathetic neuronal dysfunction in patients with idiopathic orthostatic hypertension, and reduced NE release is likely. In patients with multiple system atrophy NE clearance and apparent secretion are normal, in accord with CNS dysfunction in sympathetic regulation. Neuronal uptake of NE may not be stereoselective in man.

▶ This paper describes an interesting method for gaining information concerning neural uptake for norepinephrine. It is clear from these studies that neuronal uptake in the patients with idiopathic orthostatic hypotension was only one fourth of that with subjects without a deficient neuronal uptake, including those patients with multiple-system atrophy.

Careful studies of the autonomic nervous system and catecholamine metabolism as being carried out by this group are essential to our understanding of orthostatic hypotension. In the past few years, great advances have been made in classifying patients with the various types of orthostatic hypotension. We are not likely to have a good handle on rational treatment until these varieties are well delineated and understood.—Walter M. Kirkendall, M.D.

Hemodynamic and Humoral Effects of Caffeine in Autonomic Failure: Therapeutic Implications for Postprandial Hypotension

Jack Onrot, Michael R. Goldberg, Italo Biaggioni, Alan S. Hollister, Dawn Kincaid, and David Robertson (Vanderbilt Univ.)
N. Engl. J. Med. 313:549–554, Aug. 29, 1985   6–53

Caffeine may raise the blood pressure by blocking vasodilatory aden-

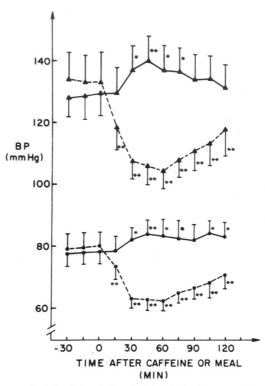

Fig 6–14.—Mean systolic *(triangles)* and diastolic *(circles)* blood pressure after caffeine alone *(solid lines)* and a standardized test meal alone *(dashed lines)* in 12 patients with autonomic failure. Blood pressure (BP) was measured with patients seated. Single and double asterisks denote $P < .05$ and $P < .01$ vs. baseline value; bars represent the SEM. (Courtesy of Onrot, J., et al.: N. Engl. J. Med. 313:549–554, Aug. 29, 1985. Reprinted by permission of The New England Journal of Medicine.)

osine receptors, suggesting its use as a pressor agent in patients with orthostatic hypotension secondary to autonomic failure. Postprandial hypotension in these patients may be related to a meal-induced shift of blood into the splanchnic circuit and a fall in central blood volume; adenosine may be an important mediator of postprandial splanchnic hemodynamics. Twelve consecutive patients with autonomic failure were given 250 mg of caffeine orally, 30 minutes before a standard meal. Five patients received 250 mg of caffeine daily for 7 days in addition to their usual treatment.

Caffeine ingestion raised the blood pressure by 12/6 mm Hg (Fig 6–14). Plasma catecholamine levels and renin activity were unchanged. Pretreatment with caffeine attenuated the blood pressure fall after eating. Caffeine treatment for 1 week continued to limit the vasodepressor response to eating. Changes in heart rate were not significant in either the acute or longer-term studies.

The pressor effect of caffeine is not mediated primarily by elevated sympathetic activity or stimulation of the renin-angiotensin system. Caffeine may prove useful in the management of autonomic failure, especially when taken before meals to attenuate postprandial hypotension. Patients presently are advised to drink two cups of coffee, containing about 200–250 of mg caffeine, with breakfast and abstain from caffeine for the rest of the day.

▶ Caffeine probably works by blocking the vasodilatation from adenosine receptors. This effect on small blood vessels beyond the nerve input makes it feasible to use caffeine in patients with several types of orthostatic hypotension, including those with multiple-system atrophy, idiopathic orthostatic hypotension, and in one patient with a paraneoplastic autonomic failure syndrome. There is no evidence that caffeine's effect is mediated by elevated sympathoadrenal discharge.

Other investigators have shown that tolerance to the pressor effect of caffeine develops with continued intake. There was no change in effectiveness after 7 days of treatment with the 250 mg daily dose used here. The authors believe that abstention for 24 hours when caffeine is used at this dose level may present the development of tolerance.—Walter M. Kirkendall, M.D.

Carotid Sinus Hypersensitivity: Evaluation of the Vasodepressor Component
Adrian Almquist, Charles Gornick, D. Woodrow Benson, Jr., Ann Dunnigan, and David G. Benditt (Univ. of Minnesota)
Circulation 71:927–936, May 1985   6–54

Attempts have failed to prevent recurrent vasodepressor-induced hypotension in patients with carotid sinus hypersensitivity. Both drugs and pacing methods were evaluated in eight men aged 49–84 years who had recurrent syncope of no apparent cause other than carotid sinus hypersensitivity. Carotid sinus massage was repeated on atrioventricular (AV) sequential pacing with an AV interval of 150 msec at a heart rate of 80, and also during muscarinic blockade with atropine and combined muscarinic and β-adrenergic blockade with atropine and propranolol. Studies also were done with norepinephrine infusion and with an oral preparation of ephedrine, the latter in a dose of 75–150 mg daily.

All patients but one had bradycardia induced by carotid sinus massage. Four patients had a unilateral response to sinus massage. Significant vasodepressor responses persisted during AV sequential pacing to maintain a constant heart rate and AV synchrony. Drug effects on the carotid sinus massage-induced vasodepressor response are shown in Figure 6–15. Administration of norepinephrine and ephedrine blunted the systolic pressure decline, but muscarinic and β-adrenergic blockade were ineffective. Two patients remained free of symptoms while taking ephedrine, but another patient had continued symptoms despite ephedrine treatment. Five patients with cardioinhibitory responses as well as vasodepressor responses received dual-chamber pacemakers and continued ephedrine therapy; they were symptom free after 5–18 months.

Mixed vasodepressor and cardioinhibitory responses may be frequent

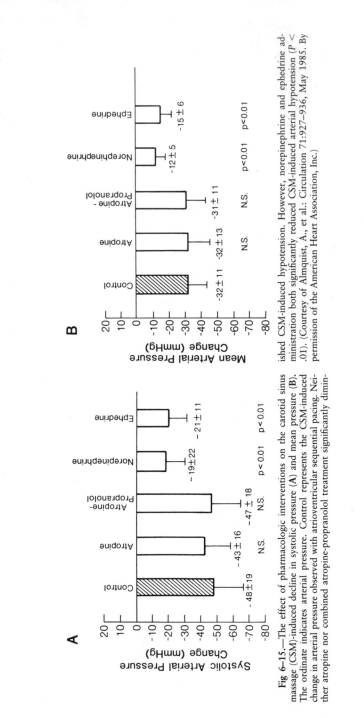

Fig 6-15.—The effect of pharmacologic interventions on the carotid sinus massage (CSM)-induced decline in systolic pressure (**A**) and mean pressure (**B**). The ordinate indicates arterial pressure. Control represents the CSM-induced change in arterial pressure observed with atrioventricular sequential pacing. Neither atropine nor combined atropine-propranolol treatment significantly dimin- ished CSM-induced hypotension. However, norepinephrine and ephedrine ad- ministration both significantly reduced CSM-induced arterial hypotension ($P <$ .01). (Courtesy of Almquist, A., et al.: Circulation 71:927–936, May 1985. By permission of the American Heart Association, Inc.)

in patients with carotid sinus hypersensitivity. Ephedrine taken orally may be a useful adjunct to AV sequential pacing in these patients, but the drug is potentially hazardous in elderly patients and those with underlying coronary artery disease.

▶ Three types of responses have been described in patients with hypersensitive carotid sinus syndromes. First is a cardioinhibitor response in which there is marked sinus bradycardia or transient atrioventricular block resulting in systemic hypotension. This can be prevented or reversed by administration of atropine. The second response is the vasodepressor one in which arterial hypotension occurs without bradycardia. This particular article is chiefly about patients with this form of the disorder. The third type of problem is one in which there is mixed response, with both cardioinhibitory and vasodepressor factors contributing.

The authors present a great deal of information concerning problems in the care of these patients. They give a well-balanced view of the value of drugs and atrioventricular sequential pacing for the treatment of these disorders.— Walter M. Kirkendall, M.D.

Renal Disease

Effect of Captopril on Blood Pressure and Renal Function in Patients With Transplant Renal Artery Stenosis

Fokko J. van der Woude, Willem J. van Son, Adam M. Tegzess, Ab J. M. Donker, Maarten J. H. Slooff, Leendert B. van der Slikke, and Steven J. Hoorntje (State Univ. Hosp., Groningen, The Netherlands)
Nephron 39:184–188, March 1985   6–55

Captopril is widely used to treat hypertension developing after renal transplantation, but captopril-induced renal insufficiency has been described in patients with graft renal artery stenosis. Nine patients with angiographically proved transplant renal artery stenosis were evaluated. All had a reduction of at least 60% in vessel diameter and hypertension, as well as a systolic murmur over the graft. All patients had cadaveric grafts. Three patients had unilateral and two had bilateral nephrectomy before transplantation. Patients initially received a diuretic, a β-blocker, and, with two exceptions, a vasodilator.

Renal function declined markedly in all nine patients when captopril was given. Two patients given acetazolamide as well as captopril became anuric. No patient had evidence of glomerulonephritis after onset of captopril therapy. Surgical reconstruction attempted in five patients, was successful in four. One patient was controlled with metoprolol alone. Another responded to discontinuance of diuretics and an augmented sodium intake.

Captopril therapy can markedly compromise graft function in patients with transplant renal artery stenosis. Detection of such stenoses is especially important in view of the possibility of effective surgical reconstruction.

Captopril may lower blood pressure in these patients, but at the same time may cause functional amputation of part of the renal parenchyma.

▶ This report documents again the reduction in renal function after captopril treatment seen in patients with either bilateral renal artery stenosis or unilateral renal artery stenosis when only one kidney is present. It was probably a coincidence that two patients given acetazolamide and captopril became anuric. I know of no pharmacologic explanation for such an association.

The adverse effect of captopril in this situation emphasizes the importance of the renin-angiotensin system in at least the initiation of hypertension in this form of blood pressure elevation. Additionally, it emphasizes the effectiveness of the currently available angiotensin converting enzyme inhibitors to block the renin-angiotensin system. It seems unlikely to me that other mechanisms that might be involved in the production of hypertension from unilateral renal artery stenosis would be so effectively countered by captopril.—Walter M. Kirkendall, M.D.

Renal Revascularization in the Azotemic Hypertensive Patient Resistant to Therapy
Christopher Y. Ying, Charles P. Tifft, Haralambos Gavras, and Aram V. Chobanian (Boston Univ. and Lahey Clinic Med. Ctr., Burlington, Mass.)
N. Engl. J. Med. 311:1070–1075, Oct. 25, 1984   6–56

Refractory hypertension in association with renal insufficiency is a common clinical presentation of bilateral atherosclerotic lesions of the renal arteries. Between 1980 and 1983, 106 patients were evaluated for refractory hypertension, which was defined as a blood pressure reading of more than 170/100 mm Hg despite treatment with 3 or more antihypertensive medications. Overall, 39 patients (37%) had renovascular hypertension. Renal insufficiency, defined as a sustained creatinine level of at least 1.5 mg/dl, was present in 21 patients (20%), 10 of whom also had renovascular hypertension. Two of the 10 were excluded because of other clinical considerations, leaving 8 patients, 3 men and 5 women whose mean age was 65.3 years. The duration of hypertension ranged from 4 years to 20 years (mean, 11.3 years). The serum creatinine level ranged from 1.8 mg/dl to 6.1 mg/dl (mean, 2.8 mg/dl). The blood pressure ranged from 175 mm Hg to 240 mm Hg systolic and from 100 mm Hg to 140 mm Hg diastolic, despite administration of 4 or more antihypertensive medications.

The intravenous pyelogram was not suggestive of renovascular disease in 3 patients. Renal vein renin levels did not lateralize in 3 patients, but these levels were elevated bilaterally. Arteriography revealed severe bilateral atherosclerotic disease in 7 patients, 6 of whom had total occlusion of a main renal artery. Acute tubular necrosis related to the use of contrast material resulted in transient elevations of the creatinine level. In-hospital medical therapy induced further deterioration of renal function despite enhanced blood pressure control. Two patients underwent percutaneous transluminal angioplasty alone, and nephrectomy or revascularization, or both, were performed in 4 patients. Blood pressure control (diastolic pressure of less than 90 mm Hg) was achieved in all patients, although each required antihypertensive medication. Renal function improved in all patients and remained stable during the follow-up period of 10–42 months.

In many patients, the relatively common presentation of refractory hypertension and renal insufficiency warrants full investigation for a renovascular cause, irrespective of the duration of hypertension. If a patient is found to have severe renovascular disease, surgical revascularization, percutaneous transluminal angioplasty, or even nephrectomy should be considered, with improvement expected in both blood pressure and renal function.

▶ It was not many years ago that it was considered poor judgment to operate on a patient with bilateral renal artery stenosis and azotemia. The improvement of operative techniques, the development of percutaneous transluminal angioplasty, and the development of better medical care for hypertensives now make it reasonable to carry out more extensive procedures for these patients. End-stage renal disease can be delayed. It is of considerable interest that renal function improved in all of these patients and was stable for up to 42 months.

The diagnosis of renal artery stenosis in patients with bilateral disease may be difficult. Performing an aortogram, preferably early on before total occlusion of a renal artery, is mandatory.—Walter M. Kirkendall, M.D.

The Prognostic Significance of Proteinuria: The Framingham Study
William B. Kannel, Meir J. Stampfer, William P. Castelli, and Joel Verter (Natl. Heart, Lung, and Blood Inst., Bethesda, Md.; Boston Univ.; Brigham and Women's Hosp., Boston; and Harvard Univ.)
Am. Heart J. 108:1347–1352, November 1985   6–57

The significance of proteinuria in asymptomatic adults remains uncertain, although many believe that isolated or intermittent proteinuria is a relatively benign finding. Morbidity and mortality during a 16-year period in the Framingham cohort were assessed in relation to proteinuria. The prevalence of definite proteinuria was variable because of the use of causal urine specimens and various tests.

Intermittent proteinuria was up to 4½ times more prevalent in hypertensive than in normotensive men. Diabetic patients and those with left ventricular hypertrophy also had an excess of proteinuria. Mortality was definitely increased in proteinuric persons at each biennial evaluation. The overall age-adjusted relative risk was 3.8 for men and 2.2 for women. Average cardiovascular mortality rates were increased by threefold in men and women with proteinuria. The increased risk was apparent at all ages. All major forms of cardiovascular disease were present in excess in relation to proteinuria, and fatal cardiovascular events were much more frequent. Noncardiovascular mortality also was increased in patients with proteinuria, by fivefold in men and 1.5-fold in women. Excessive renal disease and diabetes were also observed in these individuals.

Proteinuria is relatively uncommon in the general ambulatory adult population; however, when it occurs, hypertension, diabetes, cardiovascular disease, or overt renal disease are more likely to be present and an excess of deaths must be expected. Proteinuria seems to be a marker for cardiovascular damage and end-organ vulnerability to the effects of hypertension and diabetes.

▶ This study indicated that although proteinuria is uncommon, it frequently is, when present, a marker for hypertension, diabetes mellitus, or cardiovascular impairment. Still, the more pressing clinical problem is what is the fate of the individual without any of these diseases who presents with asymptomatic proteinuria. In this Framingham study, proteinuria under these circumstances was so uncommon that the risk could not be accurately assessed.

On the other hand, several reports have appeared that stress an excellent 5- to 18-year prognosis for asymptomatic persons with both fixed and orthostatic proteinuria.

It appears that finding patients in the general population with proteinuria is a good predictor of vascular trouble. On the other hand, if the group is defined well enough to exclude all known diseases, proteinuria apparently can be a relatively benign finding. Most of us do not live long enough to appreciate the outcome of our young patients with proteinuria. Of interest is a recent report of a 40- to 50-year follow-up of sick patients first diagnosed by Thomas Addis (Rytand. D. A., Spreiters S.: *N. Engl. J. Med.* 305:618, 1981).—Walter M. Kirkendall, M.D.

Benefits of Removal of Native Kidneys in Hypertension After Renal Transplantation
John J. Curtis, Arnold G. Diethelm, Robert G. Luke, John D. Whelchel, and Patricia Jones (Univ. of Alabama at Birmingham)
Lancet 2:739–742, Oct. 5, 1985   6–58

Six hypertensive renal transplant patients (4 men and 2 women aged 21–46 years) were investigated before and 4.5 ± 1.5 months after removal of their native kidneys. After nephrectomy, the mean arterial pressure (MAP) decreased considerably; however, renal (allograft) plasma flow increased by 77% and vascular resistance of the allograft fell by 55%. The mean transverse cardiac diameter and ECG voltage measurements of left ventricular hypertrophy both improved significantly. The rise in renal plasma flow could be induced by giving captopril, an inhibitor of angiotensin II formation, to patients who had not had their native kidneys removed. Thus, the native kidneys seem to affect the allograft via the renin-angiotensin system. The improvement in allograft plasma flow after nephrectomy was maintained for more than 1.5 years. Administration of captopril after native nephrectomy did not further change allograft plasma flow.

These results suggest that the native diseased kidneys in renal transplant patients can have marked effects on the function of the new kidney (allograft). Diseased kidneys appear to cause increased renal vascular resistance in the new kidney, which, however, maintains the glomerular filtration rate with a rise in filtration fraction. Removal of the native kidneys lowered the MAP and cardiac output, but renal blood flow increased considerably. That renal blood flow and MAP change similarly with captopril therapy, and the finding of increased plasma renin activity (PRA) before native kidney nephrectomy, suggest the following: (1) The renin-angiotensin system in the native kidneys contributes to hypertension, and (2) a response to captopril may be predictive of a good response to bilateral nephrectomy. All patients received antihypertensive therapy for the 10.2 ± 2.0 months before nephrectomy. However, the changes in heart size within 4.5 ± 1.5 months after nephrectomy suggest that the operation was more effective than antihypertensive drugs were in controlling blood pressure.

Because native kidneys apparently damage the allograft, why not revert to bilateral nephrectomy before insertion of the allograft? First, anephric patients generally do not fare well while undergoing chronic dialysis, and removal of native kidneys before transplantation is likely to increase the numbers of anephric patients returning to dialysis centers after graft failure. However, if the decision to perform a nephrectomy is postponed until about 12 months after transplantation, a much better judgment can be made of the graft's long-term function. The authors remove native kidneys only from patients who have no evidence of chronic rejection. Further, most renal transplant patients are not hypertensive a year after transplantation even if their native kidneys are left in situ. Thus, the morbidity and mortality associated with bilateral nephrectomy can be avoided by postponing the decision until after successful transplantation.

In a previous study of 32 patients with excellent allograft function while low maintenance doses of immunosuppressive drugs were taken, retained kidneys seemed to be the cause of the hypertension in 62%. It is possible that the allograft vasodilatory response to converting-enzyme inhibition would allow identification of those patients likely to benefit from native kidney nephrectomy. This response to converting-enzyme inhibition contrasts directly with the marked decline in allograft plasma flow and glomerular filtration rate observed when captopril is given to patients with functionally significant renal artery stenosis of the transplanted kidney.

▶ This digest is quite complete. It cites a considerable amount of the evidence and shows the logic behind the authors' recommendation to consider the matter of nephrectomy of the native kidneys at least a year after successful transplantation and preferably after a trial of captopril therapy.

It is to be hoped that some hypertensive patients who cannot or will not have their native kidneys removed will be followed closely with converting enzyme inhibition therapy so that we can be certain that this is effective long-term treatment.—Walter M. Kirkendall, M.D.

Subject Index

A

Abdominal compression
  for right heart assist, 252
Acetylcholine
  inotropic effect in Purkinje fibers (in
    dog), 30
Acquired immunodeficiency syndrome
  heart lesions in, 135
Adenosine
  monophosphate, cyclic, and myocardial
    contractility (in rat), 32
  myocardial contractility reduction by (in
    rat), 32
  triphosphatase, sodium-potassium (in
    rat), 282
Adolescence
  ventricular septal defect in, small,
    dynamic exercise in, 60
Adrenal
  sympatho-adrenal responses to alcohol
    drinking, 290
Adrenalectomy
  renal adaptation to potassium after (in
    rat), 282
α_1-Adrenergic blocker
  in vascular resistance in coronary artery
    disease, 165
β-Adrenergic blockers
  in coronary artery disease
    nifedipine after, 166
    vasoconstriction after, 167
Adrenergic receptors
  function, and aging, 35
α_1 Adrenergic receptors
  in beating induction and heart cell
    hypertrophy (in newborn rat), 29
β-Adrenergic receptors
  desensitization, phorbol ester- and
    diacylclycerol-mediated, 31
  regulation in heart cells (in chick), 27
  subtypes on ventricular myocytes (in
    rat), 29
β_1 Adrenergic receptors
  in beating induction (in newborn rat),
    29
Aequorin
  measurements of calcium in heart cell,
    48
Afferent responses
  interruption by transmural myocardial
    infarction (in dog), 43
Afterload
  reducing effects of milrinone, 19
Aged
  blood pressure, postural, 327

Aging
  adrenergic receptor function and, 35
AIDS
  heart lesions in, 135
Alcohol, 274 ff.
  consumption and blood pressure, 275
  hypertension and, 274
  stimulation of renin release, 290
Aldosteronism, primary, 299 ff.
  calcium channel blockade in, 299
  hypertension and sympathetic nervous
    system in, 300
Amiodarone
  in cardiomyopathy, hypertrophic,
    survival after, 124
  IV, hemodynamic and antiischemic
    effects, 214
  in ventricular tachycardia, survival
    after, 124
Anemia
  with ventricular shunt, right to left, in
    children, 61
Aneurysm
  ventricular, in myocardial infarction,
    190
Angina
  cresendo, due to plaque fissuring, 39
  pectoris
    calcium channel blocker in, 168
    hyperventilation and cold pressor test
      in, 176
    ischemia and chest pain in, 159
    monitoring, ST segment in, 161
  spontaneous, in coronary artery spasm,
    169
  unstable, mortality and survival in, 231
Angiography
  in atherosclerosis, coronary, 172
  balloon occlusion, in infant, 97
  coronary
    in coronary obstructive disease, 65
    in myocardial infarction, 189
  digital-subtraction, in renovascular
    hypertension, 298
  predicting occlusion in coronary artery
    disease, 186
  radionuclide, 205
    of biventricular performance after
      esmolol and propranolol, 26
    to predict cardiac events after
      myocardial infarction, 205
    of ventricular wall motion after
      myocardial infarction, 206
Angioplasty
  balloon, 89 ff.
    in pulmonary artery stenosis,
      congenital, 89

Index to Authors

357

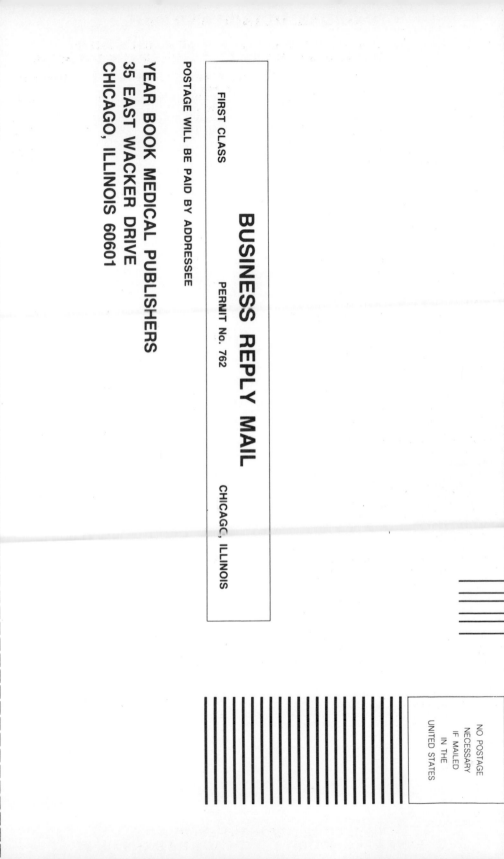

BUSINESS REPLY MAIL

FIRST CLASS   PERMIT No. 762   CHICAGO, ILLINOIS

POSTAGE WILL BE PAID BY ADDRESSEE

YEAR BOOK MEDICAL PUBLISHERS
35 EAST WACKER DRIVE
CHICAGO, ILLINOIS 60601

NO POSTAGE
NECESSARY
IF MAILED
IN THE
UNITED STATES

TO ORDER: DETACH AND MAIL

Please enter my subscription to the journal(s) and, or Year Book(s) checked below:
(To order by phone, call **toll-free 800-621-9262**. In IL., call **collect 312-726-9746**).

	Practitioner (approx.)	Resident	Institution
Current Problems in Surgery® (1 yr.)	____$49.95	____$27.50	____$65.00
Current Problems in Pediatrics® (1 yr.)	____$39.95	____$27.50	____$65.00
Current Problems in Cancer (1 yr.)	____$49.95	____$27.50	____$65.00
Current Problems in Cardiology® (1 yr.)	____$49.95	____$27.50	____$65.00
Current Problems in Obstetrics, Gynecology, and Fertility (1 yr.)	____$49.95	____$27.50	____$65.00
Current Problems in Diag. Radiology® (1 yr.)	____$42.95	____$27.50	____$65.00
Disease-A-Month® (1 yr.)	____$39.95	____$27.50	____$65.00
	Binder____$12.95 (each year)		
1986 Year Book of Anesthesia® (AN-86)	____$44.95	____$27.50	
1986 Year Book of Cancer® (CA-86)	____$44.95	____$27.50	
1986 Year Book of Cardiology® (CV-86)	____$42.95	____$27.50	
1986 Year Book of Critical Care Medicine (16-86)	____$44.95	____$27.50	
1986 Year Book of Dentistry® (D-86)	____$42.95	____$27.50	
1986 Year Book of Dermatology® (10-86)	____$45.95	____$27.50	
1986 Year Book of Diagnostic Radiology® (9-86)	____$44.95	____$27.50	
1986 Year Book of Digestive Diseases (13-86)	____$42.95	____$27.50	
1986 Year Book of Drug Therapy® (6-86)	____$44.95	____$27.50	
1986 Year Book of Emergency Medicine® (15-86)	____$44.95	____$27.50	
1986 Year Book of Endocrinology® (EM-86)	____$44.95	____$27.50	
1986 Year Book of Family Practice® (FY-86)	____$42.95	____$27.50	
1986 Year Book of Hand Surgery (17-86)	____$42.95	____$27.50	
1986 Year Book of Hematology (24-86)	____$39.95	____$27.50	
1986 Year Book of Infectious Diseases (19-86)	____$39.95	____$27.50	
1986 Year Book of Medicine® (1-86)	____$44.95	____$27.50	
1986 Year Book of Neurology and Neurosurgery® (8-86)	____$44.95	____$27.50	
1986 Year Book of Nuclear Medicine® (NM-86)	____$44.95	____$27.50	
1986 Year Book of Obstetrics and Gynecology® (5-86)	____$42.95	____$27.50	
1986 Year Book of Ophthalmology® (EY-86)	____$44.95	____$27.50	
1986 Year Book of Orthopedics® (OR-86)	____$44.95	____$27.50	
1986 Year Book of Otolaryngology-Head and Neck Surgery (3-86)	____$44.95	____$27.50	
1986 Year Book of Pathology and Clinical Pathology® (PI-86)	____$44.95	____$27.50	
1986 Year Book of Pediatrics® (4-86)	____$42.95	____$27.50	
1986 Year Book of Plastic and Reconstructive Surgery® (12-86)	____$46.95	____$27.50	
1986 Year Book of Podiatric Medicine and Surgery (18-86)	____$39.95	____$27.50	
1986 Year Book of Psychiatry and Applied Mental Health® (11-86)	____$42.95	____$27.50	
1986 Year Book of Pulmonary Disease (21-86)	____$39.95	____$27.50	
1986 Year Book of Rehabilitation (22-86)	____$39.95	____$27.50	
1986 Year Book of Sports Medicine (SM-86)	____$42.95	____$27.50	
1986 Year Book of Surgery® (2-86)	____$44.95	____$27.50	
1986 Year Book of Urology® (7-86)	____$44.95	____$27.50	
1986 Year Book of Vascular Surgery (20-86)	____$39.95	____$27.50	

*The above Year Books are published annually. For the convenience of its customers, Year Book enters each purchaser as a subscriber to future volumes and sends annual announcement of each volume approximately 2 months before publication. The new volume will be shipped upon publication unless you complete and return the cancellation notice attached to the announcement and it is received by Year Book within the time indicated (approximately 20 days after your receipt of the announcement). You may cancel your subscription at any time. The new volume may be examined on approval, may be returned for full credit, and if returned Year Book will then remove your name as a subscriber. Return postage is guaranteed by Year Book to the Postal Service.

Prices quoted are in U.S. dollars. Canadian orders will be billed in Canadian funds at the approximate current exchange rate.
A small additional charge will be made for postage and handling. Illinois and Tennessee residents will be billed appropriate sales tax. **All prices quoted subject to change.**

NAME_____ ACCT. NO._____

ADDRESS _____

CITY _____ STATE _____ ZIP _____

Printed in U.S.A.   PAY B

YEAR BOOK MEDICAL PUBLISHERS
35 EAST WACKER DRIVE   CHICAGO ILLINOIS 60601